W. R. Mann

25. viii . 78.

PHYSIOLOGICAL ASPECTS OF CLINICAL NEUROLOGY

EDITED BY
F. CLIFFORD ROSE FRCP
Consultant Neurologist, Charing Cross Hospital
Consultant Neurologist, Medical Ophthalmology
Unit, St Thomas' Hospital

BLACKWELL SCIENTIFIC PUBLICATIONS
OXFORD LONDON EDINBURGH MELBOURNE

First published in 1977

British Library Cataloguing in Publication Data
Physiological aspects of clinical neurology.
  Bibl. - Index
  ISBN 0-0632-00336-7
  1. Rose, Frank Clifford
  616.8′04′7   RC346
  Nervous system - Diseases

Printed in Great Britain
at the Alden Press, Oxford
and bound by
Mansell (Bookbinders) Ltd., Witham, Essex

CONTENTS

PART II THE MOTOR SYSTEM   155

PART III. MISCELLANEOUS   263

CONTRIBUTORS

JANE ADAM, BA *University Department of Neurology, Institute of Psychiatry and King's College Hospital Medical School, Denmark Hill, London SE5 8AF*

ROBERT B. AIRD, MD *Emeritus Professor and Chairman, Department of Neurology, University of California Medical Center, San Francisco*

E. J. ARNOTT, FRCS *Consultant Ophthalmic Surgeon, Charing Cross Hospital, London, W6*

G. BAUMGARTNER, MD *Director, Department of Neurology, University of Zurich, Kantonsspital, Ramistrasse 100, 8091 Zurich, Switzerland*

MORRIS B. BENDER, AB, MD *Henry P. and Georgette Goldschmidt, Professor and Chairman Emeritus, Department of Neurology, Mount Sinai School of Medicine, New York, N.Y.*

PROF. G. S. BRINDLEY, MD, FRCP, FRS *Department of Physiology, Institute of Psychiatry, University of London*

PAUL C. BUCY, MD *Professor Emeritus of Surgery (Neurosurgery), Northwestern University Medical School; Clinical Professor of Neurology and Neurological Surgery, Bowman Gray School of Medicine; Editor and Publisher of* Surgical Neurology

ANTONIO R. DAMASIO, MD, PhD *Associate Professor of Neurology, Department of Neurology, University of Iowa; Formerly Chief of Language Research Laboratory, Centro de Estudos Egas Moniz, Portugal, and Professor of Neurology, Department of Neurology, University of Lisbon.*

HANNA B. C. DAMASIO, MD *Instructor in Neurology, Department of Iowa.*

J. DE LEAN, MSc, MD *Senior Resident, Division of Neurology, Toronto General Hospital, University of Toronto*

DEREK DENNY-BROWN, MD *New England Regional Primate Research Center, Southborough, Mass., U.S.A.*

SIR JOHN ECCLES *Ca' a la Gra', CH 6611 Contra, Switzerland*

GEORGE ETTLINGER PhD *Professor Neuropsychology, Department of Psychiatry, Institute of Psychiatry, London SE5 8AF*

W. H. FEINDEL, MD *Director, Department of Neurosurgery, MNI*

PROF. RAGNAR GRANIT, MD DSc, For. Mem. RS *Nobel Institute for Neurophysiology, Karolinska Institute Stockholm, Sweden S-10401*

MARK HALLETT, MD *University Department of Neurology, Institute of Psychiatry and King's College Hospital Medical School, Denmark Hill, London SE5 8AF*

DR. CHRISTOPHER KENNARD MB, BS, BSc, MRCP *Registrar, Department of Neurology, Charing Cross Hospital, London, W6. Lately, Research Fellow, Division of Developmental Biology, National Institute for Medical Research, Mill Hill*

F. L. McNAUGHTON, MD *Neurologist, Montreal Neurological Institute*

PROF. C. D. MARSDEN MD, FRCP *Professor, University Department of Neurology, Institute of Psychiatry and King's College Hospital Medical School, Denmark Hill, London SE5 8AF*

W. B. MATTHEWS, DM, FRCP *Professor, Department of Clinical Neurology, University of Oxford, The Churchill Hospital, Headington, Oxford OX3 7LJ*

S. MENSE, PhD *Institute of Physiology, University of Kiel, West Germany*

P. A. MERTON, MB, BChir *The Physiological Laboratory, Downing Street, Cambridge CB2 3EG*

H. B. MORTON *National Hospital Queen Square, London WC1N 3BG*

N. B. REWCASTLE, MD *Head, Division of Neuropathology, Toronto General Hospital, University of Toronto*

J. CLIFFORD RICHARDSON, MD *Division of Neurology, Toronto General Hospital, University of Toronto*

PIERRE RONDOT MD *Professor aggregé, Faculté de Médecine Cochin Port-Royal, Centre Hôpitalier, Sainte-Anne, 1 rue Cabanis, 75674 Paris*

F. CLIFFORD ROSE, FRCP *Consultant Neurologist, Charing Cross Hospital, Consultant Neurologist, Medical Ophthalmology Unit, St. Thomas' Hospital, London.*

R. W. ROSS RUSSELL, MD, FRCP *Consultant Neurologist, National Hospital for Nervous Diseases, St. Thomas' Hospital and Moorfields Hospital*

D. N. RUSHTON PhD *MRC Neurological Prostheses Unit, Institute of Psychiatry, De Crespigny Park, London SE5 8AF*

MICHAEL SANDERS, FRCS, MRCP *Consultant Ophthalmologist, St. Thomas' Hospital, Department of Ophthalmology and MRC Hearing and Balance Unit, National Hospital, London*

PROF. R. F. SCHMIDT, PhD *Institute of Physiology, University of Kiel, West Germany*

JOHN C. SLOPER, MD, FRCP, FRCPath *Honorary Consultant Pathologist, Charing Cross Hospital. Professor of Experimental Pathology, Charing Cross Medical School, University of London*

E. G. WALSH, MA, BSc, BM, BCh, FRCP, FRSE *Department of Physiology, University of Edinburgh*

PREFACE

The basis of clinical medicine is the knowledge of normal physiology. In no field is this truism more applicable than in clinical neurology. The one person to whom modern neuro-science is perhaps most indebted is Sir Gordon Holmes on whose work the routine neurological examination is largely based. On the occasion of the centenary of his birth, a Symposium based on the theme 'The Physiological Aspects of Clinical Neurology' was held at Charing Cross Hospital, on the staff of which he served for many years. Although the happy informal atmosphere in discussions cannot be transmitted, it was strongly felt that the scientific papers, many from eminent and indeed legendary contributors, should be made known to a wider audience.

Organizing the Symposium and editing this book has made me realize just how rapidly clinical neurophysiology is advancing and each of the following contributions is a re-statement of the truism earlier mentioned.

F.C.R.

35 Harley Street,
London, W1N 1HA.
July 1976

PART I
VISION

THE DEVELOPMENT OF BINOCULAR VISUAL CONNECTIONS

C. KENNARD

The functioning of the brain involves interactions between neurones whose spatial organization and interconnections are highly ordered. This order shows a marked constancy from one member of a species to the next. Developmental processes must be able to reproduce this complex structure, so the question then arises as to whether the intrinsic genetic controls of neuronal development are capable of completing this by themselves or whether extrinsic, and hence highly variable, controls are imposed on the individual organism by its environment and experience. The role of these two contrasting control mechanisms, embodied in the terms nature and nurture, have for many years interested scientists working on the structure and function of the brain and the way in which the vertebrate binocular visual system has served to evaluate the relative roles of these two developmental mechanisms is reviewed in this chapter.

Two main problems for development are posed by binocular vision. The first, which is common to most of the major afferent projections to the brain, is that the spatial orderliness of a two-dimensional receptor surface is maintained at subcortical and cortical levels. This means in terms of the visual system that there is a fixed relationship between regions in the retina and its subcortical and cortical representation, so giving rise to a topographically ordered map. It is necessary, therefore, to discuss the developmental mechanisms which are involved in producing such a retinotopic map. Secondly, we have to consider in developmental terms the mechanisms by which higher mammals are able to localize the depths of objects and to perceive the world stereoscopically. Since the two eyes are horizontally separate they each perceive the visual world from a slightly different vantage point so that the retinal images of an object in space will be located at slightly disparate points on the two retinae. It is the integration of information registering this retinal disparity at cortical levels which locates its position in three-dimensional visual space. The setting up of the mechanism for stereopsis demands an extremely high degree of precision which may require both intrinsic and extrinsic developmental processes and will be discussed later.

The formation of retinotopic maps

In considering the first point—the development of a retinotopically ordered map at a visual centre—some concepts arising from experiments on the amphibian visual system will be used.

In amphibia the main visual pathway is the retinotectal projection. Each tectum, the phylogenetic homologue of the mammalian superior colliculus, receives fibres only from the contralateral eye which form a retinotopically ordered map over the surface (Gaze 1958); in this way, temporal ganglion cells project to rostral tectum, nasal ganglion cells to caudal tectum and the other ganglion cells project in retinotopic order across the rest of the tectum. More than 30 years ago, Sperry (1942, 1943a, b) performed a series of experiments on the retinotectal system which led him to propose a mechanism to account for the development of such an ordered map. In his chemoaffinity hypothesis of neuronal specificity (see Sperry 1951, 1963 for summary) he suggested that retinal ganglion cells are intrinsically different from one another, because during their differentiation they come to possess specific cytochemical labels. A similar process is supposed to take place in the tectum amongst the tectal cells, and the rule governing the formation of connections between the two is selective and exclusive. By this he meant that, for instance, a temporal ganglion cell would possess a specific cytochemical label and would seek out, and only synapse with, a group of tectal cells in the rostral tectum which possessed complementary cytochemical labels, ignoring all others. The chemoaffinity hypothesis is therefore separable into two main parts. Firstly, it states that cellular differentiative processes give rise to cytochemical labels, and this has so far never been proven (for reviews see Keating 1976, Keating & Kennard 1976a). Secondly, it states rules governing the formation of neuronal connections which is of particular interest in the present review.

This hypothesis allows us to predict what would happen if, in an amphibian, both eyes were made to innervate the same tectum which, normally, only receives a direct projection from the contralateral eye. The input from each eye might be expected to form a retinotopic map across the tectal surface and if the two eyes are bilaterally symmetrical it is reasonable to suppose that bilaterally symmetrical ganglion cells in each eye, such as those at the temporal pole, would bear identical cytochemical labels. If neuronal connections are formed in a selective and exclusive manner, viz. dependency on affinities between cells bearing complementary cytochemical labels, then these bilaterally symmetrical cells should terminate at the same tectal position (Fig. 1.1). Such binocular innervation of one tectum can be achieved by cutting an optic nerve, near the optic chiasma. In amphibia this often results in the nerve regenerating into the ipsilateral tectum, which is already innervated by the contralateral eye. As predicted on the basis of the

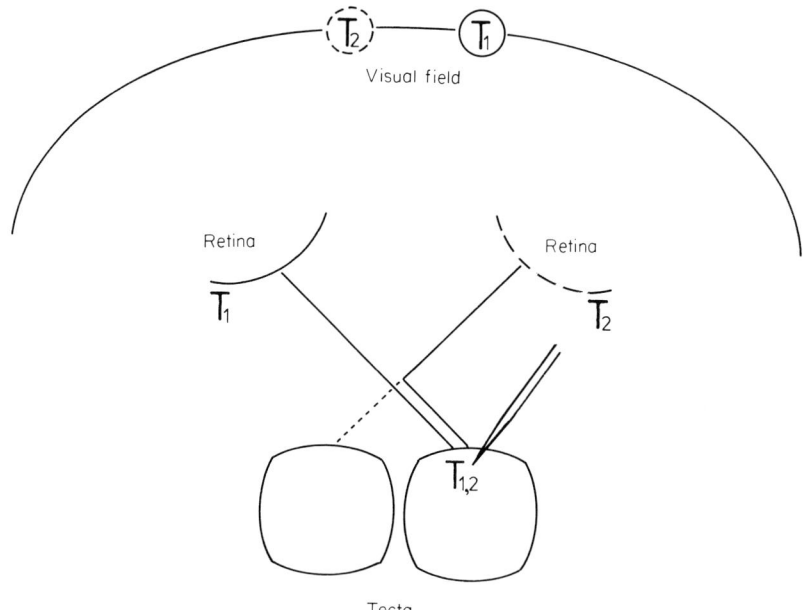

Fig. 1.1 A diagrammatic representation of the main amphibian visual pathway, the retinotectal system, in which both eyes have been experimentally induced to innervate the right tectum. Electrophysiological recording from the tectum at point $T_{1,2}$ reveals direct retinal inputs from bilaterally symmetrical points T_1 and T_2 at the temporal pole of each eye. The receptive field positions of these two retinal points lie at different positions in the visual field.

chemoaffinity hypothesis, retinotopic maps from both eyes are formed across the tectum and, indeed, bilaterally symmetrical points in the two eyes project to identical tectal regions (Sperry 1945, Gaze & Jacobson 1963, Gaze & Keating 1970). These bilaterally symmetrical retinal points are said to be equivalent. Fig. 1.1 also shows that equivalent retinal points, such as T1 and T2, have their receptive fields in very different positions in the visual field and this means that the retinotopic map of the visual world, via each eye, is reversed in relation to one another across the tectum. This is not a very useful situation from a behavioural point of view since objects at two different points in the visual world will cause activation at the same tectal position.

In mammals the lateral geniculate nucleus is normally innervated by both eyes (Fig. 1.2) but the mapping of the projections from the two eyes is somewhat different from the binocularly innervated amphibian tectum. The inputs from the two eyes are kept separate in different laminae so that the retinotopic map of the nasal half of the contralateral retina lies in lamina A above the map from the temporal half of the ipsilateral retina, which

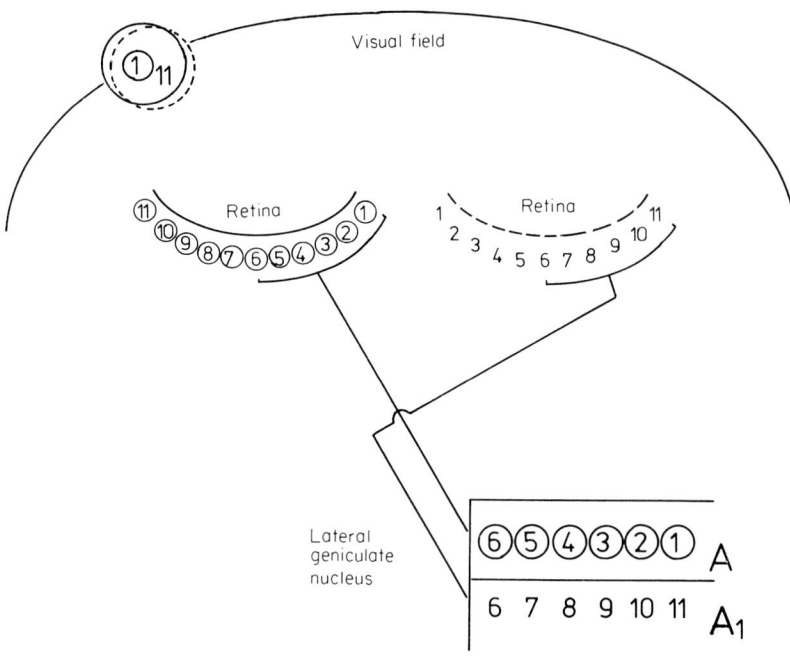

Fig. 1.2 A diagrammatic representation showing the mapping of the retinal inputs to the right lateral geniculate nucleus in a higher mammal. The nasal hemiretina, points ①–⑥ in the left retina (solid line) projects to lamina A, and the temporal hemiretina, points 6–11 in the right retina (dotted line) projects to lamina A1. Note how point ① at the nasal pole of the contralateral left eye projects to a point in lamina A which lies adjacent to the projection from the temporal pole, point 11, of the ipsilateral right eye. These two retinal points, ① and 11, are said to be corresponding since their receptive field positions lie at the same position in the visual field.

terminates in lamina A1. This means, as Fig. 1.2 shows, that points from the two retinae which are not bilaterally symmetrical, lie adjacent to one another, e.g. fibres from nasal point ① in the contralateral eye do not terminate adjacent to fibres from nasal point 1 in the ipsilateral eye, but lie adjacent to fibres from temporal point 11. The important point is that the receptive field positions of retinal points ① and 11 are found to lie at the same visual field location and these two retinal points are said to be corresponding. The nasal half-retina of one eye and the temporal half of the other receive visual information from the same hemifield, and the two inputs terminate adjacent to one another in the geniculate nucleus so that the maps of each hemifield are superimposed upon one another in register in the two laminae.

This is obviously a different method of mapping binocular inputs to that found in the amphibian when both eyes are experimentally induced to innervate one tectum, since in that case the maps of the visual world via the two eyes were reversed in relation to one another. The amphibian dorsal thalamic region normally receives direct retinal inputs from both eyes, as does the mammalian geniculate nucleus. It was of interest to see how these binocular inputs map in relation to one another since one prediction would be that equivalent retinal points in the two eyes come together, as was described above when both eyes are experimentally induced to innervate one tectum. Alternatively, these binocular inputs may map, as in the mammalian geniculate, where corresponding retinal points terminate adjacent to one another. When post-synaptic neurones, which receive direct inputs from both eyes, were recorded from electrophysiologically, it was found that the receptive fields of neurones, via the two eyes, were at identical positions in the visual field (Keating & Kennard 1976b). This means that corresponding retinal points in the two eyes are projecting to the same thalamic neurone and that, within the same animal, the retinothalamic projection maps according to a different set of rules to the phylogenetically older retinotectal projection. It is possible that the retinal ganglion cells, which project to the thalamus, and those which project to the tectum come to possess differing sets of cytochemical labels but that their connections are still selective and exclusive.

Anomalies of the visual pathways in albino mammals

To test the chemoaffinity hypothesis for the validity of the proposition that neuronal connections are selective and exclusive it is necessary to experimentally disturb the visual pathways. This can be achieved by the production of relative size disparities between the innervating retinal array and the innervated array such as the tectum or geniculate, for example, half an eye is made to innervate a whole tectum, or a whole eye is allowed to innervate a half tectum. Most of these experiments have been done on lower vertebrates such as frogs and goldfish, since they are relatively easy to operate upon as embryos and also possess regenerative abilities not found in higher vertebrates (Reviews: Gaze 1970, Hunt & Jacobson 1974, Keating & Kennard 1976a).

However, an 'experiment of nature' has provided the necessary size disparity disturbance in the developing visual system of the albino mammal. This has been found in all albino mammals so far studied including mice (Guillery *et al* 1973), rats (Lund 1965), ferrets (Guillery 1971), rabbits (Sanderson 1972), Siamese cats (Guillery 1969), and man (Guillery *et al* 1975). The abnormality common to them all is that there is a reduction in the number of ipsilaterally projecting optic nerve fibres. This is due to the fact that ganglion cells in a region of the retina, temporal to the line of decussation, instead of projecting ipsilaterally, as do the rest of the temporal ganglion cells, project contralaterally. With this anomalous decussation pattern, we have to consider, firstly, how the retinal fibres terminate in the lateral geniculate nucleus and, secondly, how the enlarged contralateral retinal representation is mapped across the visual cortex.

This abnormal decussation of optic axons does not appear to be specific to a mutation at the albino gene locus, which causes a deficiency of tyrosinase, since Sanderson *et al* (1974) have shown that the abnormality occurs in minks in which various gene combinations, involving genes other than those at the albino locus, produce a reduced retinal pigment distribution. The reduction in the size of the ipsilateral projection appears to be inversely proportional to the amount of pigment present in the pigment epithelium, indicating that a normal pigment epithelial layer in the eye is required for the normal pattern of decussation of optic nerve fibres at the optic chiasma.

Most of the studies on the abnormality of the visual system associated with albinism have been carried out on the Siamese cat, which possesses a temperature-sensitive variant of the gene product, tyrosinase, giving rise to melanin (Searle 1968). This means that the enzyme can only operate at a temperature 2° to 3°C below the body core temperature and explains why the main pigmented areas in Siamese cats are found at the cool extremities such as the paws, ears and tail. Earlier it has been explained how normally in mammals corresponding retinal points in the two eyes send fibres which terminate in the lateral geniculate nucleus in different laminae, but adjacent to one another. In Siamese cats there is a size disparity between the retina and geniculate with an enlarged contralateral retinal representation projecting to the geniculate as well as a reduced ipsilateral representation. The latter projects normally to lamina A1 but since it is reduced it leaves a vacant space (Fig. 1.3a). This is filled by the abnormally routed temporal fibres (Fig. 1.3b) from the contralateral eye (Kaas & Guillery 1973), and the question now arises as to the order in which these fibres terminate. In Fig. 1.4 the projection from retinal point ⑧ in the left retina normally terminates at point ⑧ in lamina A1 of the ipsilateral geniculate, but in the Siamese cat it crosses at the chiasma and terminates at point ⑧ in lamina A1 of the contralateral geniculate. This is its bilaterally symmetrical position in the right geniculate so that the aberrantly projecting axons from the contralateral eye terminate at the correct site, but in the wrong geniculate (Guillery, Casagrande & Oberdorfer 1974). The abnormally projecting retinal ganglion cells would appear to be properly specified for their geniculate sites of termination, but are improperly specified for their crossing at the optic chiasma (but see Lund 1975).

As a consequence of this method of mapping, the maps of the visual hemifield, generated via each eye and projecting to the two adjacent geniculate laminae, are not in register. Indeed, the anomalous projection to lamina A1 comes from a retinal region appropriate to the wrong hemifield,

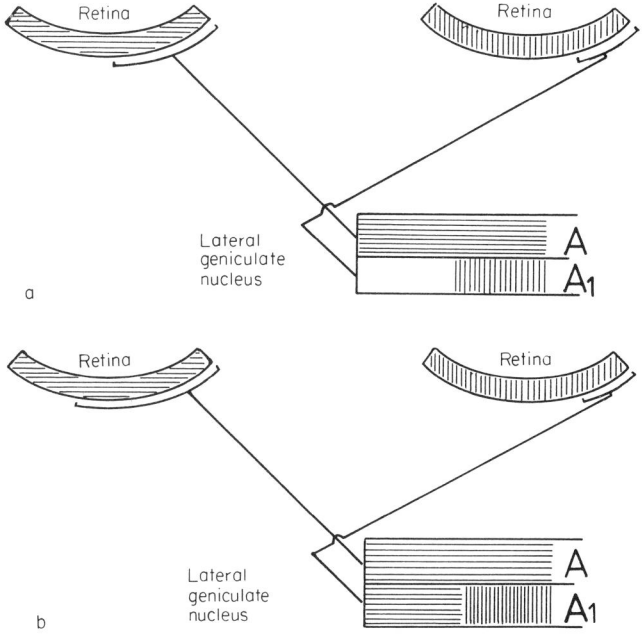

Fig. 1.3 Diagrams showing the make up of the abnormal retino-geniculate projections in albino mammals such as the Siamese cat. The projections are shown to the right lateral geniculate nucleus only.

(a) The projection from the contralateral eye to lamina A is normal, but due to the anomalous crossing of retinal axons from the temporal retina of the ipsilateral eye there is a reduced projection to lamina Al.

(b) The space left vacant by the reduced ipsilateral projection to the medial part of lamina Al is filled by the anomalous crossed projection from the temporal retina of the contralateral eye.

and its representation of the visual world is mirror-reversed in relation to the other visual field maps in the geniculate (Fig. 1.5).

Adjacent regions in each geniculate lamina, which receive projections from corresponding retinal points in the two eyes, normally project to the same group of neurones in the striate cortex (area 17). This means that in Siamese cats the anomalous representation at the lateral geniculate nucleus obviously presents considerable mapping problems at the cortical level. Firstly, how is the enlarged retinal representation from the contralateral eye (normal nasal hemiretina plus strip of temporal retina) mapped across the striate cortex; and, secondly, how is this enlarged retinal representation, which possesses a field reversal, matched with the normal but reduced retinal representation from the ipsilateral eye? These problems seem to have been solved in at least two different ways. Kaas and Guillery (1973) found that at

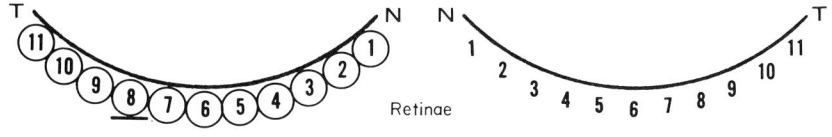

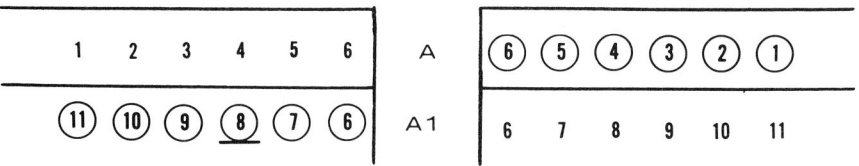

Normal cat LGN

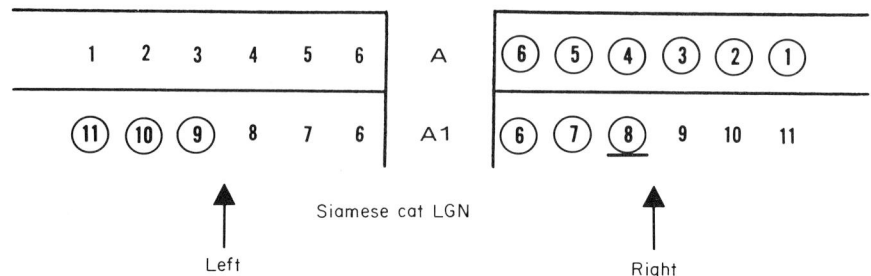

Siamese cat LGN

Left   Right

Fig. 1.4 Simplified diagrammatic representation of the retinal projection to lamina A and Al in the lateral geniculate nucleus of normal and Siamese cats based on the findings of Kaas and Guillery (1973) and Hubel and Wiesel (1971). In Siamese cats fibres which normally project to the ipsilateral side of the brain (⑥ ⑦ ⑧ and 6, 7, 8) decussate at the optic chiasma, and project to the medial part of lamina Al of the contralateral geniculate. Note how position ⑧ in the left retina projects to the correct position in lamina Al but in the wrong geniculate. (From Gaze & Keating 1972.)

cortical levels in one group of Siamese cats, rather than a matching of the inputs from adjacent geniculate laminae which receive inputs from non-corresponding retinal regions, there appeared to be suppression of both the normal and abnormal inputs projecting from lamina Al of the geniculate nucleus. This could come about by various mechanisms, for example, lamina Al may send abnormally few axonal branches to the cortex, or these axons may fail to make normal synaptic connections, or perhaps there is inhibition of these geniculo-cortical fibres at cortical levels. This pattern of connections has been called the Mid-Western pattern and may reflect the fact that lamina

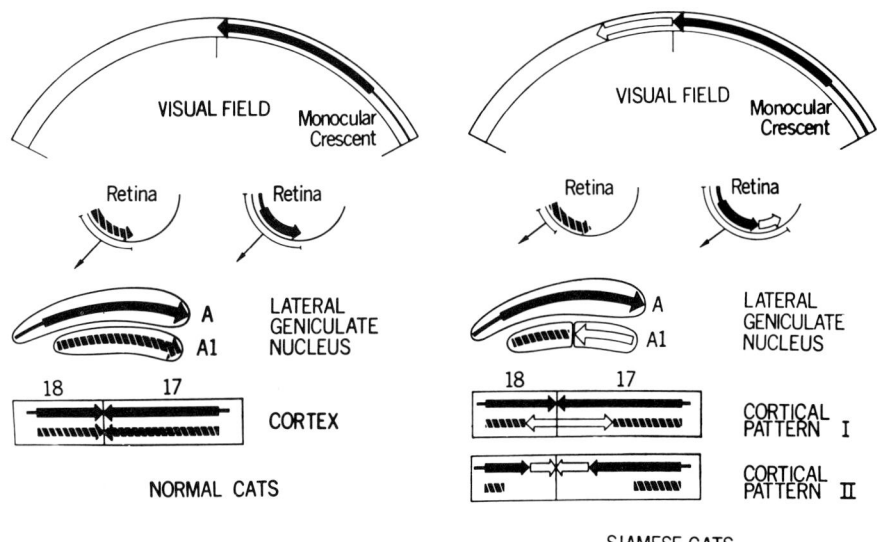

Fig. 1.5 Simplified schema of the visual pathways in the normal (left) and Siamese cats (right) showing that there is a reversal of the visual field representation in lamina A1 of the Siamese cat lateral geniculate nucleus due to the anomalous contralateral projection from temporal retina. Below is shown two possible geniculo-cortical projection patterns (I and II) for Siamese cats. Cortical pattern I shows the cortical organization that would be produced if the geniculo-cortical projection was not modified, as in the Mid-Western pattern in which the functional visual input from lamina A1 is suppressed at the cortex as described by Kass and Guillery (1973). Cortical pattern II shows the main pattern of cortical organization described by Hubel and Wiesel (1971), in which the reversal that occurs in the abnormal segment of lamina A1 (white arrow) has been corrected, so that a sequential representation of the visual field is created at the cortical level. (From Kaas & Guillery 1973.)

A1 possess a non-sequential representation of the visual field (Guillery *et al*, 1974).

The other pattern of cortical representation in Siamese cats, which has been called the Boston pattern, was found by Hubel and Wiesel (1971). They showed that the normal sequence from geniculate lamina A (via the contralateral eye) had moved away from the boundary between cortical area 17 and 18 and the abnormal sequence, also via the contralateral eye but from lamina A1, was inserted into the vacant space (Fig. 1.5). Furthermore, within this representation of the abnormal sequence a reversal is achieved, so that the mirror reversal which occurs at geniculate levels is corrected at cortical levels. Although the total area of visual cortex is not increased, 135° of the visual field is represented across it instead of 90° as is found in the normal cat; within this 135° there is an orderly sequence of cortical activation when a stimulus moves from left to right across the visual field.

There are at least two possible developmental mechanisms which could produce the Boston pattern of geniculate cortical connections. One is that these connections develop initially as in normal cats, and it is only following visual function post-natally that modifications take place due to the abnormal sequence of cortical activation. The second possibility is that the modified pattern develops innately, due to normal developmental processes, independent of visual experience. To distinguish between these two possible mechanisms it is necessary to study the pattern of connections in the newborn Siamese cat to see if the modified or normal pattern is present—such a study has so far not been reported.

The Boston pattern displays one important feature; any cortical point will receive its input, via the geniculate nucleus, from a different retinal region to normal and this suggests that the rules governing the pattern of connections of geniculo-cortical inputs are not exclusive. It suggests that the spatial order of the enlarged retinal representation from the contralateral eye to the cortex is maintained, and that competitive interactions may take place between the innervating axons to ensure that they all come to find post-synaptic sites. The important point is that these interactions must ensure that their spatial order is maintained and in the Boston pattern, since the overall input is enlarged, the ensuing map would be compressed.

This is an example of a less rigid mechanism bringing about the development of neuronal connections between two sets of neuronal arrays. Further evidence for such a mechanism, which has been given the descriptive name of systems matching by Gaze & Keating (1972), comes from studies on the development of the retinotectal pathway in amphibians (Gaze, Keating & Chung 1974) and from experiments using the size disparity paradigm which was described earlier (for reviews see Keating 1976, Keating & Kennard 1976a).

The visual pathways of the albino mammal, and of the Siamese cat in particular, have provided considerable insight into the developmental mechanisms of neuronal interconnections. They stress the importance of retinal pigment epithelium in determining ganglion cell axon decussation; they suggest that neuronal connections are not formed on an exclusive basis, and they indicate the possibility that normal sequential patterns of activation are required for the matching of inputs from the two eyes at cortical levels. Further studies using the Siamese cat as a model for the visual pathway anomaly found generally amongst albino mammals, may well provide further important clues concerning the normal development of binocular visual pathways. They may also provide possible insights into the mechanisms involved in the production of the various visual abnormalities associated with the human albino, such as strabismus and nystagmus (Duke-Elder 1963), especially since there is now strong evidence to suggest that they too possess the same abnormal decussation pattern of optic nerve fibres as do other albino mammals (Creel *et al* 1974, Guillery *et al* 1975).

The role of visual function in the development of binocular visual connections

The role of visual experience in the maturation of the visual pathways has been stressed over the past ten years (summarized by Barlow 1975). Hubel and Wiesel (1963) studied the maturation of binocular inputs at cortical levels in the cat. They found that in the visually inexperienced kitten a retinotopic map was already present, and that cortical neurones received functional binocular inputs (Hubel & Wiesel 1963). They then showed that these connections could be disrupted if normal congruent binocular visual experience was interferred with during the early post-natal months. The closure of one eye for a two-month period led to all cortical neurones receiving functional inputs from the visually experienced eye only (Wiesel & Hubel 1965). Non-congruent visual experience, experimentally induced by alternating daily monocular occlusion, or by strabismus, resulted in cortical neurones receiving functional inputs only from one or other eye, but not from both (Hubel & Wiesel 1965).

These alterations in functional visual cortical inputs can only be induced during a certain post-natal period (Hubel & Wiesel 1970a). This has been called the critical or sensitive period and in the cat extends from the third post-natal week to the third or fourth month. It is interesting that since the eye lids of cats do not open together, there is normally a period of monocular occlusion during the early post-natal period; the disruptive effect of this is obviated by the fact that the critical period does not begin until after both eye lids have opened (Blakemore & Cummings 1975). During the height of the critical period as little as six hours of monocular occlusion is sufficient to produce this disruptive effect (Peck & Blakemore 1975), yet a subsequent year of normal visual experience does little to restore the normal pattern of connections (Ganz & Haffner 1974). The possible mechanisms whereby the functional input from the deprived eye disappear are similar to those discussed in relation to the suppression of the abnormal geniculo-cortical inputs in the Mid-Western Siamese cat. Some anatomical evidence suggests that there is a withdrawal of geniculo-cortical input from the deprived eye (Thorpe & Blakemore 1975), and physiological evidence indicates that this can be restored if the monocular occlusion is reversed during the critical period (Blakemore & Van Sluyters 1974, Movshon & Blakemore 1975). Duffy *et al* (1976) have found, by reducing cortical inhibitory mechanisms with bicuculline, which causes GABA receptor blockade, that the binocular input can be restored; they deduced that the connections are in fact present, but suppressed.

The results which have been obtained from experiments on the rhesus monkey following periods of monocular deprivation and non-congruent visual experience are largely similar to those obtained from the cat under similar experimental conditions (Baker, Grigg & Von Noorden 1974,

Crawford *et al* 1975). In the rhesus monkey the critical period extends from birth to the fourth post-natal month (Von Noorden 1973).

There is a considerable amount of evidence which stresses that the normal joint usage of the two eyes may have some effect in establishing the normal orderly matching of the geniculo-cortical connections from the two eyes. This also suggests that there may be active competition taking place amongst these inputs for the available post-synaptic space, and that this competition is experience-dependent. Although these experiments indicate the animals' need for normal binocular visual experience, they also suggest that this period of neuronal plasticity appears to provide a mainly negative, potentially disruptive, role. It needs to be seen if there are any particular properties of cortical visual neurones which require a period of normal congruent visual experience for their maturation and fine tuning.

Recent evidence (Sherk & Stryker 1976, Buisseret & Imbert 1976) supports Hubel and Wiesel's (1963) original findings that in the cat the characteristics of the visual cortical neurones found in adults are mainly present at birth. This is highly surprising since anatomical evidence shows that at this time only 5% of the final number of visual cortical synapses have been formed (Cragg 1975). Some higher mammals have been found to possess a cortical mechanism for stereoscopic vision, as mentioned earlier. Cortical neurones, called disparity detectors, which are each capable of registering a particular retinal disparity, and hence the location of an object in three-dimensional visual space, have been found in both cats (Barlow, Blakemore & Pettigrew 1967, Nikara, Bishop & Pettigrew 1968) and monkeys (Hubel & Wiesel 1970b). These neurons are exquisitely sensitive in their preferred disparity and demand an extremely high degree of precision in the matching of inputs from the two eyes. It is this degree of precision which may be beyond the capabilities of innate developmental mechanisms and may provide visual experience with a true constructive role. At birth, kittens do not possess disparity detectors with the fine tuning found in the adult, and if they are reared in the dark from birth they never achieve this adult precision (Barlow & Pettigrew 1971, Pettigrew 1974). It seems that normal congruent binocular visual experience is required for the normal maturation and fine tuning of these disparity detectors. Their development may require the plasticity of neuronal connections found during the critical period in the visual cortex so that visual experience can mould their final connectivity patterns.

The development of human binocular visual pathways

We now turn to the human visual system to ascertain if there is evidence to suggest that similar mechanisms dependent upon binocular visual experience operate in its post-natal maturation.

It has been estimated that 14% of the population lack the full ability to use binocular disparities to judge depth, despite good monocular vision in both eyes and no diplopia (Richards 1972). This could be due to a reduction in the number of binocular neurones in the visual cortex, resulting from the mild degree of strabismus commonly seen during infancy which produces non-congruent binocular visual experience and possibly leads to a disruption of binocular inputs to the cortical neurones, as has been described in the cat. Evidence in favour of such a suggestion has come from the field of human psychophysics. There are a number of visual illusions such as the motion after-effect and tilt after-effects which are thought to be due to fatigue of groups of cortical neurones. Such illusions normally transfer from one eye to the other so that if the fatiguing stimulus is given to one eye, the illusion can be detected when that eye is closed and the other eye is opened. If stereoblind individuals lack binocular neurones, such transfer should be impossible, and that is precisely the result that has been obtained (Movshon, Chambers & Blakemore 1972, Ware & Mitchell 1974, Mitchell, Reardon & Muir 1975). Indeed, Hohmann and Creutzfelt (1975) have used this phenomenon to claim that the critical period for the development of binocular neurones in humans extends to the third year.

Amblyopia ex anopsia is well known to develop during infancy in humans during long periods of deprivation of normal retinal image formation, due to obstacles such as ptosis, dense corneal opacities and congenital cateracts. It is only recently that it has been shown how brief periods of eye occlusion can also cause amblyopia; if monocular occlusion in humans takes place for longer than a week during the first two years of life, then the child runs the risk of developing an amblyopia in that eye (Von Noorden & Maumenee 1968, Awaya *et al* 1973). The mechanisms involved in this are presumably analogous to those occurring in other mammals following similar brief periods of monocular occlusion during the critical period, as discussed previously. Caution must be displayed when continuous occlusion of an infant's eye is considered in the treatment of, for example, a corneal scratch or following eye surgery. Similarly, if a child who exhibits a strabismus early in life is to possess normal stereoacuity in later life it is essential that early corrective eye surgery is attempted.

Conclusions

There still remains much to be explained regarding the processes involved in the development of neuronal connections subserving binocular functions. Experimental studies in vertebrates are providing us with new insights into these processes, which hopefully will lead us to a greater understanding of some human visual anomalies and abnormalities.

The precision required for the matching of inputs from the two eyes to produce not only binocular fusion, but also stereopsis may be beyond the information content of the genome, and would be hopelessly inflexible even if it were. Instead it appears that, during a sensitive or critical period after birth, normal binocular visual experience plays an important role in ensuring the precise matching of inputs from the two eyes to cortical neurones.

Nature and nurture should not be considered as rivals in the development of the visual pathways—rather they must be considered to work in unison.

Acknowledgments

I am grateful to the Medical Research Council for their support in the form of a Training Fellowship.

References

AWAYA S., MIYAKE Y., IMAIZUMI Y., SHIOSE Y., KANDA T. & KOMURO K. (1973) Amblyopia in man, suggestive of stimulus deprivation amblyopia. *Jap. J. Ophthalmol.* **17,** 69–82.

BAKER F.H., GRIGG P. & VON NOORDEN G.K. (1974) Effects of visual deprivation and strabismus on the response of neurons in the visual cortex of the monkey, including studies on the striate and prestriate cortex in the normal animal. *Brain Res.* **66,** 185–208.

BARLOW H.B. (1975) Visual experience and cortical development. *Nature* **258,** 199–204.

BARLOW H.B. & PETTIGREW J.D. (1971) Lack of specificity of neurons in the visual cortex of young kittens. *J. Physiol.* **218,** 98–100.

BARLOW H.B., BLAKEMORE C. & PETTIGREW J.D. (1967) The neural basis of binocular depth discrimination. *J. Physiol.* **193,** 327–42.

BLAKEMORE C. & CUMMINGS R.M. (1975) Eye-opening in kittens. *Vision Res.* **15,** 1417–18.

BLAKEMORE C. & VAN SLUYTER R.C. (1974) Reversal of the physiological effects of monocular deprivation in kittens: further evidence for a sensitive period. *J. Physiol.* **237,** 195–216.

BUISSERET P. & IMBERT M. (1976) Visual cortical cells: their developmental properties in normal and dark reared kittens. *J. Physiol.* **255,** 511–25.

CRAGG B.G. (1975) The development of synapses in the visual system of the cat. *J. Comp. Neurol.* **160,** 147–66.

CRAWFORD M.L.J., BLAKE R., COOL S.J. & VON NOORDEN G.K. (1975) Physiological consequences of unilateral and bilateral eye closure in Macaque monkeys: some further observations. *Brain Res.* **84,** 150–4.

CREEL D., WITKOP C.J. & KING R.A. (1974) Asymmetric visually evoked potentials in human albinos: evidence for visual system anomalies. *Invest. Ophthalmol.* **13,** 430–40.

DUFFY F.H., SNODGRASS S.R., BURCHFIEL J.L. & CONWAY J.L. (1976) Bicuculline reversal of deprivation amblyopia in the cat. *Nature* **260,** 256–7.

DUKE-ELDER S. (1963) *System of Ophthalmology. Vol. III, Normal and Abnormal Development,* Part 2, Congenital deformities. Mosby, St Louis, Mo.

GANZ L. & HAFFNER M.E. (1974) Permanent perceptual and neurophysiological effects of visual deprivation in the cat. *Exp. Brain Res.* **20,** 67–87.

GAZE R.M. (1958) The representation of the retina on the optic lobe of the frog. *Qu. J.*

exp. Physiol. **43**, 209–14.

GAZE R.M. (1970) *The Formation of Nerve Connections.* Academic Press, London.

GAZE R.M. & JACOBSON M. (1963) A study of the retinotectal projection during regeneration of the optic nerve in the frog. *Proc. Roy. Soc. B.* **157**, 420–48.

GAZE R.M. & KEATING M.J. (1970) Further studies on the restoration of the contralateral retinotectal projection following regeneration of the optic nerve in the frog. *Brain Res.* **21**, 183–95.

GAZE R.M. & KEATING M.J. (1972) The visual system and 'neuronal specificity'. *Nature* **237**, 375–8.

GAZE R.M., KEATING M.J. & CHUNG S.H. (1974) The evolution of the retinotectal map during development in *Xenopus. Proc. Roy. Soc. B.* **175**, 107–47.

GUILLERY R.W. (1969) An abnormal retinogeniculate projection in Siamese cats. *Brain Res.* **14**, 739–41.

GUILLERY R.W. (1971) An abnormal retinogeniculate projection in the albino ferret (*Mustelo furo*). *Brain Res.* **33**, 482–5.

GUILLERY R.W., SCOTT G.L., CATTANACH B.M. & DEOL M.S. (1973) Genetic mechanisms determining the central visual pathways of mice. *Science* **179**, 1014–16.

GUILLERY R.W., CASAGRANDE V.A. & OBERDORFER M.O. (1974) Congenitally abnormal vision in Siamese cats. *Nature* **252**, 195–9.

GUILLERY R.W., OKORO A.N. & WITKOP Jr. C.J. (1975) Abnormal visual pathways in the brain of a human albino. *Brain Res.* **96**, 373–7.

HOHMANN A. & CREUTZFELDT O.D.C. (1975) Squint and the development of binocularity in humans. *Nature* **254**, 613–14.

HOLMES G. (1919) Montgomery lectures in ophthalmology. *Brit. Med. Journal* **2**, 193–9, 230–3.

HUBEL D.H. & WIESEL T.N. (1963) Receptive fields of cells in striate cortex of very young, visually inexperienced kittens. *J. Neurophysiol.* **26**, 994–1002.

HUBEL D.H. & WIESEL T.N. (1965) Binocular interaction in striate cortex of kittens reared with artificial squint. *J. Neurophysiol.* **28**, 1041–59.

HUBEL D.H. & WIESEL T.N. (1970a) The period of susceptibility to the physiological effects of unilateral eye closure in kittens. *J. Physiol.* **206**, 419–36.

HUBEL D.H. & WIESEL T.N. (1970b) Stereoscopic vision in the Macaque monkey. *Nature* **225**, 41–2.

HUBEL D.H. & WIESEL T.N. (1971) Aberrant visual projections in the Siamese cat. *J. Physiol.* **218**, 33–62.

HUNT R.K. & JACOBSON M. (1974) Neuronal specificity revisited. *Curr. Top. Dev. Biol.* **8**, 203–59.

KAAS J.H. & GUILLERY R.W. (1973) The transfer of abnormal visual field representations from the dorsal lateral geniculate nucleus to the visual cortex in Siamese cats. *Brain Res.* **59**, 61–95.

KEATING M.J. (1976) The formation of visual neuronal connections—an appraisal of the present status of the theory of 'neuronal specificity'. In: Gottlieb G. (Ed.) *Studies on the Development and Behaviour of the Nervous System. Vol. 3. Development of Neural and Behavioural Specificity.* Academic Press, New York.

KEATING M.J. & KENNARD C. (1976a) The amphibian visual system as a model for developmental neurobiology. In: Fite K. (Ed.) *The Amphibian Visual System—A Multidisciplinary Approach.* Academic Press, New York.

KEATING M.J. & KENNARD C. (1976b) Binocular visual neurones in the frog thalamus. *J. Physiol.* **258**, 69–20.

LUND R.D. (1965) Uncrossed visual pathways of hooded and albino rats. *Science* **149**, 1506–7.

LUND R.D. (1975) Variations in the laterality of the central projections of retinal ganglion cells. *Exp. Eye Res.* **21**, 193–203.

MITCHELL D.E., REARDON J. & MUIR D.W. (1975) Interocular transfer of the motion after-effect in normal and stereoblind observers. *Exp. Brain Res.* **22**, 163–73.

MOVSHON J.A. & BLAKEMORE C. (1974) Functional reinnervation in kitten visual cortex. *Nature* **251**, 504–5.

MOVSHON J.A., CHAMBERS B.E.I. & BLAKEMORE C. (1972) Interocular transfer in normal humans and those who lack stereopsis. *Perception* **1**, 483–90.

NIKARA T., BISHOP P.O. & PETTIGREW J.D. (1968) Analysis of retinal correspondence by studying simple units in cat striate cortex. *Exp. Brain Res.* **6**, 353–72.

PECK C.K. & BLAKEMORE C. (1975) Modification of single neurones in the kitten's visual cortex after brief periods of monocular visual experience. *Exp. Brain Res.* **22**, 57–68.

PETTIGREW J.D. (1974) The effect of visual experience on the development of stimulus specificity by kitten cortical neurones. *J. Physiol.* **237**, 49–74.

RICHARDS W. A. (1971) Anomalous stereoscopic depth perception. *J. Opt. Soc. Am.* **61**, 410–14.

SANDERSON K.J. (1972) Normal and abnormal retinogeniculate pathways in rabbits and minks. *Anat. Rec.* **172**, 398.

SANDERSON K.J., GUILLERY R.W. & SHACKLEFORD R.M. (1974) Congenitally abnormal visual pathways in mink (*Mustela vision*) with reduced retinal pigment. *J. Comp. Neurol.* **154**, 225–48.

SEARLE A.G. (1968) *Comparative Genetics of Coat Colour in Mammals.* Academic Press, New York.

SHERK H. & STRYKER M.P. (1976) Quantitative study of cortical orientation selectivity in visually inexperienced kittens. *J. Neurophysiol.* **39**, 63–70.

SPERRY R.W. (1942) Reestablishment of visuomotor coordinations by optic nerve regeneration. *Anat. Rec.* **84**, 470.

SPERRY R.W. (1943a) Effect of 180° rotation of the retinal field on visuomotor coordination. *J. exp. Zool.* **92**, 263–79.

SPERRY R.W. (1943b) Visuomotor coordination in the newt (*Triturus viridescens*) after regeneration of the optic nerve. *J. Comp. Neurol.* **79**, 33–55.

SPERRY R.W. (1945) Restoration of vision after crossing of optic nerves and after contralateral transplantation of eye. *J. Neurophysiol.* **8**, 15–28.

SPERRY R.W. (1951) Mechanisms of neural maturation. In: Stevens S.S. (Ed.) *Handbook of Experimental Psychology*, pp. 236–80. Wiley, New York.

SPERRY R.W. (1963) Chemoaffinity in the orderly growth of nerve fibre patterns and connections. *Proc. natn. Acad. Sci. U.S.A.* **50**, 703–10.

THORPE P.A. & BLAKEMORE C. (1975) Evidence for a loss of afferent axons in the visual cortex of monocularly deprived cats. *Neuroscience Letters* **1**, 271–6.

VON NOORDEN G.K. (1973) Experimental amblyopia in monkeys. Further behavioural observations and clinical correlations. *Invest. Ophthalmol.* **12**, 721–6.

VON NOORDEN G.K. & MAUMENEE E.A. (1968) Clinical observations on stimulus deprivation amblyopia (amblyopia ex anopsia). *Am. J. Ophthalmol.* **65**, 220–4.

WARE, C. & MITCHELL D.E. (1974) On interocular transfer of various visual after effects in normal and stereoblind observers. *Vis. Res.* **14**, 731–4.

WIESEL T.N. & HUBEL D.H. (1965) Comparison of effects of unilateral and bilateral eye closure on cortical unit responses in kittens. *J. Neurophysiol.* **28**, 1029–40.

A PHYSIOLOGICAL CLASSIFICATION OF NYSTAGMUS

E. J. ARNOTT

Nystagmus is the term applied to any involuntary rhythmical movement of the eyes.

The velocity, frequency and amplitude may be measured by electro-nystagmography or infra-red reflection techniques. It may be looked upon as an abnormality of the ocular posture and as such can be caused by any of the factors, physiological or pathological, which govern the ocular subsystems and their central and peripheral connections. This can be subdivided into four divisions:

(1) the fixation and smooth pursuit mechanism which is centred in the occipital cortex;
(2) the gaze or saccadic mechanism, centred in the precentral gyrus;
(3) the vestibular mechanism with its central and peripheral locations;
(4) the vergence mechanism centred in the midbrain.

The fixation mechanism

The ocular movements which occur in fixation, either examining or pursuing an object, are smooth and of low velocity. The fixation mechanism is centred on the fovea and is devoted to detailed visual analysis through the foveal mechanism and subserved by small X ganglion cells. From the fovea impulses are referred via the neurones to the striate cortex. The nervous impulses for smooth pursuit movements probably originate in the visual association areas of the occipital cortex and are transmitted by the occipito-mesencephalic tract. This tract passes lateral to the ventricles and medial to the optic radiation to terminate in the paramedian pontine reticular formation and the pretectal and superior collicular nuclei. The occipital cortex controls pursuit movements to the same side. This mechanism is fundamental to and maintains visual stabilization. As with the other visual motor systems, nystagmus, associated with the fixation mechanism, may be physiologically or pathologically induced. Physiological fixation nystagmus may be induced

19

by opticokinetic testing, oculonystagmography or the Pendular Eye Tracking Test (PETT).

Opticokinetic nystagmus has recently gained in importance in a test to localize the site in homonymous hemianopia and also as a means of testing visual acuity in an infant. Rotation of a moving object in front of the eyes produces a slow movement in the same direction and a rapid compensatory movement in the opposite direction. The stimulus may be presented as a striped tape, a scarf with red and black stripes some 6 mm wide, or a rotating drum with white and black stripes.

Both phases of this optically elicited nystagmus, resulting from the movement of an object in the other direction, are mediated through the same side of the cerebral hemisphere. The slow movement is initiated in the occipital lobe, the saccadic or fast phase is initiated in the precentral motor area of the frontal lobe with nervous impulses using the fronto-pontine pathways. Opticokinetic dissociation may be of great localizing value as to the site of a cerebral lesion. In the presence of a homonymous hemianopia opticokinetic nystagmus will be abnormal in a parietal but not in an occipital lobe lesion (Kestenbaum 1930). This helps to differentiate a lesion of the striate cortex from that of the second and third part of the optic radiations.

Vertical opticokinetic nystagmus can be induced by vertical rotation of the drum. Absence of the fast phase of vertical opticokinetic nystagmus indicates bilateral lesions of the fronto-bulbar pathways. Opticokinetic testing is valuable in patients with vertical elevator palsy for the attempt to perform upward saccades as with a downward rotating drum produces retraction or convergent nystagmus, a pathognomonic feature of pretectal involvement (Sanders & Bird 1970).

The opticokinetic nystagmus test has been used as a means of testing visual acuity in infants in whom no subjective visual responses can be obtained. An assessment of the visual acuity is made by determining the minimum size of a moving object that just elicits opticokinetic nystagmus.

The opticokinetic reaction may be varied in patients with ocular disturbance but can help to differentiate between fixation gaze and vestibular nystagmus. Rotation of the drum towards the side of the lesion will potentiate the jerk nystagmus in a vestibular and gaze type lesion whilst in fixation nystagmus there is no change in the nystagmus or inversion.

The pendular eye tracking test (PETT)

This utilizes the electrical field generated by the standing corneo-scleral potential of the eye. Skin electrodes are placed at the medial and lateral canthi. As the cornea moves towards an electrode, relative positivity is induced and recorded as a deflection from the straight ahead position. Eye movements can be induced by using the Barany drum or pendular tracking. In the pendular eye tracking test (PETT) the patient follows a target which moves horizontally in a pendular way.

Three different deformations of the PETT have been observed:

(1) a normal-shaped curve with superimposed fast movements;
(2) a deformed curve;
(3) the absence of sinusoidal tracing.

In diseases of the inner ear the PETT usually shows a normal curve which can sometimes be modified by the appearance of small fast movements.

The PETT can be useful in localizing disease of the central nervous system. The normal curve with superimposed fast movements tends to be associated with cerebellar disease; the deformed curve often appears in connection with more widespread lesions of the brain stem while the disappearance of the curve is usually due to a lesion in the oculomotor pathway in the tegmentum of the pons and midbrain.

Pathologically induced fixation nystagmus

This nystagmus almost invariably presents with nystagmus in forward gaze and may be associated with defects in the visuo-sensori-motor pathways subserving the fixation mechanism. Pathologically induced fixation nystagmus may be associated with defects of the afferent part of the fixation mechanism or defects of the efferent pathway and central connections of the fixation mechanism.

Defects of the afferent part of the fixation mechanism constitutes the so-called ocular fixation nystagmus, which is normally present from early infancy and apart from the associated embarrassment of visual function is usually of no serious clinical significance. Ocular nystagmus from early infancy is pendular and symmetrical in the central or paracentral zone changing to a jerk nystagmus on dextro- or laevo-version of the eyes; there may be a slight rotatory component. The primary cause of the visual defect is usually apparent, such as cataract, optic atrophy or changes in the vitreous. The nystagmus is very rarely vertical, and ceases when the eyes are closed; there is a decrease of the nystagmus in fixation on a near object.

Included in the ocular fixation subsystem are hereditary jerk nystagmus, latent nystagmus, spasmus nutans, occupational or Miner's nystagmus and uniocular pendular nystagmus.

Hereditary jerk nystagmus is rare; it is usually sex-linked, occurring only in males. It is a pendular jerk nystagmus, the fast phase being in the direction of lateral gaze and is bidirectional. The reduction in acuity due to the nystagmus is proportional to the nystagmus intensity (the product of amplitude and frequency at a given gaze angle). The attempt to fixate is the driving stimulus for the nystagmus. The classification of congenital nystagmus into two basic wave forms, pendular and jerk, is an oversimplification and oculographic studies of congenital nystagmus reveal several types of wave form. A pendular sinusoidal wave form in one position of gaze may become distorted as the gaze angle changes. A probable cause for the departure from pure sinusoidal wave forms in most cases of congenital nystagmus is relative to the desirability of prolonged target foveation. This may result in flattening of the peak of the oscillation at which the target is foveated (Dell Osso 1972, Young 1963, Dell Osso *et al* 1974).

There is a neutral position, central or off-central to one side of gaze, in which the nystagmus is minimal, absent or only slightly pendular in type. A compensatory head turn may be adopted so the neutral position is placed in the straight ahead viewing position. The compensatory head position can be corrected by symmetrical muscle surgery to place the neutral position in the primary position of gaze or by prisms. It is probable that this type of nystagmus is due to instability in the oculo-motor system of the fixation mechanism, classically referred to as the pursuit system.

Latent nystagmus occurs in susceptible subjects when one eye is occluded with jerking of both eyes in the fast phase towards the non-occluded eye. In this condition, if one eye is lost from injury, permanent nystagmus occurs in the remaining eye. Latent nystagmus can make occlusion in an amblyopic eye difficult, and if occlusive therapy needs to be carried out atropine occlusion is preferable.

Spasmus mutans is a self-limiting condition occurring in impoverished under-fed infants between the ages of 6 and 18 months, living under conditions of poor lighting. This type of nystagmus is now rarely seen. The nystagmus is usually binocular, horizontal and pendular, but may be uniocular with vertical or rotatory elements. Head nodding, if present, tends to be compensatory for the nystagmus and is in a direction opposite to that of the ocular movement.

Miner's nystagmus used to be seen commonly in English coalmines when the miner worked for long hours on the ceiling at the coal face in a semi-squatting position with poor illumination. The nystagmus occurred only on upward gaze with movements of small amplitude (0·5 mm) and high frequency. The movements were horizontal or vertical, usually mixed, and pendular or jerk in type.

Uniocular pendular nystagmus may occur in an amblyopic eye associated with a strabismus, high refractive error or astigmatism.

Another type of fixation nystagmus may occur due to defects of the efferent pathway and central connections of the fixation mechanism. This may occur at any period of life and is of serious clinical significance, being usually associated with lesions in the posterior fossa (Norton 1969). In this type of nystagmus, which occurs in patients with brainstem dysfunction, e.g. multiple sclerosis or vertebro-basilar insufficiency, the patient is aware of movement of the outside environment. As in the congenital type of fixation nystagmus it may be pendular becoming jerk on horizontal gaze with the fast component in the direction of gaze. On upward gaze it usually becomes a vertical nystagmus.

Other types of neurological fixation nystagmus may include ocular flutter and ocular dysmetria, as described by Cogan (1954). These types of nystagmus are associated with an ataxia of the fixation mechanism and are signs of cerebellar disease.

See-saw nystagmus is a rare form of pendular rotatory dysjunctive nystagmus first described by Maddox; as one eye elevates and extorts, the other depresses and intorts. This type of nystagmus is normally associated with a bitemporal hemianopia. As the underlying lesion is usually a middle cranial fossa lesion, associated brain stem involvement cannot be ruled out as a cause of the nystagmus. Like other types of fixation nystagmus, it diminishes or ceases when the eyes are closed.

Periodic alternating nystagmus is a disturbance of the fixation mechanism in which there is a horizontal jerk nystagmus which changes direction at set intervals. The usual sequence is a jerk nystagmus to one side lasting for 90 seconds, a neutral phase of 10 seconds, followed by a 90-second phase with nystagmus in the opposite direction. This basic pattern continues during the waking hours and sometimes during sleep. The responsible lesion usually involves the lower part of the brain stem and it has been seen with a wide variety of aetiological factors (David & Smith 1971).

Positional nystagmus can occur in either brain stem or vestibular disease. The nystagmus occurs when the susceptible patient is rapidly changed from a sitting to a supine position or vice versa. This is subdivided into peripheral and central types.

The peripheral type is associated with marked vertigo, occurs after a short latent period, lasting usually for a minute, and disappears after repetition of the movement; this is not associated with severe neurological disease.

The central type occurs without a latent period and does not show fatiguability or habituation. The central type is more often associated with brain-stem or cerebellar disease.

The gaze or saccadic mechanism

The second of the ocular subsystems is the gaze or saccadic mechanism centred in the precentral gyrus. This system is responsible for high velocity movements which may be produced voluntarily with impulses mediated from the frontal cortex (area 8 of Brodmann), or in response to auditory or eccentric visual stimuli. They also occur in the rapid eye movement phase of sleep, and in the fast saccadic phase of vestibular and opticokinetic nystagmus. The anatomical pathway passes from the frontal cortex via the anterior limb of the internal capsule, to the subthalamic region and zona incerta. For control of vertical movements it terminates in the pretectal region, and for horizontal movements in the paramedian pontine reticular formation after decussation in the midbrain (Brucher 1966). The final common pathway for horizontal conjugate movements lies in the paramedian pontine reticular formation, which is situated ventral to the longitudinal fasciculus at the level of the abducens nucleus.

This cellular organization is responsible for all conjugate horizontal movements and functions as a pulse generator (Robinson 1972). Conjugate horizontal gaze pathways from the PPRF convey excitatory impulses to the ipsilateral abducens nucleus and via the median longitudinal fasciculus to the contra-lateral mesencephalic medial retus nucleus which is situated ventrally in the oculo-motor complex (Warwick 1953). Simultaneously, inhibitory impulses pass to the contra-lateral abducers and ipsilateral medial rectus nuclei.

The fixation and gaze systems subserve focal and ambient vision (Trevarthen 1968), distinguishing between 'what' and 'where'.

With the gaze mechanism, the saccadic or 'noticing' aspect detects movements, achieves spatial orientation and brings objects seen by the periphery of the retina on to the fovea. This is carried out by the rods in the retina and large Y ganglion cells which transmit impulses via relatively large nerve fibres to the cerebral cortex and superior colliculus where a retinotopic map is also situated (James 1892). Saccadic movements utilize fast twitch fibres situated centrally in the occular muscles innervated by rapid conduction neurones, small peripheral tonic muscle fibres maintain sustained activity (Bach-y-Rita 1971).

Gaze nystagmus can be physiological or pathological. Physiological and point nystagmus occurs in about 60% of patients in extreme lateral gaze, the nystagmus occurring after a latent period of some 30 seconds. Another type of physiological end point nystagmus occurs without a latency period. This type of nystagmus occurs within 1–2 mm of the end-point position of gaze occurring usually in nervous patients who are otherwise healthy.

Pathological gaze-type nystagmus occurs in several conditions. There may be a gaze-type nystagmus, not strictly a gaze nystagmus, or a true gaze nystagmus. Gaze-type nystagmus can occur in an ocular palsy with paresis of an extra ocular muscle, nystagmus occurring when the gaze is in the direction of action of the paralysed muscle.

Another type of gaze-type nystagmus is that associated in the syndrome of the medial longitudinal fasciculus with involvement of the sixth nerve nucleus.

This is often called ataxic nystagmus. As is well known in this condition, on attempted version of the eyes to one side, there is little movement of the adducting eye and the abducting eye has a jerk nystagmus towards the direction of gaze. This type of nystagmus may occur in lesions involving the brain stem. Cogan 1968 has stated that if unilateral, it is likely to be due to disseminated sclerosis, while if bilateral, a vascular lesion should be considered.

True gaze nystagmus may be either horizontal symmetrical or horizontal asymmetrical. Gaze paretic nystagmus is characterized by a slow frequency of less than 2 cycles per second. It represents a manifestation of a gaze or saccadic paresis associated with a lesion in the fronto-mesencephalic system or the PPRF. In this type there is no nystagmus on forward gaze, but it develops on deviation with the fast component varying as to the direction of gaze. If gaze nystagmus develops due to a lesion of the fronto-mesencephalic system, as for instance with occlusion of the middle cerebral artery, the nystagmus is usually of short duration and associated with a definite weakness of horizontal gaze to that side. Continued pathological gaze nystagmus is usually associated with defects of the PPRF. Aetiological factors include drug toxicity, demyelinating disease, degenerative disease, vascular disease, focal infection or tumour.

Included in this category of gaze nystagmus are a number of conditions with a gaze-evoked nystagmus which are not a true gaze nystagmus in the accepted meaning. These have no localizing value other than implying disease or dysfunction of brain stem structures, and include up-beat nystagmus and down-beat nystagmus.

Up-beat nystagmus is a jerk nystagmus of large amplitude in the primary position, with the fast phase upwards, increasing on elevation, but decreasing on down gaze. It may very rarely be congenital, or drug induced, but is usually associated with dysfunction of the anterior vermis of the cerebellum (Daroff & Troost 1973).

Down-beat nystagmus may arise with several posterior fossa conditions, but especially signifies disorders at the cranio–cervical junction (Cogan 1968). Prominent down-beat nystagmus on lateral gaze correlates with compressive lesions at the level of the foramen magnum, such as meningioma, basilar invagination, and the Arnold–Chiari malformation (Hart & Saunders 1970). This site is caudal to the major brain stem areas, and may be the one type of nystagmus due to an impairment of the spino-vestibular input.

The vestibular mechanism

The third of the ocular subsystems consists of the labyrinth, the peripheral end organ, the vestibular nerve, the vestibular nuclei and their central connections. Vestibular nystagmus occurs when one vestibular apparatus is affected so that it is either less or more irritable than the vestibular apparatus on the other side. The normal functioning of the vestibular system produces ocular stability in relation to head, body and environmental movement. This is achieved by close integration of vestibular, neck muscle and cervical afferents with pontine and cerebellar complexes. Neither disturbance of the otolith system nor tonic neck reflexes play a major role in the production of nystagmus in man, and in lesions of the labyrinth it is disturbance of the semi-circular canals which produces the classical picture of peripheral vestibular nystagmus. As with the other ocular subsystems, vestibular nystagmus may be physiological or pathological. It is a jerk nystagmus.

Physiological vestibular nystagmus occurs in normal subjects with some degree of vertigo when the labyrinth (end organ) is stimulated by rotation, with warm or cold water in the meatus (as in caloric testing) or galvanic stimulation.

The mechanism of per-rotary and post-rotary nystagmus, caloric nystagmus and galvanic (electrical) nystagmus are well known and will not be enumerated.

Pathological spontaneous vestibular nystagmus may be peripheral or central, and can be identified by certain characteristics. It is always a jerk and there is usually in addition a fine rotatory component. Vestibular nystagmus may be first, second or third degree.

Peripheral vestibular nystagmus (due to a lesion of the labyrinth or branch of the auditory vestibular nerve). Irritative pathological lesions of the labyrinth do occur but are subclinical in their manifestations. In clinical practice diseases of the vestibular end organ cause 'destructive' effects. Conditions affecting the labyrinth end organ include Ménière's disease and diffuse or circumscribed labyrinthitis. Peripheral vestibular nystagmus is a jerk nystagmus and is always directed towards the side opposite to that of the lesion. The nystagmus is always horizontal, with usually a superimposed rotatory element; purely vertical nystagmus is never found in this condition. In association with this unidirectional jerk nystagmus there is vertigo, in the direction of the nystagmus, with past pointing and a fall towards the side of the lesion with the eyes closed (Romberg's sign). Within ten days after the onset of the lesion the nystagmus shows a decrease in intensity and finally ceases. If at a later date a lesion destroys the other labyrinth, for a few days there appears a nystamus whose direction is towards the side of the labyrinth first destroyed. Peripheral vestibular nystagmus is always associated with some acoustic disturbance.

In a lesion of the labyrinth or vestibular nerve, post-rotatory nystagmus to the side of the lesion is at first much shorter to the side opposite the lesion, and later is a little shortened to both sides. The warm and cold tests are ineffective at the ipsilateral ear, while absence of the galvanic reaction on one side indicates a lesion of the nervous pathway.

Central vestibular nystagmus due to a lesion involving the vestibular nuclei or their central connections is usually horizontal rotatory but may be vertical. The superior or cephalic portion of Deiter's nucleus seems to be related to vertical nystagmus, its middle portion to horizontal nystagmus and its inferior (caudal) part to rotatory nystagmus. The central vestibular nystagmus may be first, second or third degree in type and, in contradistinction to peripheral vestibular nystagmus continues as long as the causative lesion remains. The nystagmus may be bi-directional, the fast phase being to the left on gaze to the left, and right on gaze to the right. The direction of the fast phase does not localize the site of the lesion. With central vestibular lesions the direction of past pointing, vertigo and Romberg fall, while being present, may be variable in direction and will not help to localize the side of the central lesion. Both peripheral and central vestibular nystagmus have a frequency of 3 to 6 beats per second. In central vestibular nystagmus there may be no associated acoustic disturbance or vertigo. Post-rotatory nystagmus may be normal, and the caloric test may show a 'readiness for nystagmus' or a prevalence to one side.

The vergence mechanism

The fourth ocular motor subsystem is the vergence mechanism. The vergence system produces, in contrast to the other ocular subsystems, movement of each eye in opposite directions, a dysjunctive nystagmus. A phylogenetically recent addition, this system is dependent on the neuro-mechanism of binocular depth perception and specific cells for this purpose have been found in area 18 of the cortex (Hubel & Wiesel 1970). The vergence system produces slow dysjunctive movements that keep the target on the fovea of the eye. As with the other subsystems the vergence mechanism may be associated with physiological or pathological nystagmus.

Physiological vergence nystagmus includes the hysterical and voluntary nystagmus which has the highest frequency of all types of nystagmus, being 1000 cycles per minute. With this fast frequency there is a small amplitude. Voluntary nystagmus can only be maintained for a few moments, and cannot be held when the position of gaze is changed. The nystagmus may be horizontal, conjugate and pendular in type, but there is usually a superimposed convergent and divergent element.

Pathological vergence nystagmus is characterized by convergent movements of the eyes, exaggerated by attempts to converge or look upwards. When the nystagmus becomes more severe there is actual retraction of the globe, associated with the convergent movements, so-called nystagmus retractorius. There is usually an associated disturbance of convergence with a palsy of upward gaze. The phenomenon may be explained by clonic spasms of convergence with contraction of all the horizontally acting recti muscles. The syndrome of the sylvian aquaduct may show this type of nystagmus with upward or downward gaze palsy, convergence spasms and movements, vertical upward or downward jerk nystagmus, pupillary disturbances and paresis of one or more of the extra-ocular muscles.

In this chapter one has attempted to classify nystagmus on an anatomical and physiological basis. There are, however, in this classification, a few ends which cannot be satisfactorily tied, and certain unclassified 'nystagmoid' movements must be mentioned, which do not fit into any of the former ocular sub-groups. These include:

Ocular myoclonus

Unilateral or bilateral slow pendular vertical movements, often occurring in synchrony with movements of other midline structures, particularly the palate (Daroff & Waldeman 1965).

Opsoclonus

First described in children as 'myoclonic encephalopathy' (Kinsbourne 1962). Rapid involuntary conjugate saccadic movements of a chaotic nature may occur with encephalitis, post-encephalitic syndromes or neoplasms, particularly in association with neuroblastoma.

Ocular bobbing

This refers to a downward, maybe dysconjugate, jerk of both eyes, followed by a slow drift upwards to the primary position. The eyes may remain deviated for several seconds before returning to the normal position. This condition is usually associated with a comatose patient who has extrapontine compression or an extensive destructive lesion of the pons (Fisher 1964).

Square wave jerks

These are small (2°) horizontal jerks from and back to the mid-position, associated with a degenerative cerebellar disease (Jung & Kornhuber 1964).

Superior oblique myokymia

A rare condition, occurring in otherwise normal patients. This consists of rapid, small amplitude, intermittent, uniocular phasic contractions of the superior oblique muscle, causing oscillopsia (Hoyt & Keane 1970).

References

BACH-Y-RITA P. (1971) *The control of eye movements.* Academic Press, New York.

BRUCHER J.M. (1966) *Int. J. Neurol.,* **5,** 262.

COGAN D.G. (1954) Ocular dysmetria; flutter-like oscillations of the eyes and opsocionus. *Arch. ophth.* **51,** 318–35.

COGAN D.G. (1968) *Canad. J. Ophthal.* **2,** 4.

DAROFF R.B. & TROOST, B.T. (1973) *J. Amer. med. Ass.* **225,** 312.

DAROFF R.B. & WALDEMAN A.L. (1965) *J. Neurol. Neurosurg. Psychiat.* **28,** 375.

DAVID D.G. & SMITH J.L. (1971) *Amer. J. Ophthal.* **72,** 757.

DELL OSSO L.F. (1972) Eye movement recordings as a diagnostic tool in a case of congenital nystagmus. *Amer. J. Ophthal.,* **49,** 3–13.

DELL OSSO L.F., FLYNN J.T. & DAROLL R.R. (1974) Hereditary congenital nystagmus. *Arch. ophth.,* **92,** No. 5, 366.

FISHER M. (1964) *Arch. Neurol.* **11,** 543.

HART K.D. & SAUNDERS M.D. (1970) *Trans Ophthal. Soc. U.K.* **90,** 483.

HOYT W.F. & KEANE J.R. (1970) *Arch. Ophthal.,* **84,** 461.

HUBEL D.J. & WIESEL T.N. (1970) *Nature (Lond.),* **225,** 41.

JAMES W. (1892) *Textbook of Psychology,* Macmillan, London.

JUNG R. & KORNHUBER H.H. (1964) *The Oculomotor System* (Bender, Harper & Row, New York) 428.

KESTENBAUM A. (1930) *Arch. F. Ophthal.,* **124,** 113.

KINSBOURNE M. (1962) *J. Neurol. Neurosurg. Psychiat.,* **25,** 271.

NORTON E.W.D. (1969) *Neuro-ophthalmology Symposium,* Smith 1, 288.

ROBINSON D.A. (1972) *Invest. Ophthal.,* **11,** 497.

SANDERS M.D. & BIRD A.C. (1970) *Trans Ophthal. Soc. U.K.* **90,** 433.

TREVARTHEN C.B. (1968) *Psychol. Forsch.,* **31,** 299. (1969) *Science* **163,** 895

WARWICK R. (1953) *J. comp. Neurol.,* **98,** 449.

YOUNG L.R. (1963) Measuring eye movements. *Amer. J. Med. Electronics,* **2,** 300–307.

DISTURBANCES OF OCULAR MOVEMENTS IN CEREBELLAR DISEASE

M. D. SANDERS

Cerebellar disease and disorders of ocular movements provided a life-long source of interest for Sir Gordon Holmes which is reflected in the fact that he wrote an equal number of papers on each subject. His contributions on ocular movements laid the foundations for our understanding of disorders of ocular movements in diseases of the central nervous system. He appreciated that ocular movement abnormalities were of relatively minor significance in cerebellar disease but emphasized the frequency of nystagmus, the occurrence of gaze paresis, and described skew deviation after acute destructive lesions of the cerebellum.

In this chapter, the experimental evidence for the functions of the cerebellum in the control of ocular movements are reviewed and then related to the clinical situation in man.

The division of ocular movement control into 4 separate subsystems provides appropriate sections for the consideration of the role of the cerebellum. These include:

(1) saccadic system;
(2) pursuit system;
(3) oculo-vestibular system;
(4) vergence system.

The role of the cerebellum will be discussed in relation to the first three subsystems.

1. Saccadic system

Cortical representation of voluntary conjugate eye movements is attributed to frontal area 8 of Brodman on anatomical evidence (Astruc 1971) though physiological evidence has not been conclusive (Bizzi & Schiller 1970); clinical evidence supports the concept of the frontal region for control of voluntary saccadic movements. Pathways from this region descend via the anterior limb of the internal capsule, with many synapses in the basal ganglia

(Astruc 1971) before passing into descending pathways to the midbrain and pontine nuclei. Termination of these fibres occurs at the pretectal nuclei for the control of vertical gaze, and in the paramedian pontine reticular formation for the control of horizontal gaze.

The cerebellum has extensive connections with the superior colliculus, the pontine nuclei and the nucleus prepositus hypoglossi, all of which are thought to play a significant role in the supranuclear control of ocular movements. A recent extensive study of eye movements evoked by cerebellar stimulation in the alert monkey (Ron & Robinson 1973) showed that saccades could be elicited from stimulation of the vermis (lobe V, VI and VII) with a latency of 15–35 m sec. Hemispheric stimulation, particularly of Crus I and II and the lobulus simplex, also produced saccadic movements, and these occurred in all directions but were dependent on electrode position. Rebound saccades were also seen at the end of stimulation. Single-cell recordings from Purkinje cells reveal an inverse relationship between Purkinje-cell activity and saccadic amplitude (Llinas 1974). There is abundant experimental and clinical evidence that saccades are not generated in the cerebellum but in the paramedian pontine reticular formation (Daroff & Hoyt 1970), so that the cerebellum serves probably to monitor the precision and accuracy of saccades.

2. Pursuit system

Stimulation of the cerebellum also produces slow pursuit movements (Ron & Robinson 1973). These were elicited by stimulation of the cerebellar hemisphere (Crus I and II and lobulus simplex) and the velocity could be increased with an increase in all stimuli parameters. Visual texture decreased the velocity of pursuit movements, and the latency of movements was 10–15 m sec.

In order to function satisfactorily in visual pursuit, visual sensory information would seem an essential prerequisite. Evidence for this has been produced by a climbing fibre input in the rabbit (Maekawa & Simpson 1973), and also a mossy fibre input to the flocculus (Maekawa & Takeda 1975). Buchtel *et al* (1973) demonstrated units in the cerebellum that were directionally sensitive and whose discharge rate was proportional to target velocity. Confirmation of a visual input to the flocculus in primates has recently been provided (Fuchs, Lisberger & Miles 1975) so that the cerebellum is well equipped to provide a role in the pursuit subsystem.

3. Oculo-vestibular movements

Possibly the most important function of the cerebellum is in monitoring the oculo-vestibular reflex. This reflex has been intensively studied by Ito (1972) who described two reflex pathways; a direct pathway with a tri-neuronal chain consisting of primary vestibular afferents, vestibulo-ocular relay neurones and ocular motor neurones and an alternative pathway linked with the flocculus by primary vestibular neurones which terminate in the cerebellar cortex as a mossy fibre input. The Purkinje cells in the flocculus then project to the vestibular neurones and so inhibit the vestibulo-ocular relay neurones.

This system was further investigated in some interesting experimental work (Robinson 1975) where reversing prisms were placed on cats and the oculo-vestibular reflex studied. The gain in the oculo-vestibular reflex could by adaption be reduced by 88% but, on removal of the vestibulo-cerebellum, the adaptive changes were completely abolished. This suggests that the cerebellum plays an important role in adapting the gain of the oculo-vestibular reflex, which serves to produce compensatory eye movements in relation to head or body movements.

Cerebellectomy and hemicerebellectomy

Though the effects of cerebellectomy on ocular movement control are contradictory, there is evidence that all the ocular motor subsystems for conjugate gaze may be involved. Saccades have been found to be normal in several reports (Westheimer & Blair 1973, Burde *et al* 1975), though hypometric saccades have been reported (Ashoff & Cohen 1971). Abnormalities of the pursuit system with the development of 'cogwheel pursuit' has been described (Westheimer & Blair 1973, Burde *et al* 1975). An abnormal response to vestibular stimulation has also been reported (Burde *et al* 1975) with a decreased latency in response and prolonged continuation of nystagmus induced by calorie stimulation.

The cerebellum has been accorded many functions including a role as computer, an inline corrective filter, a spatio-temporal translator, and a motor repair shop. This diversity reflects the complex role of the cerebellum and our difficulty in understanding its function, but, in relation to ocular movement control, it appears to be concerned in monitoring all types of conjugate ocular movement.

Clinical disorders of ocular movements in man

The magnitude of the cerebellar connections with the brain stem makes the clinical demarcation between cerebellar and brain stem disease almost impossible and a spectrum emerges of primary cerebellar disease, cerebellar pathway disease and brain stem disease. Experimental and clinical work has defined accurately the purely brain stem disorders but current investigations are attempting to define disorders of the cerebellum and its pathways. Further complexity is added by the extensive anterograde, retrograde and transneuronal degeneration that occurs after cerebellar excision in man (Smith 1975).

The list of clinical disorders attributable to disorders of the cerebellum or cerebellar system is given below and represents a modification of the classification suggested by Daroff (1975).

(1) Ocular dysmetria
(2) Hypo- or hyper-metric saccades
(3) Cogwheel pursuit
(4) Nystagmus   a horizontal   i gaze paretic
                                          ii rebound

                        b upbeat
                        c downbeat
(5) Square wave jerks
(6) Ocular flutter
(7) Macro-oscillations
(8) Opsoclonus

Other conditions which may relate to a cerebellar system disorder include periodic alternating nystagmus, ocular myoclonus and skew deviation. Clinical definition of these varied disorders has induced terminological, technical and geographical confusion and further discussion is available in recent reviews (Daroff 1975, Hoyt 1975).

Some of these disorders are described and illustrated in the following case histories, the first example a disorder essentially of the cerebellar hemisphere.

Case history

A 23-year-old man (A75311) was admitted to the Maida Vale Hospital under the care of Dr R. Kocen with severe headache, vomiting and right cerebellar signs.

At the age of 15 years he developed a severe headache with vomiting. Investigations at another hospital by angiography showed a right-sided cerebellar angioma which was deemed inoperable and he was subsequently treated by radiotherapy. At 18 years a further severe headache, neck stiffness and vomiting developed but this subsided after one week.

The present episode again commenced with severe occipital headache, and examination showed vertical, rotary and horizontal nystagmus and right cerebellar signs. Vertebral angiography demonstrated a right cerebellar angioma (Fig. 3.1). Operation by Mr Lindsay Symon resulted in complete removal of the right cerebellar hemisphere, but the vestibulo-cerebellum was not removed. Post-operatively there were no brain stem signs and a post-operative angiogram showed complete removal of the angioma (Fig. 3.1).

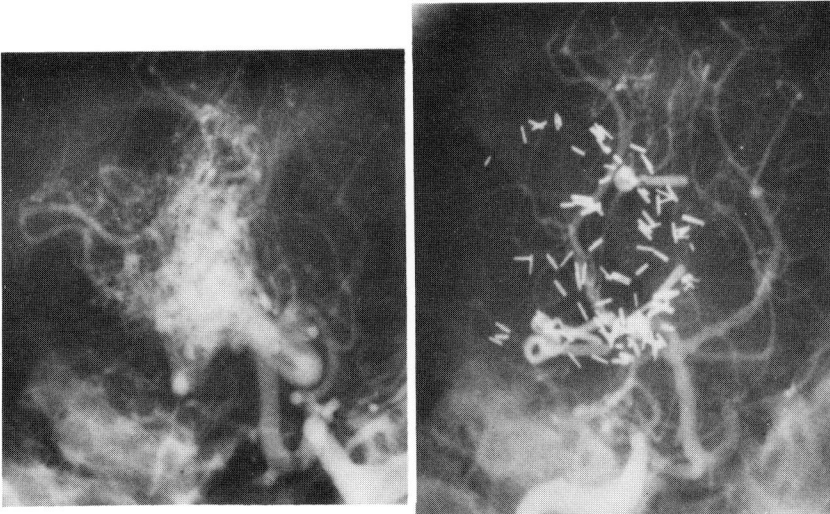

Fig. 3.1   (a) Right cerebellar angioma pre-operatively (left), and (b) post-operatively (right).

Examination at one month and two years post-operatively showed right cerebellar signs. Ocular movement examination revealed the following abnormalities:

(1) ocular dysmetria;
(2) rebound nystagmus;
(3) cogwheel pursuit.

There was no abnormality of vertical gaze, saccades were normal and convergence intact.

Oculographic recordings using silver–silver chloride electrodes and the D.C. system were performed in the M.R.C. Hearing and Balance Unit. In addition to the clinical findings already described square wave jerks were also demonstrated in the primary position (see Figs. 3.2, 3.3, 3.4, 3.5).

The ocular motor signs in this patient can therefore be attributed to the cerebellar ablation, though concomitant damage to, or micro-angiomatous involvement of, the cerebellar peduncles or brain stem cannot be entirely eliminated.

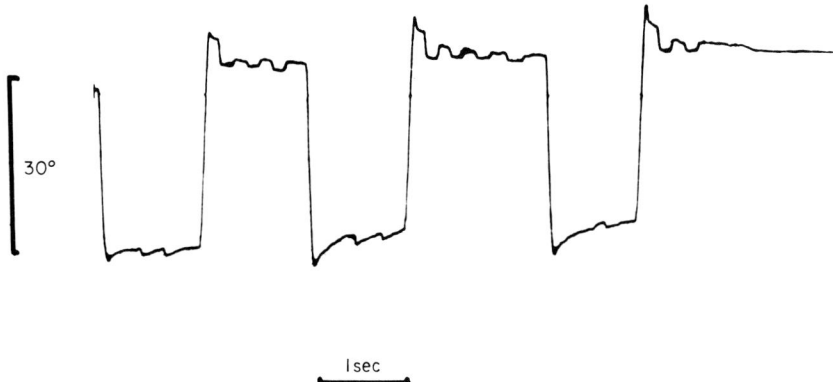

Fig. 3.2 *Ocular dysmetria.* Hypermetric saccades are seen on right gaze (upward deflection) after a 30° saccade. The saccade is of normal velocity and after a short latency a corrective saccade is initiated to be followed by square wave jerks. On left gaze (downward deflection) nystagmus to the left is seen.

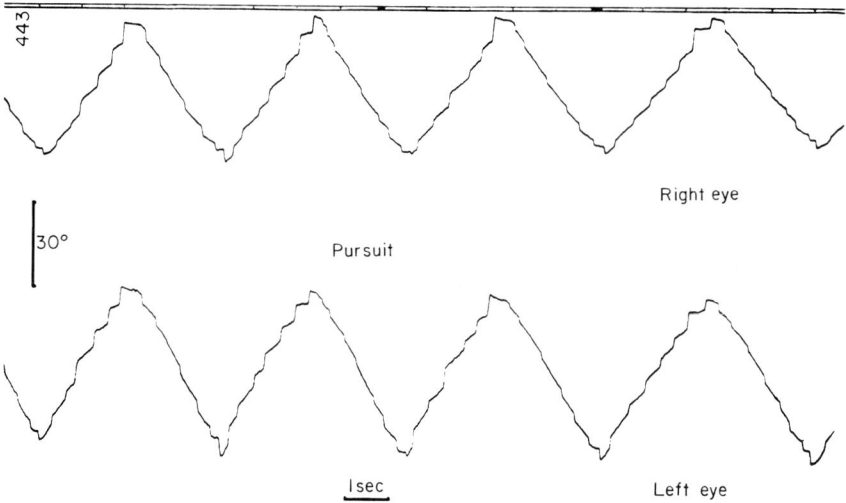

Fig. 3.3 *Cogwheel pursuit.* Slow pursuit movements show the interposition of small amplitude saccadic movements, which are present on right gaze (upward deflection) more than on left gaze (downward deflection).

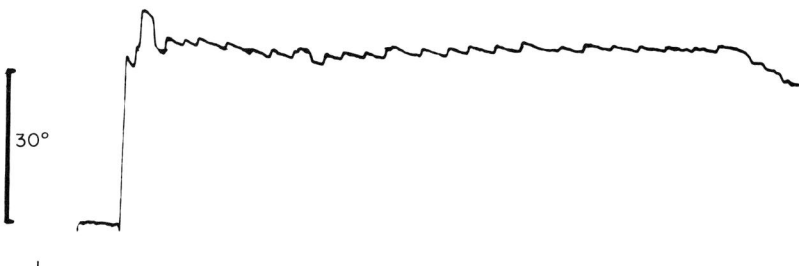

30°

L

Fig. 3.4 *Rebound nystagmus.* After maintaining left gaze (L) the nystagmus gradually fades and, after a saccade to the mid line, nystagmus to the right commences.

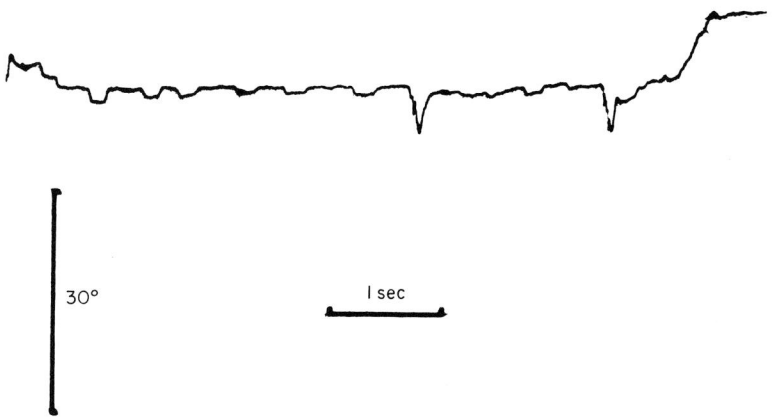

30°   I sec

Fig. 3.5 *Square wave jerks.* On primary position in the dark the patient demonstrated small saccades of 3° amplitude to the left, which were followed after a short latency by a corrective saccade. These movements were not visible on clinical examination.

Oscillating eye movements

In increasing degrees of severity the oscillatory eye movements recorded with cerebellar disease are:

(1) square wave jerks;
(2) ocular flutter;

(3) macro-oscillations;
(4) opsoclonus.

1. *Square wave jerks* have been demonstrated and when they interrupt fixation, have been attributed to cerebellar disease (Daroff 1975).

2. *Flutter-like oscillations* are attributed to cerebellar disease because of the associated truncal ataxia seen on neurological examination (Winkler *et al* 1966). The ocular movements consist of rapid intermittent horizontal bursts of saccades of varying amplitude between 8 and 12°.

Case history

A 23-year-old girl under the care of Dr C. J. Earl at The National Hospital developed mild cerebellar signs and ocular flutter (Fig. 3.6a, b). These

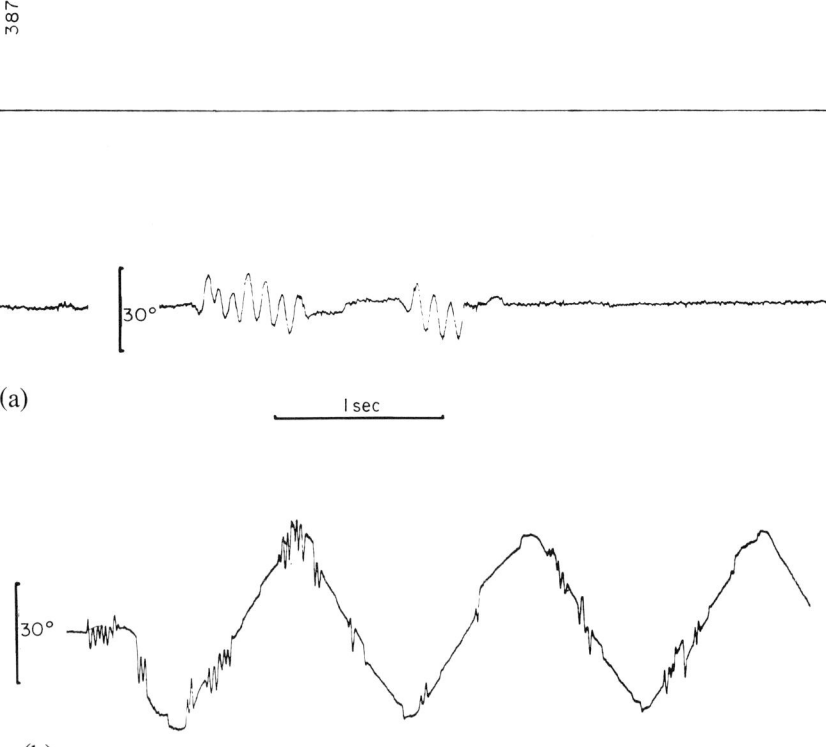

Fig. 3.6 *Flutter-like oscillations.* Bursts of horizontal saccadic movements are shown which are present in the primary position (a) and enhanced by visual fixation and pursuit (b).

occurred maximally with visual fixation and were associated with rapid movements of the head and eyelids. Examination of the C.S.F. showed a lymphocytosis and over the period of a year resolution gradually occurred.

3. *Macro-oscillations* consist clinically of large amplitude low velocity, saccadic movements, and precise definition by oculographic techniques is being undertaken in several centres (Dell Osso *et al* 1975, Selhorst *et al* 1976).

Case history

An 11-year-old girl with right-sided cerebellar signs and a hypoplastic cerebellum was referred by Dr J. Wilson at the Hospital for Sick Children, London. Conjugate gaze to the left was normal but on gaze to the right fixation could not be maintained and large pendular macro-oscillations were elicited.

4. *Opsoclonus* consists of frequent, irregular, rapid, multidirectional conjugate eye movements and clinical and pathological evidence has suggested cerebellar disease (Ellenberger & Netsoky 1970).

Down beat nystagmus

Vertical nystagmus with the fast phase downwards in the primary position was described by Cogan (1968) in 27 patients with low brain stem or cerebellar disease. Recognition of this condition in 2 families with familial degeneration of the cerebellum has suggested that it may be included in the cerebellar system disorders of ocular movements. Of particular interest is a recent paper which suggested that this was a pursuit nystagmus and that down velocity information could not be transmitted to the neural integrator that generates smooth eye movements in response to visual system commands (Zee *et al* 1974).

Case history

A 30-year-old female under the care of Professor Marshall at The National Hospital had down-beat nystagmus in the primary position with accentuation on eccentric lateral gaze (Fig. 3.7). There was no family history of cerebellar dysfunction and no neurological signs of cerebellar disease. An air encephalogram showed cerebellar atrophy with no sign of the Arnold–Chiari malformation. Oculographic records showed square wave jerks in addition to the down-beat nystagmus.

There is no doubt that the sophisticated recording of eye movements in patients and experimental animals is introducing a new era in our

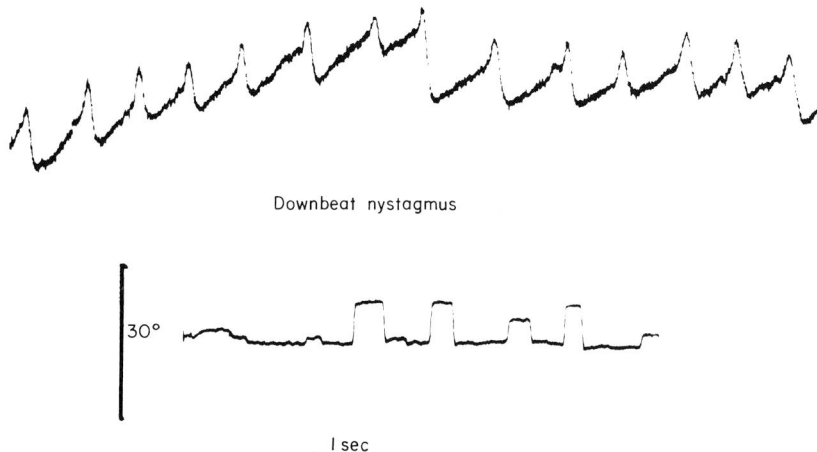

Downbeat nystagmus

30°

I sec

Fig. 3.7 *Downbeat nystagmus.* Vertical recording (top) to show nystagmus with a fast component downwards. Also present were square wave jerks (lower tracing) with an amplitude of 12° in this patient.

understanding of the role of the cerebellum in the control of ocular movements.

Acknowledgments

I would like to thank Dr R. Kocen, Mr Lindsay Symon, Dr C. J. Earl and Professor J. Marshall at The National Hospital and Dr J. Wilson at The Hospital for Sick Children, Gt Ormond Street for allowing me to study their patients. I am indebted to Dr D. Hood of the M.R.C. Hearing and Balance Unit at The National Hospital for the oculographic tracings and Mr J. Leech. My thanks to Miss G. Hopkins for secretarial help and Mr Prentice and Mr Sennhenn for photographic assistance.

References

ASCHOFF J.C. & COHEN B. (1971) Changes in saccadic eye movements produced by cerebellar cortical lesions. *Exp. Neurol.* **32**, 123–133.

ASTRUC J. (1971) Cortico-fugal connections of area (8) frontal eye fields in *Macaca mulatta. Brain Res.* **33**, 241.

BIZZI E. & SCHILLER P.H. (1970) Single unit activity in the frontal fields of unanaesthetised monkeys during head and eye movements. *Exp. Brain Res.* **10**, 151.

BUCHTEL H.A., RUBIA F.J. & STRATE P. (1973) Cerebellar unitary responses to moving visual stimuli. *Brain Res.* **50**, 463.

BURDE R.M., STROUD M.H., ROPER HALL G., WIRTH F.P. & O'LEARY J.L. (1975)

Ocular motor function in total and hemi-cerebellectomised monkeys. *Brit. J. Ophth.* **59,** 560.

COGAN D.G. (1968) Downbeat nystagmus. *Arch. Ophth.* **80,** 757–768.

DAROFF R.B. & HOYT W.F. (1971) Supranuclear disorders of ocular control systems in man. In BACH-Y-RITA P., COLLINS C.C. & HYDE J.E. *The control of eye movements.* New York, Academic Press. 175–235.

DAROFF R.B. (1975) Summary of clinical presentations. In *Basic mechanisms of ocular motility and their clinical implications.* LENNERSTRAND G. & BACH-Y-RITA P. Pergamon Press, Oxford and New York.

DELL'OSSO L.F., TROOST B.T. & DAROFF R.B. (1975) Macro square wave jerks. *Neurology, Minneapolis.* **25,** 975–979.

ELLENBERGER C. Jr. & NETSBY M.G. (1970) Anatomic basic and diagnostic value of opsoclonus. *Arch. Ophth.* **83,** 307–310.

HOYT W.F. & FRISEN L. (1975) Supranuclear ocular motor control: Some clinical considerations. In BACH-Y-RITA P. *Basic mechanisms of ocular motility and their clinical implications.* Pergamon Press, Oxford and New York.

ITO M. (1972) Neural design of the cerebellar motor control system. *Brain Res.* 40, 81–84.

LLINAS R. (1974) Motor aspects of cerebellar control. *The Physiologist* **17,** 19–46.

LISBERGER S.G. & FUCHS A.F. (1974) Response of flocculus Purkinji cells to adequate vestibular stimulation in the alert monkey. Fixation vs compensatory eye movements. *Brain Res.* **69,** 347–353.

MAEKAWA K. & TAKEDA T. (1975) Mossy fibre responses evoked in the cerebellar flocculus of rabbits by stimulation of the optic pathway. *Brain Res.* **98,** 590–595.

MAEKAWA K. & SIMPSON J.I. (1973) Climbing fibre response evoked in vestibulo-cerebellum of rabbit from visual system. *J. Neurophys.* **36.** 649–666.

ROBINSON D.A. (1975) The neural basis for pontine and cerebellar control of eye movements. *Jap. J. Ophthal.* **19,** 25–28.

RON S. & ROBINSON D.A. (1973) Eye movements evoked by cerebellar stimulation in the alert monkey. *J. Neurophys.* **36,** 1004–1022.

SELHORST J.B., STARK L., OCHS A.L. & HOYT W.F. (1976) Disorders in cerebellar ocular motor control. *Brain Res.* **99,** 509–522.

SMITH M.G. (1975) Histological findings after hemicerebellectomy in man: Anterograde, retrograde and transneuronal degeneration. *Brain Res.* **95,** 423–442.

WESTHEIMER G. & BLAIR S.M. (1973) Oculomotor defects in cerebellectomised monkeys. *Invest. Ophthal.* **12,** 618–621.

ZEE D.S., FRIENDLICH A.R., ROBINSON D.A. (1974) The mechanisms of downbeat nystagmus. *Arch. Neurol.* **30,** 227–237.

SPASM OF VISUAL FIXATION

D.DENNY-BROWN

Case I

In early 1930 it was my great privilege and good fortune to be able to assist Gordon Holmes investigate a patient, W.M., aged 56, who had suffered from a difficulty in speech and swallowing for one year. The difficulty had begun after a sudden but mild ictus but had become much worse after another six months. He was obviously suffering from pseudobulbar paralysis, such that by the time of admission to hospital he was unable to articulate, nod or shake his head, close his eyes or open his mouth on request, but could communicate fairly well by writing. He could sit up, put on his glasses and walk well if assisted, though he tended to fall backwards if unaided. He presented a fixed staring expression (Fig. 4.1a) owing to retracted eyelids. He could read and understand simple words and phrases. The most remarkable sign was an immobility of his eyes, which he was unable to move up or down, or to the right on request. On attempting to look to the right he would turn his head to the right but his eyes continued to look at the examiner. When, however, his eyes were fixed on any moving object they would follow movements to either side or up or down, provided the movement was slow and uniform. If the object approached his eyes he could converge well. If his head was moved while he fixed an object a relative compensatory movement of the eyes was easily obtained in any direction (Fig. 4.1c). He tended to advance the lips towards, and to suck, any object approaching the lower part of his face.

Only when fixation was abolished by placing an opaque screen in front of the eyes, or by holding the lids closed (which the patient could not do himself) or by taking him into a dark room, was it possible for the patient to move his eyes freely in any direction. Vestibular reactions produced by irrigation of the auditory canals, or by anodal current were reduced to small and slow deviations without nystagmus, but in a dark room normal nystagmus occurred. The rapid phase and full deviation had been reduced by fixation on his surroundings.

The importance of overactive fixation in limiting voluntary eye movement was fully discussed by Holmes (1930). In previous reports of Parinaud's syndrome there had been many references to inconsistency in the pattern of paralysis. The patient W.M. was also observed from time to time to look

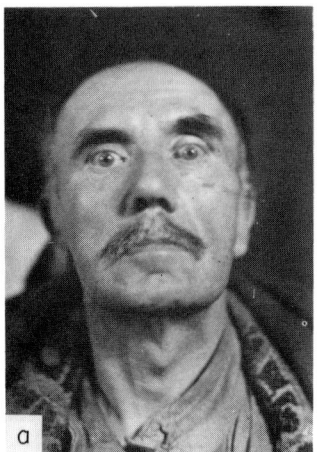 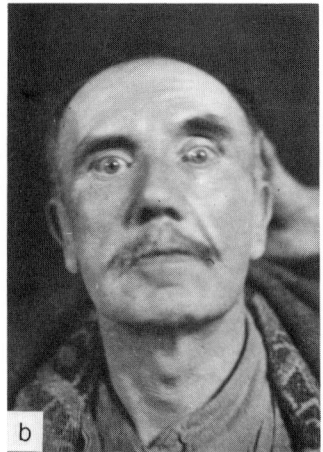 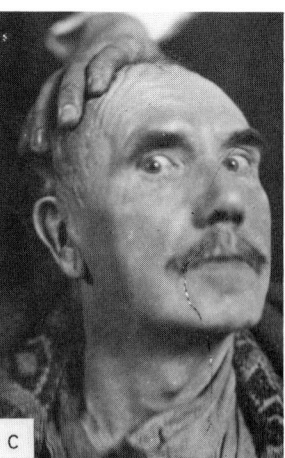

Fig. 4.1 Holmes' patient W.M. a, natural expression looking forward. b, slightly greater retraction of the upper eyelids when asked to look upwards, or to the right. c, relative movement of the eyes to the right when his head was passively turned to the left.

about him in the hospital in a way that he could not in response to request. Tiling (1874), Ballet in the discussion of the case of Crouzon (1900) and Babinski (1900), Cantonnet and Landolt (1907) and Roux (1910) all mention this phenomenon, which they attributed to 'automatico-reflex movements' as when the eyes are attracted by the sudden appearance of a bright light in the periphery of the visual field. Holmes (1930) drew attention to the abnormal intensity of fixation as cause of the defect, and the presence of the examiner in front of the patient was enough to bring about fixation. He cited the early observation of Gowers (1879) on similar spasm of fixation, which Gowers likened to reflex spasticity. However, the condition described by Gowers was the great slowing of deviation of the eyes seen in familial spinocerebellar degeneration, which is not abolished by blocking fixation. Holmes returned to the subject in 1936, and in his Horsley lecture in 1938, and came to the conclusion that the frontal lobes explore space and direct the turning of the eyes towards any object of interest and, in so doing, inhibit or control the maintenance of fixation on a point, managed by the occipital centres which were concerned with binocular convergence and fusion. Conversely, he maintained, damage to the occipital mechanism caused the eyes to oscillate about the object they try to fix in a manner similar to the 'opsoclonus' of Orzechowski (1927). Patients with this disorder complained of difficulty in seeing and could not follow letters or lines, particularly objects in motion, owing to failure of fixation. Holmes mentioned two cases he had seen but did not specify them. Cases 2 and 3 of his 1918 paper were described as not being able to accommodate and being unable to bring the object into central vision. The lesions in these two were not verified, but in 1938 he states that in two further cases the lesions 'involved the dorsal portion of the thalamus, including the pulvinar'. Holmes thought that such loss of fixation must be due to loss of the cortico-tectal pathways from the occipital cortex.

This difficulty in fixation thus described briefly by Holmes and equated with loss of occipital control has been confused with the disorders of eye movements related to disturbance of visual orientation, also described by Holmes (1918) and Holmes and Horrax (1919). The patient could see the object but could not locate it in space. Central vision was intact, and quite small objects, once located, could be recognized. There was inability to see more than one object at once. In addition there was often an 'ocular apraxia', an inability to move the eyes to command. We shall return to this problem later in our discussion.

In relation to the spasm of fixation seen in pseudobulbar paralysis we would like to emphasize some additional features shown by two of our own patients of whom we made a cinematographic study in 1956 and 1957.

Case II

D.P., a man aged 63, had a slowness in walking and a difficulty in reading for one year. He said he had trouble seeing objects below the level of his shoulders. The visual fields were full to confrontation (finger movements) as also in the patient W.M. He presented a mild pseudobulbar syndrome with rigidity, slowing of gait with small steps and a minimal difficulty in articulation and swallowing. There was paralysis of downward gaze and slowing of lateral eye movements. At times he could look upward well to order (Fig. 4.2a) but if asked to follow movement of the finger down he did so only as far as the horizontal (Fig. 4.2b,c). If then one tilted his head back a downward movement of the eyes resulted (doll's head phenomenon). If asked to follow movement of the finger upward the eyes ceased to follow above the horizontal (Fig. 4.2d). For some minutes thereafter no upward movement could be obtained, though he could look to right and left and now had good downward movement to order (Fig. 4.2d,e). Downward movement was then associated with blepharospasm (Fig. 4.2f) if it was maintained more than a few seconds (a downward spasm with convergence). After a rest for a few minutes the patient could again look up to order, then down to horizontal. Once again, if the patient was asked to look down the eyes did not move, though the eyelids lowered.

It was obvious that some factor other than persistent fixation was interfering with movement. This variability in the limitation of eye movement in the absence of any obvious fixation spasm was also well shown by the following patient.

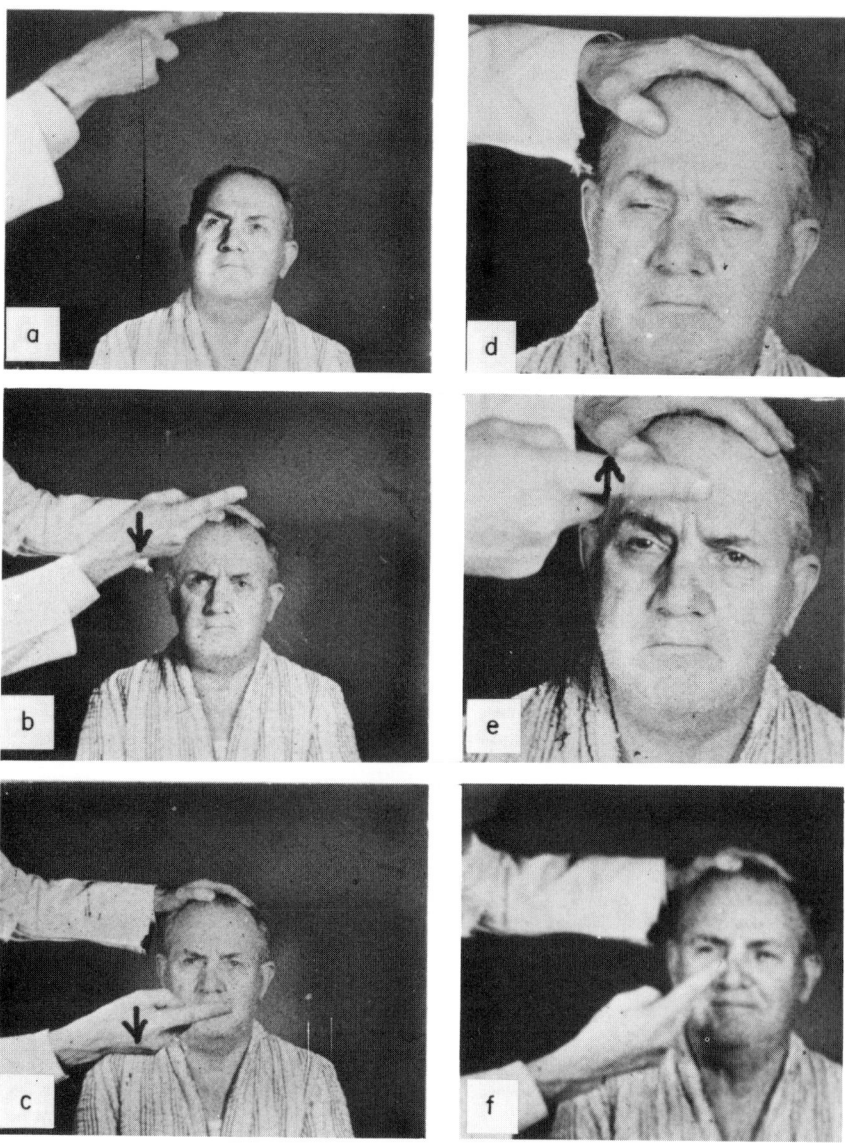

Fig. 4.2 The patient D.P. described in the text. a, looking up to the examiner's finger, on request. b, following the finger down. c, as the finger gets below the horizontal the eyes cease to follow. d, after a doll's head manoeuvre the patient could look down to request, but after a few seconds developed blepharospasm. e, now as the eyes follow the finger up, they do not go *above* the horizontal. f, convergence.

Case III

F.C., a man of 67 years who complained that he had not been able to see properly for 6 months. He had some slowness in gait with occasional falls since a mild 'stroke' 10 years earlier. The most obvious sign was his staring expression (Fig. 4.3). He was alert but stared straight in front of him. He was at first unable to look up to order and had some limitation of voluntary movement to both sides. His memory was poor but he had no difficulty in speaking or swallowing. On repeated examination his ability to make eye movements was quite variable. For example, on one occasion he was at first unable to look up or down, but could look well to the right and then to the left (Fig. 4.3a). When he was asked to look to the right again the eyes swung to the median position (Fig. 4.3b) where they remained for 30 seconds before he could get them to the right. On later occasions the halt occurred in moving the eyes from right to left. He showed a full range doll's head movement up and down. After getting his eyes up by doll's head manoeuvre he could get his eyes fully up to order (Fig. 4.3c), and down again to horizontal (Fig. 4.3d), but not below. If now he was asked to converge downward movement was associated with the resulting convergence (Fig. 4.3f). He could close his eyes to order, but took many seconds to open them again because of blepharospasm. He walked with a gait *à petits pas*, but had only very slight rigidity, with increased reflexes.

In these two patients each deviation of the eyes from midposition was a separate event which was influenced by preceding deviations, and which for a time facilitated deviation in the same direction and impaired it in the opposite direction. Also one had the impression that visual attention remained for a time focused on the centre of gaze, whether it was directed centrally or peripherally. Both of these patients were suffering from mild pseudobulbar paralysis, probably due to lacunar degeneration, as was the patient reported by Alajouanine and Thurel (1931) who was later found to have multiple small softenings affecting the globus pallidus and internal capsule on one side and the lenticular nucleus on the other, without subthalamic lesion.

In this condition, the variability of response indicates the operation of some process that interferes with ability for willed movement, rather than the loss of some specific pathway for vertical or other movement. That the eyes are locked in fixation under some circumstances and not in others is only part of the explanation. There is in fact little evidence of spasm, and the eyes are not always convergent at the critical moment. Even when fixation is prevented by opaque screen or other means the response, though greatly improved, is usually still slow and limited. Nor is it necessarily movement in one direction that is affected, for as Steinert and Bielschowsky (1906) first noted in a patient with apparent loss only of upward movement, once having obtained upward deviation by passive movement of the neck he was unable to

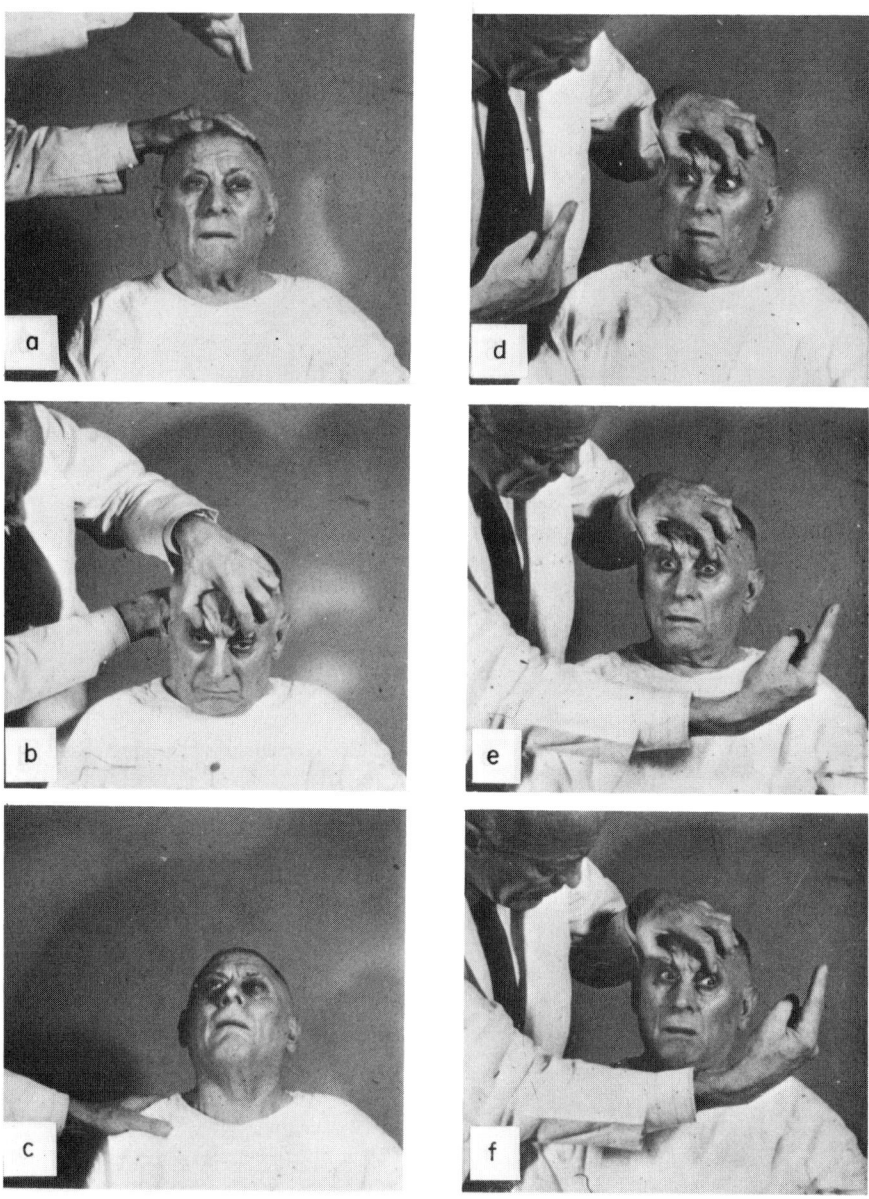

Fig. 4.3 The patient F.C. a, unable to look up at the observer's finger. b, with passive forward movement of the head the eyes move up (doll's head phenomenon). c, now he can look up to order, even without a specific target. d, he looks to order to the examiner's finger at his right side. e, when told to look to the examiner's finger to his left the eyes swing to the midline and stop. Note lid retraction. f, after some 30 seconds the eyes turn to the left.

lower them by effort of will, though he could do so from the primary position. Alajouanine *et al* (1926) relate the defect in movement to the presence of rigidity, rather than a true paralysis. The survival of 'automatico-reflex' movements has been regarded by some, particularly Alajouanine and Thurel (1931), and Morax (1937) as peculiar to pseodobulbar types of Parinaud's syndrome. The absence of automatico-reflex movement such as following, doll's head movement and Bell's phenomenon are held by these authors to be characteristic of lesion at mesencephalic or tegmental level. This distinction is not in fact very well founded. Verified tegmental lesions, as in the case of André-Thomas *et al* (1933) and that of Angelerques *et al* (1957) showed some reduction in associated reflex vertical movements but not a total loss. Movements in following an object or in association with passive movement of the neck were defective, but so also was convergence which, as Schuster (1921) pointed out, is necessary for these reactions. Bell's phenomenon on the other hand was not affected. Most such patients have been confused and disoriented but the case of André-Thomas *et al*, followed for a long period, developed some spasm on looking up as well as a primary defect looking down. A particularly interesting feature of the case of André-Thomas was that if, after downward movement of the eyes had been obtained by passive extension of the neck, one then told the patient to 'look downwards' the eyelids lowered, without further movement of the eyes. The lesion in both these verified cases was a bilateral infarct dorsomedial to the red nucleus, extending towards the aqueduct. The posterior commissure was totally spared in the case of André-Thomas *et al*. In the patient of Angelergues *et al*, the nucleus of Darkschewitsch and the interstitial nucleus of Cajal were destroyed, but the posterior commissure remained intact. Such lesions are in the focal zone of the territory of the mesencephalic (tubero-thalamic) artery (Segarra 1970), more complete occlusion of which can indeed destroy aqueductal grey matter and the whole third nerve complex (Castaigne *et al* 1962).

Thus, the dissociation of paralysis of voluntary vertical movement and of reflex conjugate eye movements is not purely a pseudobulbar phenomenon. The case of Tiling (1874) is cited as evidence that bilateral lesions of frontal cortex can produce loss of voluntary vertical eye movement, but the lesions in this case involved underlying white matter and the putamen. Tournier (1898) also reported an excellent case of this kind with complete loss of voluntary eye movements and retention of reflex deviations. There is no evidence that cortical lesions can produce Parinaud's syndrome. We have encountered several cases of bilateral middle cerebral artery lesions with no apparent ability to move the eyes, yet who opened the mouth automatically and visually directed the lips to a morsel of food that was offered (Fig. 4.4a, c). They could turn the head and eyes rapidly towards an unusual sound (Fig. 4.4b). This phenomenon was also present in Holmes' case, W.M. The

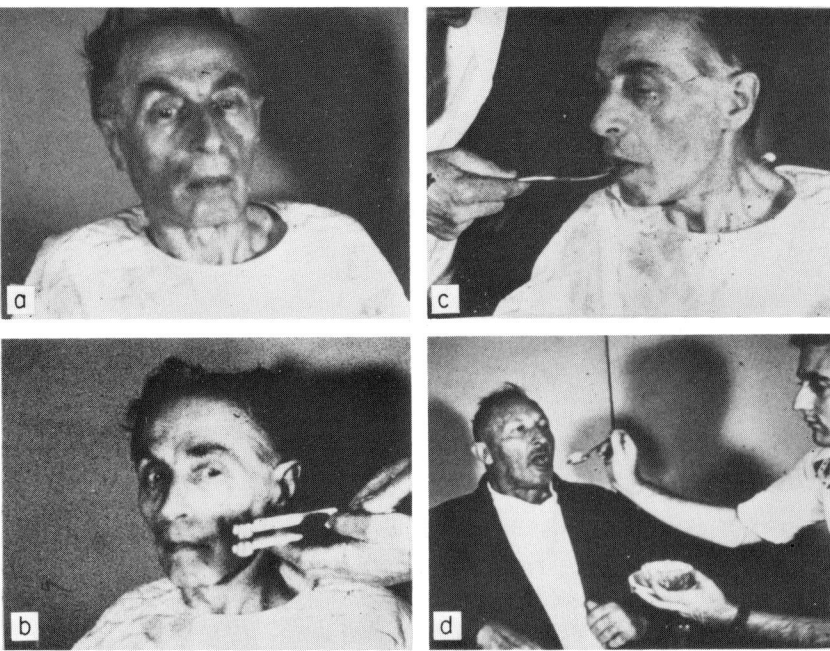

Fig. 4.4 The patient M.D., at rest, a, unable to look up, down, or to either side to order. b, yet he immediately turned his head to look at the source of the noise made by a tuning fork to his left side. c, he lowered his eyelids and advanced his lips to an object approaching his mouth. d, the patient W.K. unable to turn his eyes in any direction by willed effort, opened his mouth and advanced his lips to an approaching spoon.

phenomenon was also very striking in one of our patients 10 days after severe carbon monoxide poisoning with presumed pallidal lesions (Fig. 4.4d) in spite of complete inability to deviate the eyes to request, or when an object was introduced into the periphery of the visual field. On the other hand Parinaud's syndrome has a well-known association with paralysis agitans (Janischewsky 1909) and postencephalitic parkinsonism (Bollack 1922, Bouttier *et al* 1922). Retracted eyelids and relative fixity of central gaze are a commonplace in all types of parkinsonism. The frequent need to blink before transferring fixation from one point to another, also noted by Kinnier Wilson (1940), indicates a difficulty in relaxing fixation.

In postencephalitics, Parinaud's syndrome is frequently associated with prolonged spasms of involuntary conjugate deviation of the eyes called oculogyric crises. Such spasms are now becoming uncommon, but were a frequent association with parkinsonism from 1920 to 1940 (McCowan & Cook 1928, Jelliffe 1932). They were most commonly upward, but could be lateral, downward or forward in the primary position (Van Bogaert 1928,

Holterdorf 1928). They were usually provoked by a strong deviation of the head in a direction opposite to the usual direction of spasm, and could be overcome temporarily by passive rotation of the head in the direction of spasm (Garcin *et al* 1932), thus demonstrating special reflex sensitivity. We ourselves showed the provocation of a crisis by attraction of fixation into the sensitive field (Denny-Brown 1962, p. 100).

Case IV

One of our postencephalitic patients, M.H., suffering from general rigidity and tremor, with mild dystonic tilt of the head to the left, was liable to severe oculogyric crises with deviation of the eyes to the left and upward, associated with blepharoclonus, lasting an hour or longer. An attack could be provoked by rotating an optokinetic drum so that the stripes entered the right side of her visual field, carrying her eyes to the left (Fig. 4.5). On rotation of the drum in the opposite direction only a normal optokinetic nystagmus resulted.

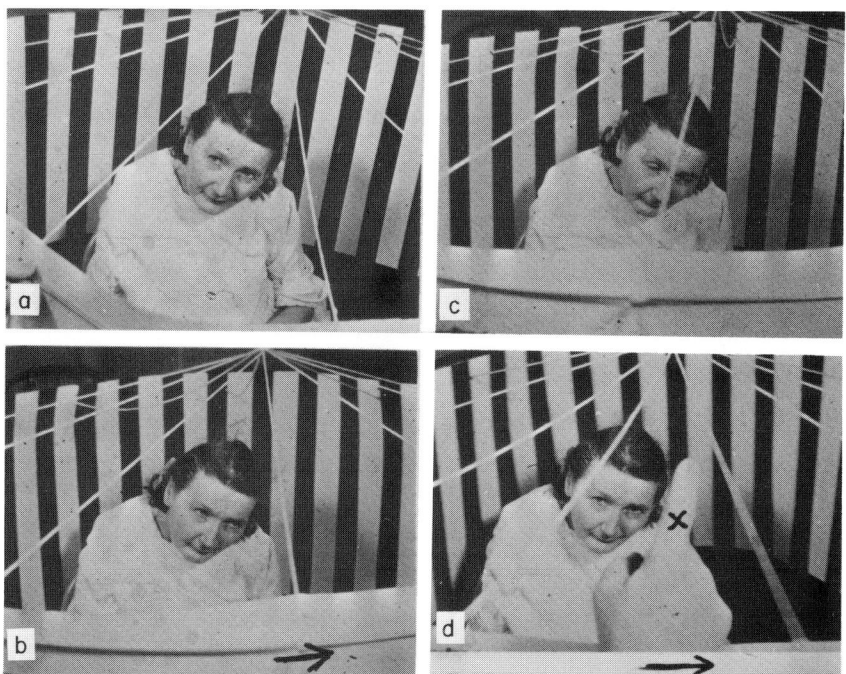

Fig. 4.5 The patient M.H., a parkinsonian in her natural posture surrounded by a stationary optokinetic drum (a). b, when the drum was rotated to her left her eyes followed far to the left. c, an oculogyric spasm of forced deviation to the left then occurred and lasted many minutes, though the drum ceased rotating. d, when she was asked to fix on the examiner's finger (x) rotation of the drum to the left failed to precipitate an oculogyric attack.

If the patient was made to fix forwards on the observer's finger (Fig. 4.5c) rotation of the drum right to left no longer evoked spasm. In this patient here was some slowness and limitation of voluntary movement of the eyes to the left side where reflex following movement was overactive.

In some patients there was complete loss of voluntary movement in the direction of liability to crisis, as in the case of Lhermitte, de Massary and Kyriaco (1928), indicating the reflex nature of the attraction to the peripheral field released from the mechanism of return of the eyes to central position.

Oculogyric crises therefore represent a spasm of ocular movement, sometimes of convergence, that is related to difficulty in voluntary conjugate deviation of the eyes, in the sense of a reflex release phenomenon. Though they were almost pathognomonic of postencephalitic syndromes, crises have been observed in other conditions such as multiple sclerosis (Duke Elder 1949); they were severe in the case of Parinaud's syndrome reported by Babinski (1900), and are related to the convergence spasm associated with tumours and cysts in the neighbourhood of the aqueduct of Sylvius.

Experimental dissociation of conjugate eye movement

It has been a fundamental assumption that in mammalian forms the striate cortex is essential to any visually determined behaviour. Though anatomical studies, and more recently electrical recording, have established that primary visual impressions are relayed to the superior colliculus there has been no evidence that this structure alone can direct behaviour in mammals. More recently Straschill and Hoffmann (1969) have shown that primary impressions are also relayed to the pretectal region in the cat, which is identified with the regulation of the pupillary reflex to light (Magoun *et al* 1936). The accessory optic tract and nucleus (Giolli 1963) also relays some visual information to the cerebellum via the brain stem. Alone this pathway provides some sensitivity to luminosity, but does not account for ocular movement (Pasik & Pasik 1973).

Decortication

Like others we have had great difficulty in maintaining survival of completely decorticate monkeys after the first week. The operation was done in two stages of suction removal of all cortex except that covering the insula. Our longest survivals have been 14, 23 and 84 days after removal of the second cortex. As TerBraak (1936) first reported in the decorticate monkey, our animals showed good optokinetic nystagmus, with both fast and slow phases, in the first week to the side opposite the first cortical removal. Gradually in the second week, corresponding to the development of

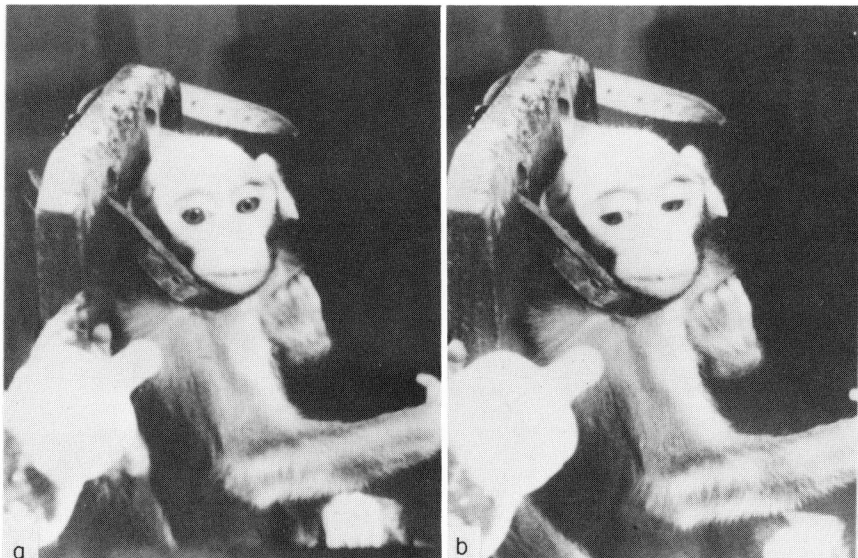

Fig. 4.6 Monkey CAB 46, bilaterally decorticate for 5 weeks, looking towards a silently approaching food syringe.

dystonic rigidity in the limbs, the rapid phase lessened, leaving only a steady movement of the eyes following the moving stripes of the drum. In the first month visual reactions were limited to avoiding, blinking and stilling on exposure to bright light. Beginning in the fourth week rooting of the lips on contact with a feeding nipple appeared, together with great facilitation of sucking movement. In the fifth week the animal was observed to look towards a silently approaching feeding bottle on the right side (left cortex removed before right, 162 days earlier) (Fig. 4.6). The divergent eyes look approximately at the feeding bottle and follow its movements. (The remaining visual reactions of this animal, given in a preliminary paper by Denny-Brown and Yanagisawa at the International Congress in Barcelona, will be reported elsewhere.)

For the present discussion it may be concluded that subcortical structures can mediate attraction of the eyes and following movement in the young decorticate Macaque monkey.

Cortical dissociation of visual perception

In a recent paper we have made a full report (Denny-Brown & Chambers 1976) on the successful removal of area 17 of Brodmann on both sides with survival of the greater part of areas 18 and 19 in three Macaques, reported

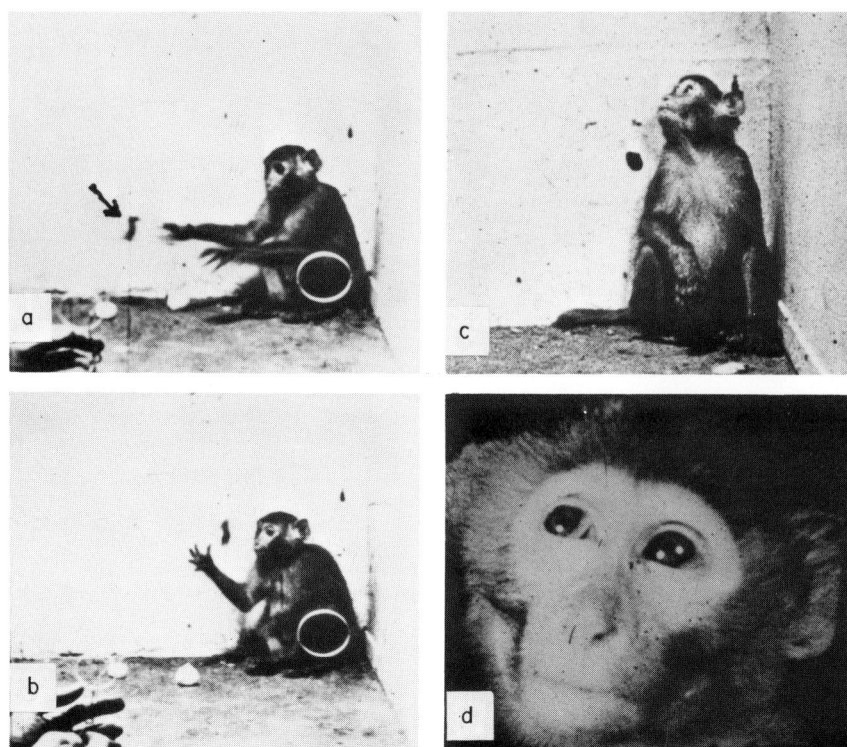

Fig. 4.7 Monkey COR 16, with bilateral ablation of area 17, a, reaching for small dark target (arrow) introduced silently on a wire, and b, capturing the object, though not looking directly at it. c, the same animal 5 weeks after section of both 8th nerves, sitting in habitual resting posture. Note upward direction of gaze. d, close-up of the upward directed, divergent eyes.

briefly in 1955. These animals, with complete degeneration of the lateral geniculate nuclei, had an almost completely intact inferior pulvinar, which is thought to be the simian equivalent of the medial interlaminar nucleus which projects to areas 18 and 19 in the cat (Kinston *et al* 1969, Campos-Ortega *et al* 1970, Mathers & Rapisardi 1973, Trojanowsky & Jacobson 1975). These animals had facile visual placing and spatial orientation. Though their eyes were slightly divergent they looked at any object that moved in the periphery of their visual field, and could reach and grasp it fairly accurately (Fig. 4.7). They were unable to perceive a still object by vision, and identified all objects by feel and smell. Though Hubel and Wiesel (1970) have found cortical cells in area 18 of the monkey that respond selectively to binocular convergence, no such convergence was observed by us in animals lacking area 17, even in survivals of 6 and 7 months. On the other hand judgement of depth is an important feature of panoramic vision. Perception was greatly improved in dim light but, even then, was least or absent in the centre of the visual field, as if they had a large central scotoma. They were expressionless and mute, and investigated other animals by smell. After the first week there was a very active optokinetic response in all directions. If areas 18 and 19 were removed in addition to area 17 on both sides these visual responses did not develop even after 3 months of survival.

In the same paper we have also reported two Macaque monkeys with almost complete removal of the peristriate areas 18 and 19, leaving 17 intact except for its edges. The operation necessarily damages the borders of area 17 and leaves an isthmus of white matter connecting the remaining occipital lobe with the rest of the brain, which results in patchy damage to the radiation. Nevertheless, wedges of surviving cells in the lateral geniculate nuclei attested to survival of large segments of geniculo-calcarine projection for as long as $4\frac{1}{2}$ months. The inferior pulvinars showed severe degeneration. These animals had excellent vision for still objects, sorting out edible from inedible fragments without the use of smell. They exhibited the facial grimacing and calling of natural simian visuo-social behaviour and regained visual placing, but this was slow and tentative. They stopped short of collision with walls or falls from edges if they were allowed to move slowly and confirm visual impressions by reaching. If hurried, they collided with walls and table legs and had many falls from edges. They appeared to have no ability to judge relative distance and, though they could reach accurately for an object within arm's length, they had a staring expression and looked

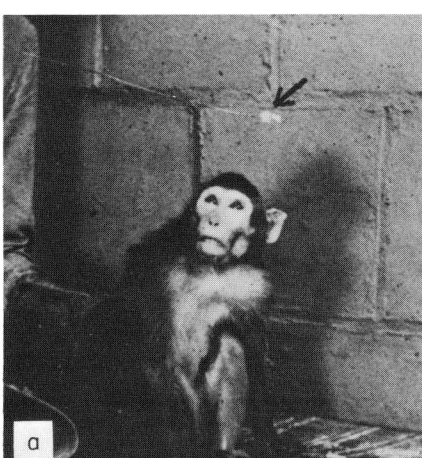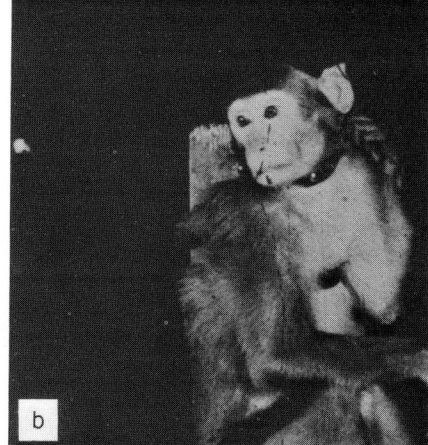

Fig. 4.8 Monkey TM 26 following bilateral ablation of areas 18 and 19 (Denny-Brown & Chambers 1976) converging on a white cotton object descending from above, as it entered the central field. b, converging on a white object coming into the left margin of the figure.

fixedly at the examiner, seemingly unaware of an approaching object. When they looked to an object the eyes converged (Fig. 4.8). All this performance was most remarkable considering the absence of any known projection of area 17 to cortex other than area 18 and 19. Our attention was, therefore, drawn to subcortical representation of the striate and peristriate visual cortex, and their downward projections.

The collicular system

In our Sherrington Lecture to the Royal Society of Medicine in 1962 we reported a remarkable degree of depression of visual perception following bilateral removal of the superior colliculus in the monkey (Denny-Brown

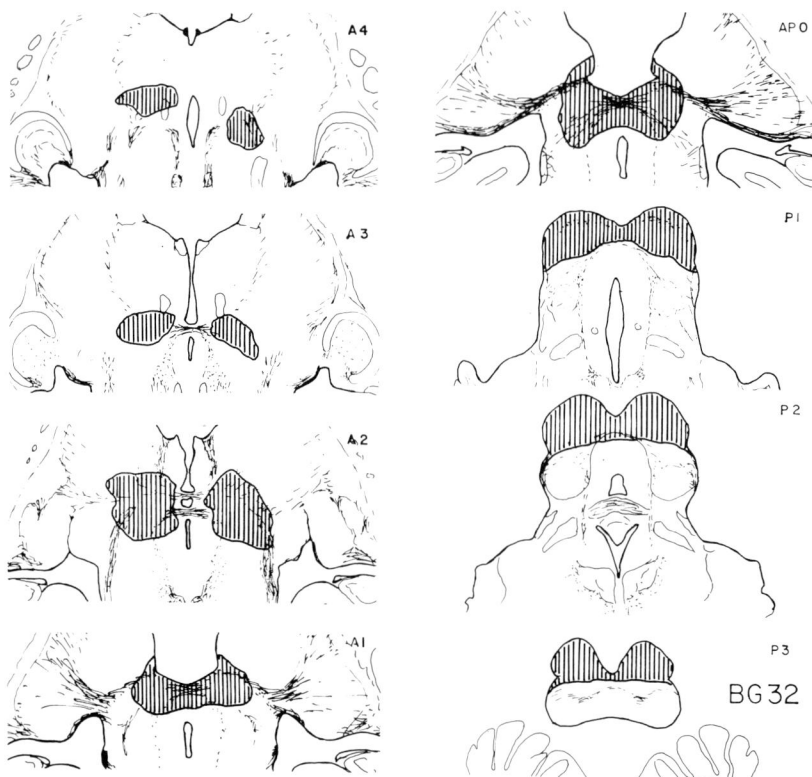

Fig. 4.9 Chart of lesions in the animal BG 32 plotted from serial sections in the stereotaxic plane onto standard outlines of midbrain and thalamus prepared from the Snider–Lee Atlas (1961) at 1 mm intervals from 3 mm caudal to interaural plane (P3), to 4 mm rostral (A4). (From Denny-Brown & Fischer 1976.)

1962b). Some recovery of vision for movement and for visual placing occurred in all segments of the periphery of the visual field after 4 to 6 weeks, after an initial severe depression of perception. In one animal, BG 25, there was some recovery of vision for still objects in one field after 5 weeks, but this was subsequently found to be due to the sparing of a small band of cortico-mesencephalic fibres, crossing from the pulvinar to a small segement of spared superior colliculus in this animal. In 6 other animals the entire cortico-mesencephalic fibre system was interrupted and the superior colliculus removed, as in the chart of one animal, BG 32, shown here in Fig. 4.9. In these 6 animals there was no recovery of vision for still objects in survivals of 1 to 5 months (Denny-Brown & Fischer 1976). The eyes were slightly divergent, and the pupils reacted well to light except in one animal, BG 32, in which the pretectal nucleus was destroyed in the most rostral edge of the

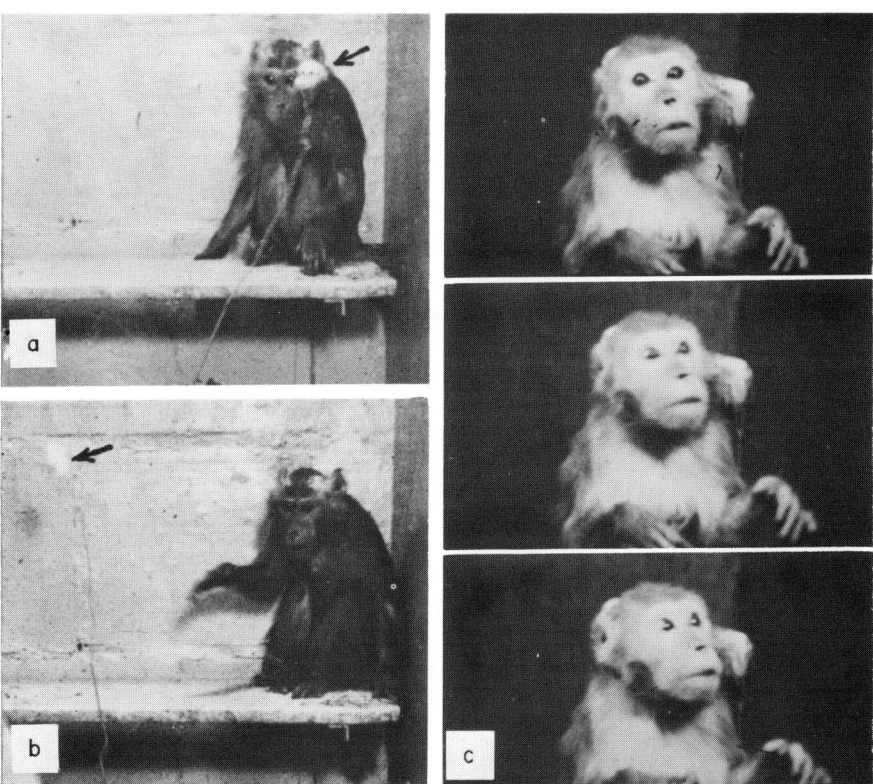

Fig. 4.10 The animal BG 32, with ablation of superior colliculus and section of cortico-mesencephalic tracts, has no reaction to white object (arrow) in front of his eyes at a, but begins to reach for it as it passes into his peripheral field in b. c, shows three frames of the attraction of his eyes to an object entering his left visual field. Note the divergent eyes.

lesion. Visual placing and orientation were accurate as soon as vision for moving objects returned but tended to become catatonic. Once visual attention was gained the object was followed well (Fig. 4.10) unless it entered the central field where it was lost; reaching and grasping were facile (Fig. 4.10b); there was no fixation. The tecto-interstitial fibres upon which convergence is assumed to depend, were completely degenerated. These reactions were inhibited by bright illumination. Although there was severe degeneration of the posterior commissure good upward movement was present in response to a moving target in the upper field, and occasionally as a spontaneous inspection of the surroundings. In spite of intact lateral geniculate nuclei and area 17 and easily recorded cortical-evoked potentials to flash, visual perception in these animals was reduced to that following removal of area 17.

Trevarthen (1968) has proposed two mechanisms for vision in primates, the one focal, depending on foveal and parafoveal retina and the primary visual area of cortex, the other an ambient appreciation of surrounding space, dependent upon colliculus and midbrain. The experiments we have described are in favour of different mechanisms for a similar division of visual function. It was evident that some structure other than the colliculus must serve peripheral vision and its associated visuo-spatial reactions that we call 'panoramic vision'.

The tegmental system

In relation to discussion of the neurological lesions responsible for dystonia we have already described the distortion of posture of head and eyes produced by pretectal lesions (Denny-Brown 1962a, b). More recently, by means of serial electrolytic stereotaxic coagulations in Macaque monkeys we have determined that the minimal lesion to produce lasting distortion of head posture was one that lay close to the midline just rostral to the third nerve nucleus and 5 mm rostral to the posterior commissure (Denny-Brown & Fischer 1976). It is immediately dorsal and medial to the red nucleus. The essential structure is the large-celled nucleus of the deep tegmental grey matter of Crosby *et al* (1962) (Fig. 4.11, TG), called the *nucleus interstitialis tegmentalis commissurae posterioris* by Kuhlenbeck and Miller (1949); in many atlases it is called, simply, *area tegmentalis*. It is distinguished by its large cells with long dendrites (Fig. 4.11), and lies in the most medial extension of the field H2 of Forel (lenticular fasciculus). It receives fibres from the basal ganglia through the lenticular fasciculus and from the pretectal area. It has two commissures with its fellow on the opposite side, one forms the most ventral bundle of the posterior commissure, the other is the ventral commissure of Forel, passing under the most rostral oculomotor

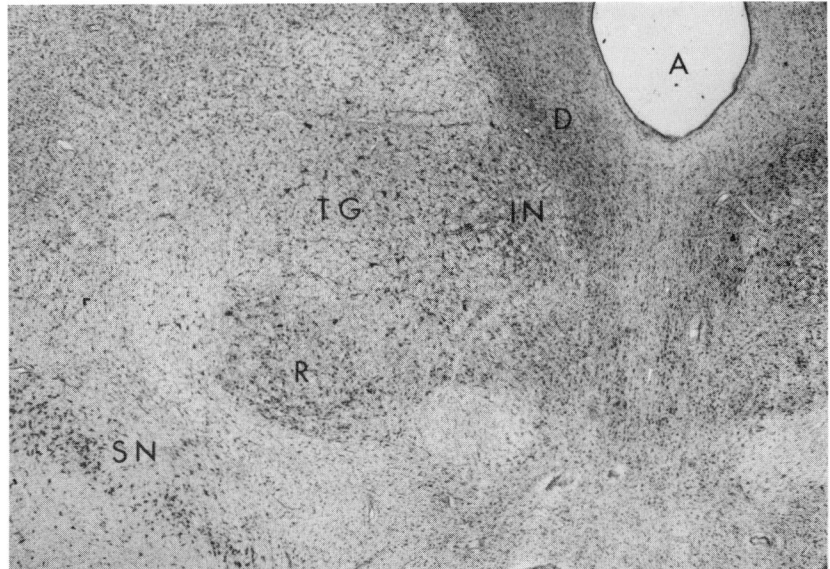

Fig. 4.11 Section of the mesencephalic tegmentum of a chronic decorticate macaque monkey, stained by Nissl method, to show the aqueduct (A), nucleus of Darkschewitsch (D), interstitial nucleus of Cajal (IN), the large-celled nucleus of the deep tegmental grey matter (TG) and small-celled part of the red nucleus (R). (×16.)

nucleus and lying dorsal to the most rostral part of the decussation of Forel (Figs. 4.12, 4.13). With the interstitial nucleus of Cajal this large-celled tegmental nucleus forms a capsule surrounding the most rostral part of the nuclear complex of the third nerve. A well-placed lesion spares the greater part of the interstitial nucleus of Cajal and its related tecto-interstitial fibres and causes degeneration of the most rostral part of the central tegmental tract (Figs. 4.14, 4.15).

The effect of lesion in this structure was investigated in 40 *Macaca mulatta* at the New England Regional Center in the years 1968–70 and has been reported by Denny-Brown and Fischer (1976). We obtained lesions satisfactory for long-term study in 16 adult *Macaca mulatta* and 7 infants. Since our interest here is chiefly in the disorder of fixation we shall base our description chiefly on two typical animals.

A unilateral tegmental lesion such as that shown in Fig. 4.14 produced a pronounced and lasting tilt of the head of the opposite shoulder (Fig. 4.16a) which was not affected by subsequent section of the 8th nerves, but was completely abolished by blindfolding (Fig. 4.16b). The tilted posture was therefore visually determined; an attempt to compensate for a tilted, distorted visual field. If the head was held straight by the observer the eye on the side of the lesion was turned slightly up and in, that on the other side down and in

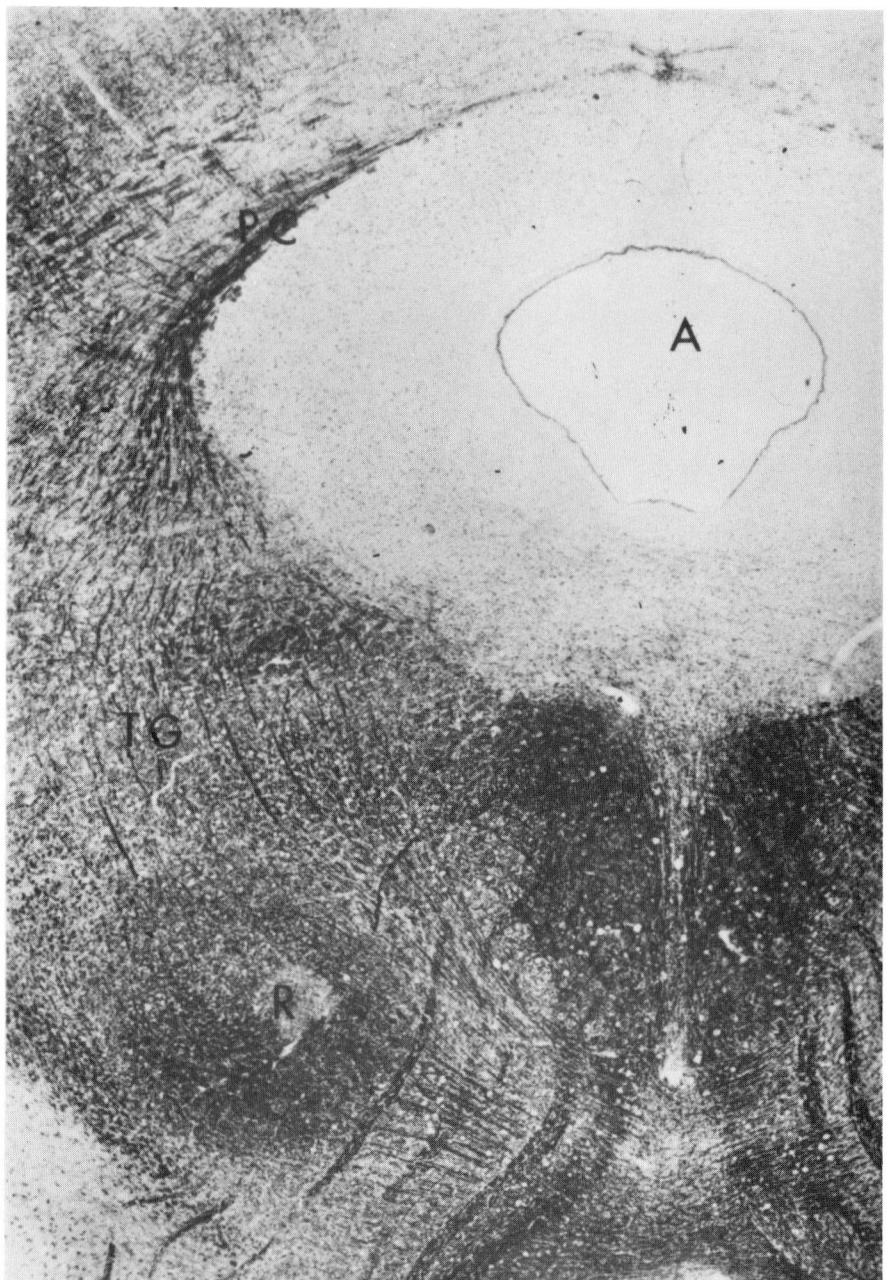

Fig. 4.12 Section of decorticate midbrain tegmentum 2 mm caudal to that in Fig.
4.11, Gros–Bielschowsky stain to show most ventral bundle of posterior commissure
(PC) above, terminating in deep tegmental grey (TG), and ventral commissure of
Forel taking origin in the same area and crossing between the oculomotor nucleus and
the decussation of Forel, below. (×18.)

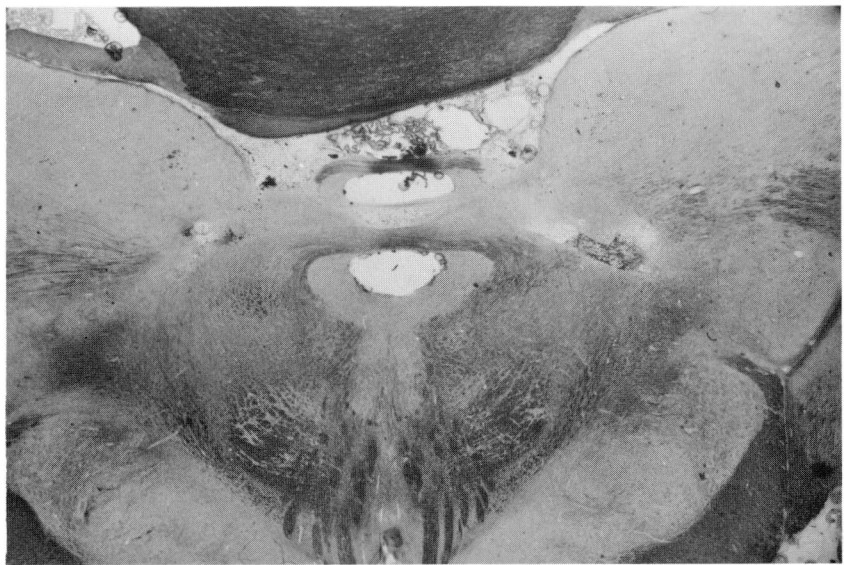

Fig. 4.13 The most rostral part of the lesion in BG 34, an animal with complete section of cortico-mesencephalic tracts and ablation of superior colliculi, similar to that charted in Fig. 4.9, to show the dorsal tegmental commissure, lying in the most ventral part of the otherwise degenerated posterior commissure. The tecto-interstitial bundles, important for convergence, have degenerated. Loyez stain. (× 16.)

(skew deviation). Immediately the head was released the head again tilted and the eyes became parallel. If the animal lay on a surface the head was not righted from lying on the side opposite the lesion. These reactions, which we have illustrated elsewhere (Denny-Brown & Fischer 1976) were associated with inability to deviate the eyes upwards in response to a new stimulus entering the periphery of the upper visual fields, or in natural cage behaviour, as well as severe restriction in downward movements, and also at first to the side opposite the lesion. Movement of the eyes upward could be obtained by forward passive flexion of the neck, or by getting the animal to fix on an object and then moving the object upward. Convergence was not affected. (Some compensation occurred in following weeks, which need not concern us here.)

If *bilateral* lesions were made in the same situation (Fig. 4.17) no tilt of the head resulted (if the lesions were made at the same time) but a complete absence of conjugate upward and downward movement occurred, and in the first days a great limitation in lateral deviation. At first it was not possible to obtain vertical deviations by doll's head manoeuvre or in following an object, probably owing to a complete absence of convergence. There was no response of any kind to quite large objects moved silently in the upper visual

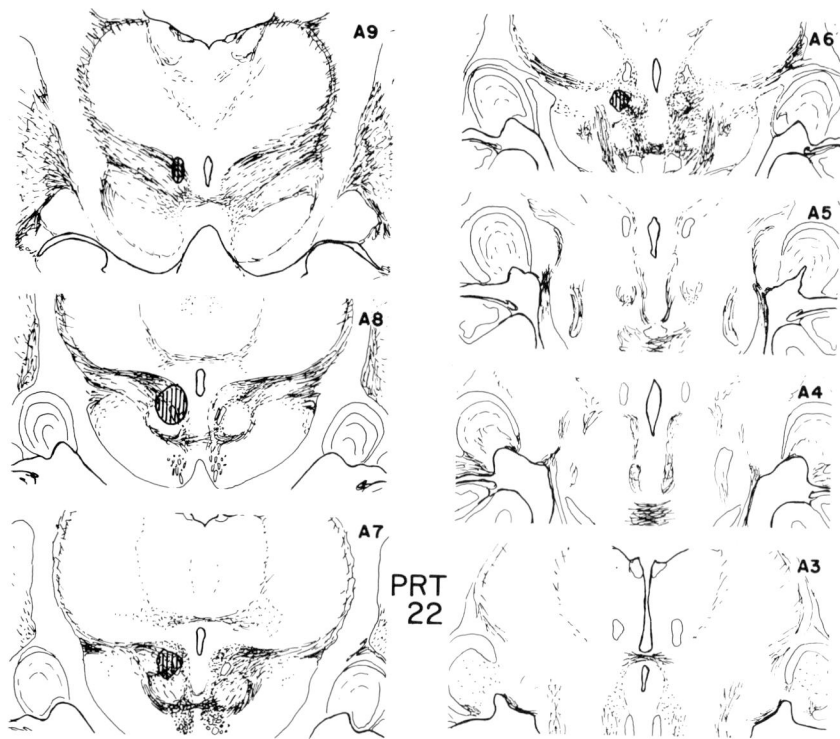

Fig. 4.14 Chart of lesion in the left side of the tegmentum of monkey PRT 22, plotted on standardized outlines of sections 1 mm apart in the stereotaxic plane, as in Fig. 4.9.

field (Fig. 4.18a), and the response occurred only when the target came to the centre from below, or near the centre from the side (Fig. 18d). At first the posture of the head was unstable, particularly in one animal that had both 8th nerves sectioned before the bilateral tegmental lesion. The head would fall forward thus indicating a defect in optic righting of the head. The animals did not right the head from a lying position on either side, but got upright by rolling onto the abdomen and pushing up, raising the head only with positive limb supporting.

After 2 weeks the eyes could converge on an object directly in front of the animal (Fig. 4.19a, b), and the eyes could then follow the object downwards a short distance, and very well in lateral movements. A fixed object could be followed up only by dorsiflexing the neck. The eyelids were always slightly retracted in forward gaze, and the axes of the eyes parallel but slightly below the horizontal. The animal charted in Fig. 4.17 did not regain spontaneous movement of the eyes upward in a survival of 2 years. Four others showed no

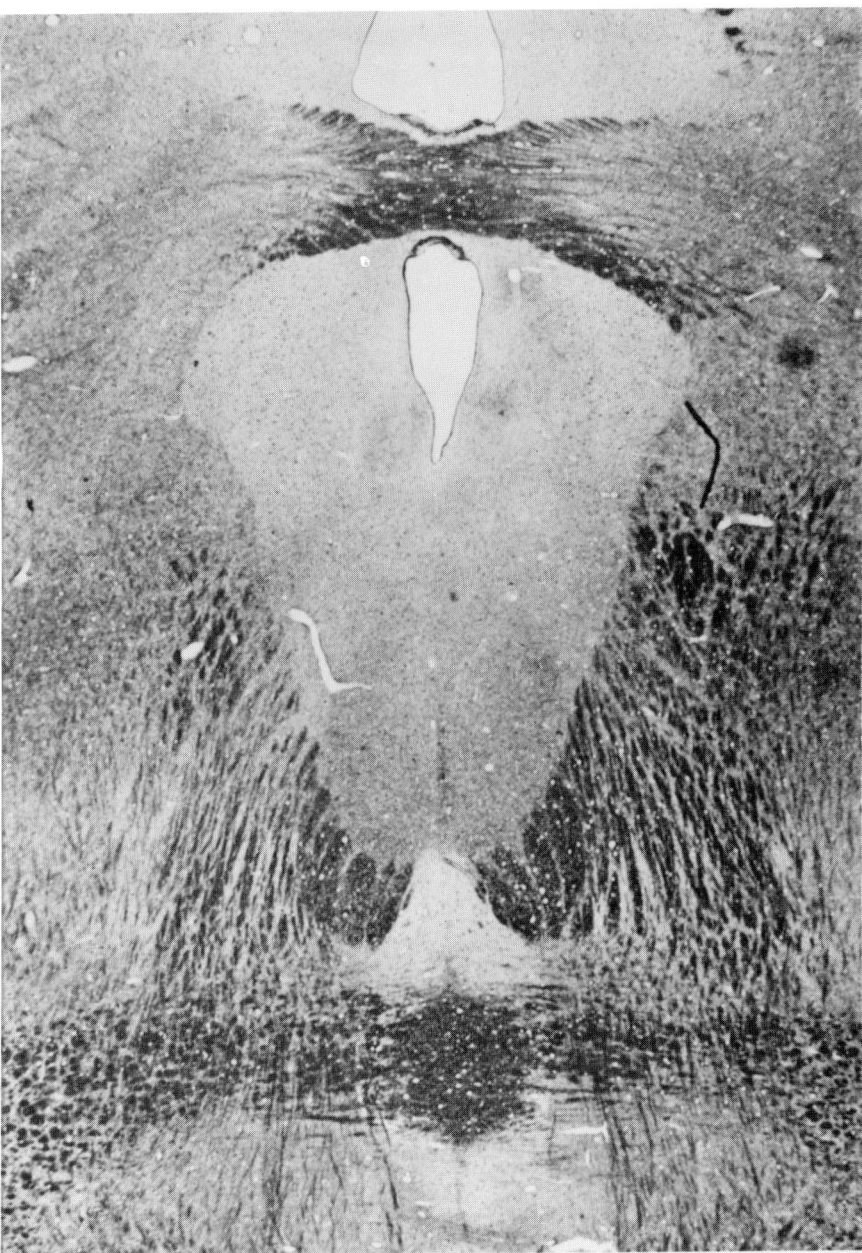

Fig. 4.15 Section at the level of the posterior commissure of monkey PRT 13 killed 410 days after a unilateral tegmental lesion identical with that shown in Fig. 4.14, to show pallor of central tegmental tract on the left. Note intact medial longitudinal fasciculus and posterior commissure. Luxol Fast Blue. (× 13).

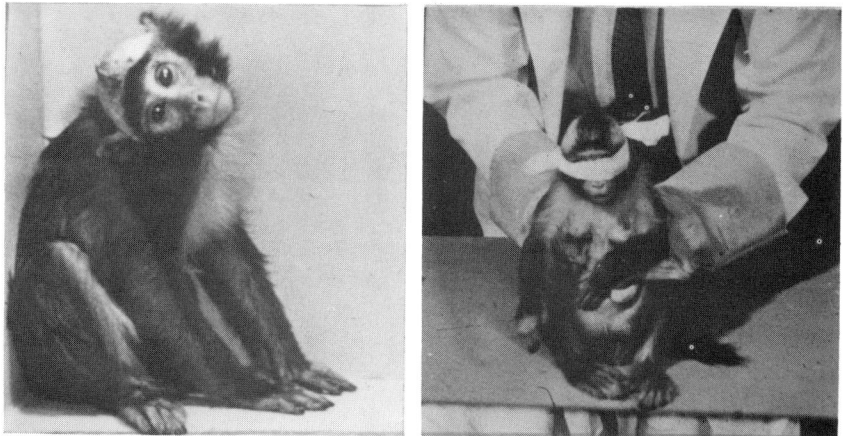

Fig. 4.16 The monkey PRT 22, with unilateral tegmental lesion, showing the head tilt in a, and its abolition by blindfolding, b.

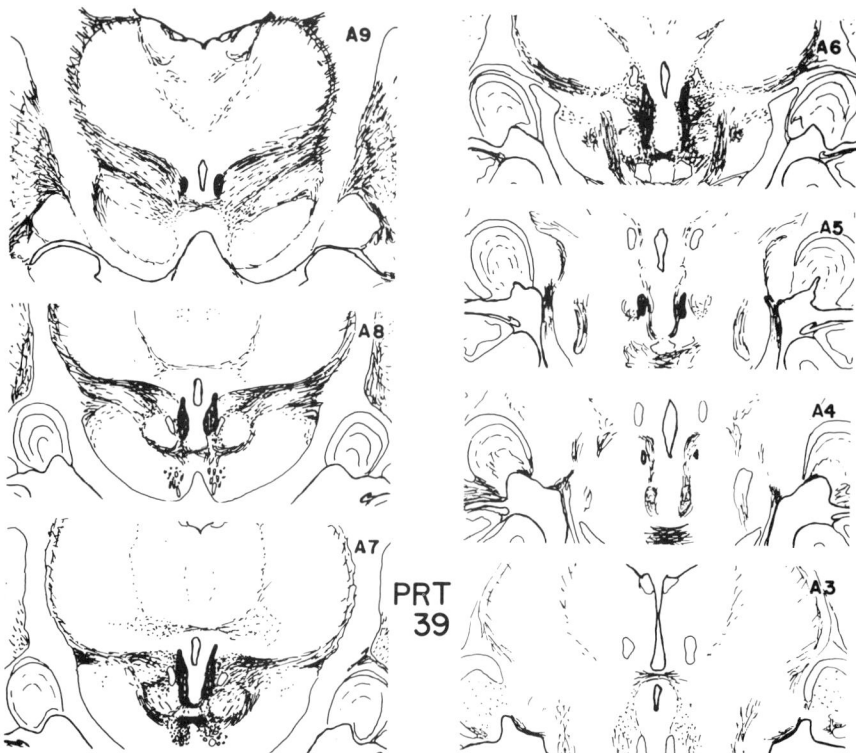

Fig. 4.17 Chart of the bilateral tegmental lesions in the monkey PRT 39, plotted on outlines at intervals of 1 mm from A3 to A9 in Figs. 4.9 and 4.15.

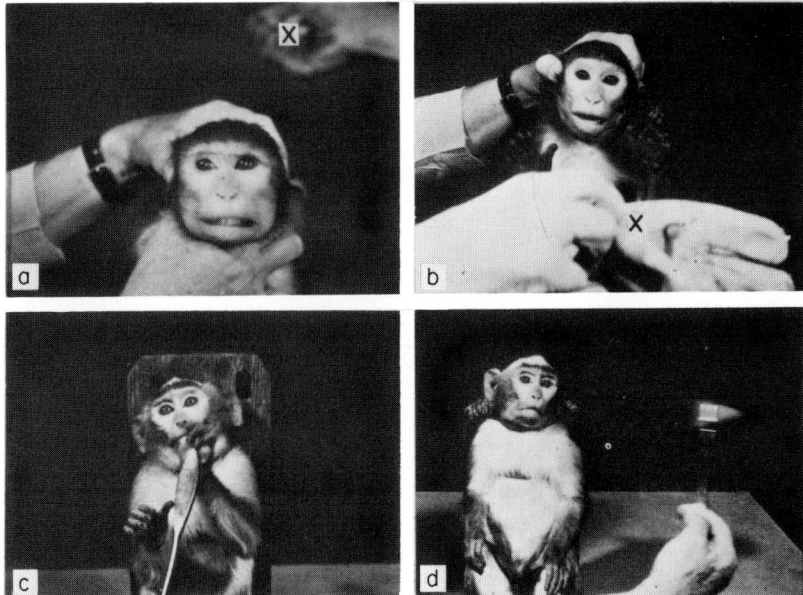

Fig. 4.18 The animal PRT 39, with bilateral tegmental lesions for over two years, showing, in a the absence of any reaction to the hand of the observer (x) above. Note retracted eyelids. b, no reaction to hand holding a large object (x) coming up from below. In c, he reaches for an object as it comes within approximately 20° below fixation point, without looking at it. d, one week after the production of the bilateral lesion the animal failed to react to moving objects more than 20° to either side of the fixation point.

recovery in 9, 9, 10 and 18 months. In others some downward movement recovered but was abolished for 30 seconds to 1 minute following an upward movement induced by neck flexion. Conversely, 1 animal that showed most commonly an absence of downward movement also lost spontaneous and following upward movement for a period of many minutes after a downward movement had been elicited by neck extension.

After 3 months the animal, PRT 39 had regained visual placing, and showed no behaviour that could be interpreted to result from loss of spatial orientation. He had a staring expression, and walked on two legs with head held back (Fig. 4.19a). He could now reach below the horizontal for objects, without lowering the eyes. He still had poor head righting. If an object was brought slowly into the visual field from above he gave no sign of reaction until the eyes suddenly converged upon it just as it came below the horizontal, and about 5° below the horizontal if it came from below (Fig. 4.20). Once converged on the object he would reach for it or push it away. If it came from the side convergence occurred a little further away from the

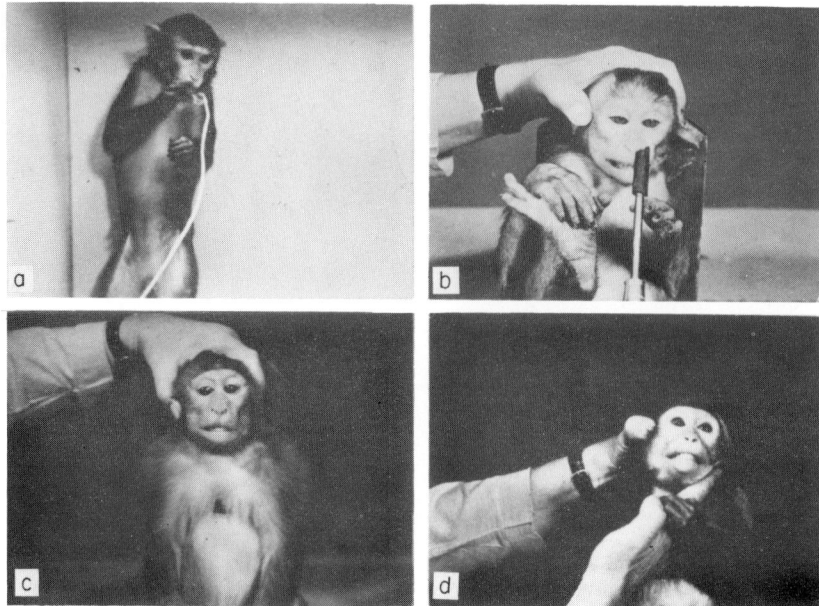

Fig. 4.19 Monkey PRT 39, two years after lesion, in a, standing reaching for an object on a wire that has come into his central field. b, shows the animal converging on a near object. c, shows persistent downward oculogyric spasm one minute after downward movement had been induced by dorsiflexion of neck. Note absence of convergence. d, oculo-gyric upward spasm of the eyes induced by passive ventral flexion of the neck, persisting after release of the passive movement.

centre of the field, about 10–15°. Thus the effective visual field for convergence was in the shape of a small horizontal slit. In following months the lateral and downward extent of the effective field for the elicitation of visual response enlarged a little but after a year it was only an estimated 20° below, and 30–40° laterally (Fig. 4.21). Within this field convergence could not be maintained for more than a few seconds, following which runs of rapid (3 to 4 a second) side-to-side opsoclonic movements occurred. In rapid movie frames it was clear that these movements, as in opsoclonus in man, were a rapidly alternating fixation, first by one eye, then the other. At this time there was a facile optokinetic response to movement of a striped drum from right or left, but none to stripes entering the field from above or below. Vertical movement of the stripes strangely produced a horizontal opsoclonus.

This limitation of eye movements continued through the second year after making the lesions. The animal was never able to look up, except as a result of passive movement of the head on the neck. The eyes then tended to stay up in spasm for many seconds before he could get them down to horizontal (Fig. 4.19d). Similarly, after passive movement of the head upwards the eyes

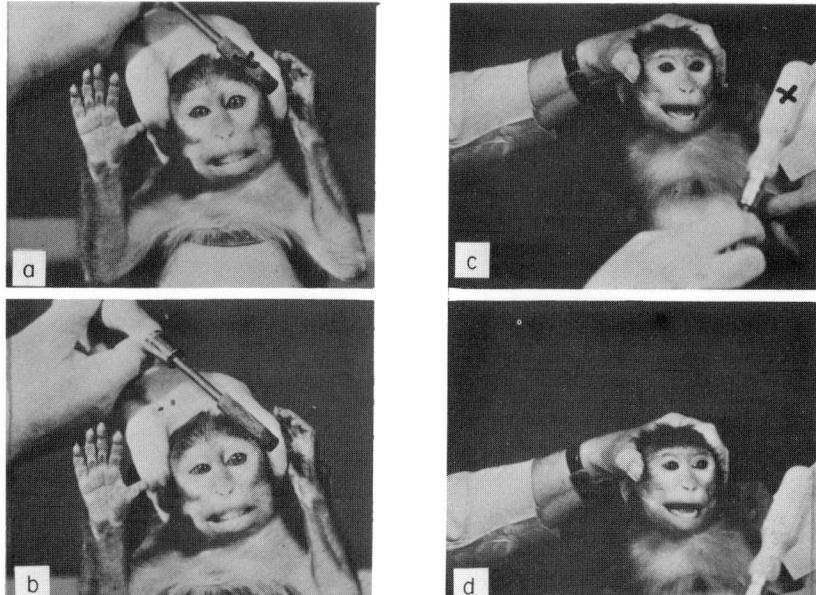

Fig. 4.20 Monkey PRT 39, two years after production of the lesion, showing the lack of reaction to an object (x) coming down from above a, and b, sudden convergence on the object, in less than $\frac{1}{16}$ of a second, as it enters the central field (frames a and b consecutive). c, shows an object coming up from below and in the next frame, d, sudden convergence on it.

would often remain in spasm downwards after the head had returned to horizontal (Fig. 4.19c). In such spasms the eyes were slightly divergent. They were due to abnormal reaction to movement in the panoramic field, and were not spasms of fixation. These spasms persisted unchanged after section of both 8th nerves. Lateral movements became more facile, but the animal could not transfer the eyes directly from right to left without a pause in middle position, and often a blink before beginning the remainder of the transfer (Fig. 4.21). Also, if the examiner stood directly in front of the animal,

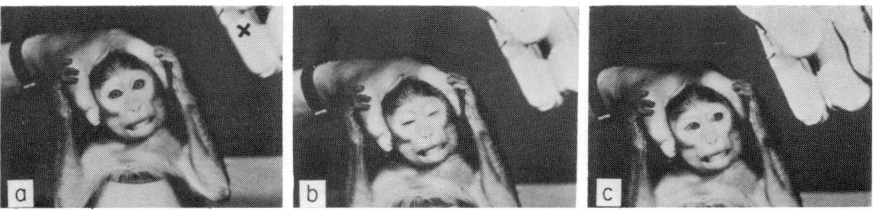

Fig. 4.21 Monkey PRT 39, two years after lesion, inattentive to an object coming from his left, until at b he blinks, and in c, converges on the object at approximately 30°.

or some other large stimulus confronted him there was for a time no reaction to an object introduced to any part of the visual field. The animal then continued his original fixation, as if mesmerized, for many seconds. If an object of special interest, such as a pin, was brought close to his eyes a spasm of convergence would then occur, lasting as long as 30 seconds after the stimulus had been withdrawn.

Thus it was clear that the mechanism of fixation, not only in the sense of binocular convergence, but also in terms of centring of conjugate eye movement, was indeed overactive.

Discussion

The complex physiology underlying the process of binocular fixation and fusion has recently been admirably reviewed by Bishop (1973) and we have nothing new to report on this aspect of the subject. Our own observations relate to the physiological setting in which fixation occurs, and the reasons for its overactivity in some circumstances and absence in others. Our animal experiments showed that discrete lesions in the tegmentum of the midbrain could create the same phenomena that are observed in patients with pseudobulbar syndromes. The overactivity of fixation was clearly present, with the same limitation of conjugate eye movements, particularly vertical deviations. The disorder affected all conjugate eye movement in the beginning, and also convergence. In addition there was a severe depression of all visual perception which we would view as the primary disorder. In the human patient it is a truism to say that there must be looking before seeing (Holmes 1936). Undue persistence of fixation became evident only when central vision recovered. Our earlier experiments on cortex and colliculus had shown that peripheral vision, and attraction of the eyes to the periphery of the visual field have a mechanism independent of the geniculo-calcarine system, even of the colliculus. This panoramic system utilizes the inferior pulvinar and tegmental grey muclei and, because of its depression by bright light, is probably derived from the scotopic (dark adapted) vision, served by the rods in the retina. The two systems relate to the posterior thalamic nuclei and parietal cortex through the extensive interconnections now demonstrated between these structures and the pulvinar nuclei (Mathers & Rapisardi 1973, Trojanowski & Jacobson 1975). The overlap of the visual fields of panoramic and macular vision is large, but the effect of loss of geniculo-calcarine vision is a central scotoma, with loss of form vision, closely resembling the visual defect described in patients with amblyopia *ex anopsia* (Heine 1905, Wald & Burian 1944). Conversely, loss of panoramic vision results in an overactivity of fixation, defective attraction to the periphery and poor spatial orientation. It was clear that overactive central fixation could interfere with eye movements even in the absence of convergence. The eyes would stare at any large target, even when slightly divergent. In these experiments binocular convergence and accommodation related exclusively to the presence of small objects of special interest in the central field, e.g. a needle, or the tip of a feeding syringe. To this extent, convergence behaved as the most intense form of fixation, not otherwise separable as a behavioural mechanism by our methods of examination.

Animals with some recovery of peripheral vision would still present evidence of overactive fixation. Persistent fixation in the presence of some peripheral vision was described in parkinsonians by Janischewsky (1909), and we have found it to be a prominent sign in experimental simian lesions of the putamen (Denny-Brown & Yanagisawa 1976). The pathways for control of visual orientation descend from the cortical frontal and parietal eye fields through the putamen and globus pallidus to reach the field of Forel. The anatomical pathway from the putamen has been clearly defined (Johnson & Clemente 1959, Nauta & Mehler 1966). We found that extensive lesion of the putamen greatly limited or abolished the peripheral responses characteristic of panoramic vision. Any such response that remained required facilitation by neck reflexes (doll's head phenomenon) and then tended to be prolonged as a released oculogyric spasm, usually upwards (Denny-Brown & Yanagisawa 1976). Thus, oculogyric spasm belonged to the spectrum of disorders of panoramic vision, sometimes allied with, but not directly related to, overactive visual fixation.

Optic apraxia

The disorder called visual disorientation described by Holmes (1919) and Holmes and Horrax (1919), resulting from bilateral parietal war wounds was also associated with difficulty in voluntary conjugate eye movement. The patients were unable to look towards, or to fix objects outside the central field. This type of defect was also described by Bálint (1909) in other types of bilateral parietal lesion. Of the several components of the syndrome, Holmes emphasized the loss of visual orientation, Bálint the defect in eye movement. Hécaen and de Ajuriaguerra (1954) have reported cases with differing emphasis on these factors, with excellent discussion. The patients have not only a great difficulty in directing the eyes but also in locating any object in the visual field in reference to any other object, to the vertical meridian or, indeed to their own body. Central vision, convergence and accommodation were intact. The eyes, once fixed, could be made to move in any direction by contrary movement of the head (doll's head phenomenon). Following a moving object with the eyes was possible only with very slow movement. Even when fixed on an object, the eyes resisted deviation from the median position. When the fixed object was moved the eyes followed, but when it came back across the midline the eyes ceased to follow past the midpoint. When the eyes ceased following the patient reported that the object had disappeared from vision. Holmes (1921) called the disorder 'ocular apraxia', and described the associated difficulty in perceiving two objects at once, unless they were very close together. He likened this aspect to tactile and visual inattention associated with unilateral parietal lesions. Hécaen and de Ajuriaguerra note that in their patients there was 'a kind of concentric narrowing of the field of attention'. This is precisely the disorder of perception exhibited by the monkey following tegmental lesion, and in some degree by the patients D.P. and F.C. Such pseudobulbar patients exhibit a more general disorientation, and complain less of specific defects in spatial localization than the patients of Holmes, but the restriction of the visual field is of the same type. Thus in one of Roth's patients with pseudobulbar syndrome (Roth 1901) it is stated that the patient, in addition to being unable to look up, could not indicate objects such as window or door in his upper field. It is evident that a perceptual defect must be an important element in the inability for voluntary eye movement in all these states.

The special vulnerability of upward movement

The greater vulnerability of eye movement in the vertical plane is the most striking feature of pseudobulbar and tegmental lesions. The explanation lies, not in the presence of some special pathway for such movement, but in the fact that the righting (anti-gravity) responses for head and eyes are the chief function of the pathway from globus pallidus to the tegmental grey matter both in monkey and man. Thus, with the onset of the very restricted bilateral tegmental lesion in the case of André-Thomas *et al* (1933) it is stated that the head fell forward and the patient was unable to raise it. This is also the case with our monkeys with bilateral lesion of outer globus pallidus (Denny-Brown 1962) in whom there was also an inability to raise the eyes above the horizontal (Fig. 4.22) with inability to right the head. Conversely, when optic righting is overactive, as it is in animals after bilateral 8th nerve lesion following removal of area 17, the animal tends to sit with the head and eyes directed upwards for minutes at a time (Fig. 4.7c). In such animals blindfolding caused the head to fall forward.

   We find no evidence for separate mechanisms for reflex and voluntary movement of the eyes. Rather the ability to deviate the eyes by effort of will depends on summation of facilitations by a number of factors including the perception of a target in the visual field, the ability to abolish fixation already in operation, the posture of the head in relation to optic as well as labyrinthine and neck reflexes and to the contactual orientation of the body to ground. Absence of one or more of these will impair the ability to make a purely voluntary vertical eye movement. This important principle was

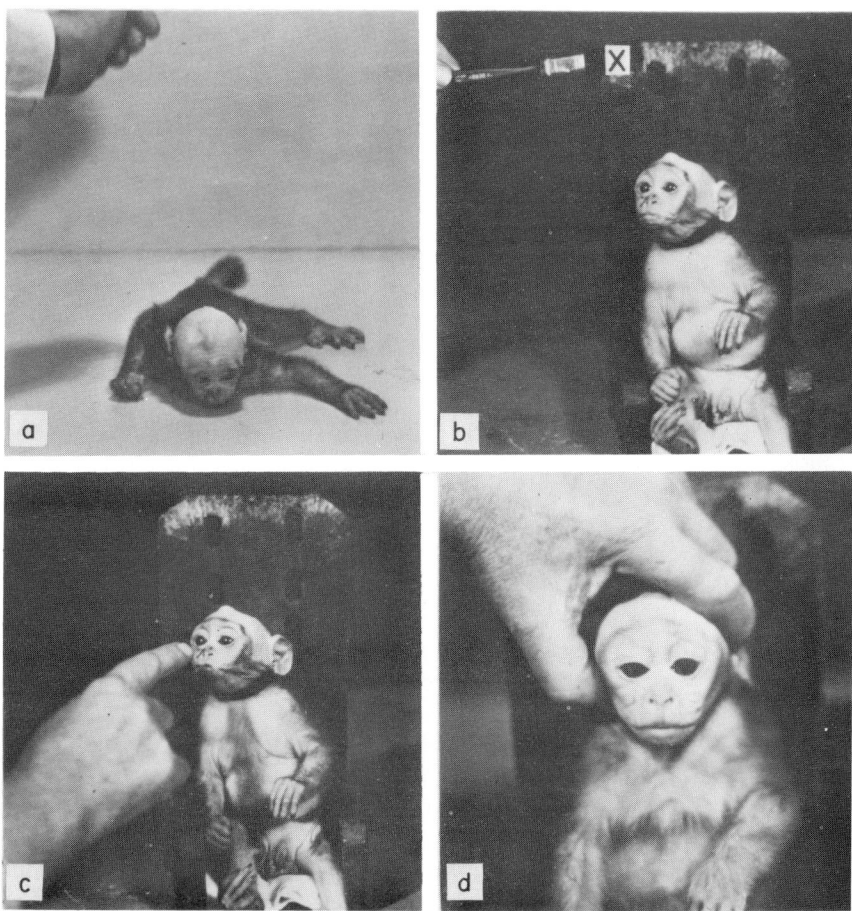

Fig. 4.22 Monkey PUT 24, an infant with bilateral lesions of putamen that encroached on the outer globus pallidus, causing inability to right the head, a, and absence of upward movement of the eyes to an object (x) in b. In c, the lips are protruded toward the approaching finger of the examiner. d, shows convergence downward, with accommodation. Lateral eye movements were not restricted.

particularly evident in the experimental animal, PRT 22, whose lesion is shown here in Fig. 4.14 three weeks after unilateral tegmental lesion when he had recovered convergence and when he had regained some ability to look upwards. At that time both 8th nerves were sectioned, and in the following week he had again lost all ability for upward movement and convergence. Indeed, for a few days he exhibited independent eye movements. In this period also he had no optic head righting. Compensation by the other tegmentum then gradually occurred. In the distortion of spatial reference

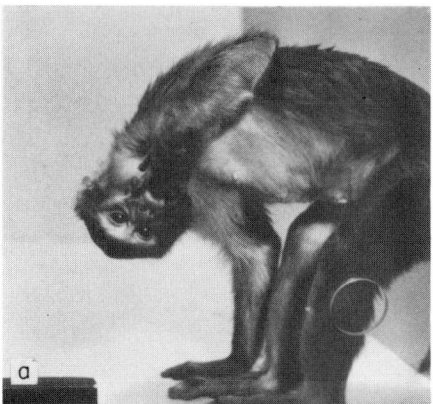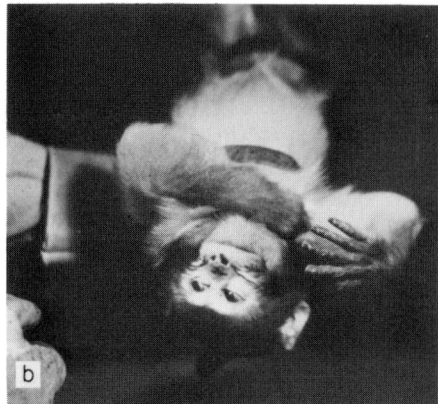

Fig. 4.23 a, monkey PRT 38 unable to look up for eighteen months occasionally looked at the examiner upside down, but when held upside down, b, developed an intense and very prolonged oculogyric spasm upward.

following tegmental lesion the labyrinth must serve to stabilize the central point of visual perception in relation to which all projected eye movement is programmed. Thus, some animals with bilateral tegmental lesions always preferred to look at the examiner upside down (Fig. 4.23a) and others, when held upside down developed intense upward oculogyric spasm in spite of not having had any ability for upward movement for many months (Fig. 4.23b).

Although our experimental studies do not put the same emphasis on direction of visual attention by the frontal lobes, they strongly support the main conclusion of Gordon Holmes that visual fixation is secondary to, and independent of direction of gaze to a new object (Holmes 1936, 1938). Though fixation is overactive following most lesions of the panoramic system, perception is impaired, so that large enough bilateral lesions of the basal ganglia result in reduction of visually directed behaviour to reflex mouthing associated with akinetic mutism. In this condition of total optic apraxia, the whole geniculo-striate-collicular system ceases to influence perception or behaviour. After a long period some additional panoramic vision recovers, as in the decorticate monkey.

Conclusions

(1) Hyperactivity of visual fixation, as described by Holmes in 1930, is an important factor in the restriction of eye movements in Parinaud's syndrome.
(2) The restriction of movement of the eyes is not the result of loss of a pathway or separate organization for upward movement or downward movement as such, but arises from impairment of conjugate deviations from

the primary, central position toward the periphery in general, with only a relative directional preponderance.

(3) Each such deviation is a separate event, requiring not only cancellation of existing fixation, or pre-existing deviation, but also a background perceptual reference or gestalt with reflex stabilization by optical, labyrinthine and body righting.

(4) A tegmental organization of peripheral, dark-adapted (scotopic) vision, 'panoramic vision', can function independently of geniculo-calcarine, photopic vision and of the colliculus. Panoramic vision can provide magnetic attraction to movement and lines of contrast, enabling spatial perception, following of moving objects, and direction of approximate but effective limb movement.

(5) Panoramic vision is controlled by pathways descending from the frontal and parietal cortical eye fields, facilitated by the basal ganglia, through the lenticular fasciculus and tegmental grey matter.

(6) Macular fixation and form vision are dependent on the integrity of the geniculo-calcarine system and superior colliculus.

(7) There must normally be an equilibrium between macular fixation and panoramic vision, for loss of one leads to overactivity of the other.

(8) A special vulnerability of upward eye movement is related to the altered vertical reference for fixation associated with defective panoramic vision.

(9) Defect in the organization of panoramic vision at any level can lead to overactivity of proprioceptive (neck reflex) facilitation of peripheral deviation in the form of oculogyric spasms.

(10) The midbrain tegmentum and the pathways controlling it play an important part in the initiation of visual perception.

References

ALAJOUANINE T., DELAFONTAINE P. & LACAN J. (1926) Fixité du regard par hypertonie, prédominant dans sens vertical, avec conservation des mouvements automatico-réflexes, associé à un syndrome extrapyramidal avec troubles pseudobulbaires. *Revue neurol.* **42,** 410–18.

ALAJOUANINE T. & THUREL R. (1931) Révision des paralysies des mouvements associés des globes oculaires. *Revue neurol.* **47,** 125–69.

ANDRÉ–THOMAS, SCHAEFFER H. & BERTRAND I. (1933) Paralysie de l'abaissment du regard, paralysie des inférogyres, hypertonie des supérogyres et des releveurs des paupiéres. *Revue neurol.* **49,** 535–42.

ANGELERGUES R., DE AJURIAGUERRA J. & HÉCAEN H. (1957) Paralysie de la verticalité du regard d'origine vasculaire. *Revue neurol.* **96,** 301–19.

BABINSKI J. (1900) Sur la paralysie du mouvement associé de l'abaissment des yeux. *Revue neurol.* **8,** 525–7.

BÁLINT R. (1909) Seelenlähmung des 'Schauens', optische Ataxie, räumliche Störung des Aufmerksamkeit. *Mschr. Psychiat. Neurol.* **25,** 51–81.

BISHOP P.O. (1973) Neurophysiology of binocular single vision and stereopsis. In:

Jung R. (Ed.) *Handbook of Sensory Physiology*, Chap. 4, Vol. VII/3, Central processing of visual information, Part B, Springer Verlag, Heidelberg.

BOLLACK J. (1922) Paralysie des mouvements associés des yeux postencéphalitiques. *Revue neurol.* **38**, 75–7.

BOUTTIER H., ALAJOUANINE T. & GIROT (1922) Paraplegie en flexion avec état parkinsonien et syndrome de Parinaud. *Revue neurol.* **38**, 1514–19.

CAMPOS-ORTEGA J.A. HAYHOW W.R. & CLÜVER P.F. DE V. (1970) A note on the problem of retinal projections to the inferior pulvinar nucleus of primates. *Brain Res.* **22**, 126–30.

CANTONNET A. & LANDOLT M. (1907) Paralysie de l'élévation des globes oculaires pour les mouvements voluntaires avec intégrité des mouvements automatico-réflexes. *Revue neurol.* **15**, 1205–6.

CASTAIGNE P., BUGE A., ESCOUROLLE R. & MASSON M. (1962) Ramollissement pédonculaire médian tegmento-thalamique avec ophthalmoplégie et hypersomnie. *Revue neurol.* **106**, 357–67.

CROSBY E.C., HUMPHREY T. & LAUER E.W. (1962) *Correlative Anatomy of the Nervous System*. Macmillan, New York.

CROUZON O. (1900) Tic d'elevation deux yeux. *Revue neurol.* **8**, 54–5.

DENNY-BROWN D. (1962a) *The Basal Ganglia and their Relation to Disorders of Movement*. Oxford University Press, London.

DENNY-BROWN D. (1962b) The midbrain and motor integration. *Proc. R. Soc. Med.* **55**, 527–38.

DENNY-BROWN D. & CHAMBERS R.A. (1955) Visuo-motor responses related to the peristriate cortex of the monkey. *Arch. Neurol. Psychiat.* (Chicago) **73**, 566–7.

DENNY-BROWN D. & CHAMBERS R.A. (1976) Physiological aspects of visual perception. I. Functional aspects of visual cortex. *Archs Neurol.* (Chicago) **33**, 219–227.

DENNY-BROWN D. & FISCHER E.G. (1976) Physiological aspects of visual perception. II. The subcortical visual direction of behaviour. *Archs Neurol.* (Chicago) **33**, 228–242.

DENNY-BROWN D. & YANAGISAWA N. (1976) The role of the basal ganglia in the initiation of movement. *Res. Publs Ass. Res.*

Nerv. Ment. Dis. **55**, 115–147.

DUKE-ELDER W.S. (1949) The neurology of vision, Vol. IV of *Textbook of Ophthalmology*. Mosby, St Louis.

GARCIN R., ISRAEL & BLOCH-MICHEL (1932) Crises oculogyres postencéphalitiques. Influence de la position de la tête dans l'espace sur le relâchement transitoire du spasme oculaire. *Revue neurol.* **1**, 730–8.

GIOLLI R.A. (1963) An experimental study of the accessory optic system in the cynomolgus monkey. *J. comp. Neurol.* **121**, 89–108.

GOWERS W.R. (1879) Note on a reflex mechanism in the fixation of the eyeballs. *Brain* **2**, 39–41.

HÉCAEN H. & DE AJUROAGUERRA J. (1954) Bálint's syndrome (psychic paralysis of visual fixation) and its minor forms. *Brain* **77**, 343–400.

HEINE L. (1905) Ueber das zentrale Skotom bei der kongenitalen Amblyopie. *Klin. Mbl. Augenheilk.* **43**(1), 10–40.

HOLMES G. (1918) Disturbances of visual orientation. *Br. J. Ophthal.* **2**, 449–68, 506–16.

HOLMES G. (1921) Palsies of the conjugate ocular movements. *Br. J. Ophthalmol.* **5**, 241–50.

HOLMES G. (1930) Spasm of fixation. *Trans. Ophthal. Soc. U.K.* **50**, 253–62.

HOLMES G. (1936) Looking and seeing. *Ir. J. med. Sci.* **129**, 565–76.

HOLMES G. (1938) The cerebral integration of the ocular movements. *Br. med. J.* **2**, 107–12.

HOLMES G. & HORRAX G. (1919) Disturbances of spatial orientation and visual attention with loss of stereoscopic vision. *Arch. Neurol. Psychiat.* (Chicago) **1**, 385–407.

HOLTERDORF A. (1928) Uber die paroxysmalen tonischen Blickkrämpfe bei der chronisch-myastatischen Enzephalitis. *Münch. med. Wschr.* **75**, 1118–21.

HUBEL D.H. & WIESEL T.N. (1970) Cells sensitive to binocular depth in area 18 of the macaque monkey cortex. *Nature* **225**, 41–2.

JANISCHEWSKY A. (1909) Un cas de maladie de Parkinson avec syndrome pseudo-bulbaire et pseudo-opthalmoplegique. *Revue neurol.* **17**, 823–31.

JELLIFFE S.E. (1932) *Psychopathology of Forced Movements and the Oculogyric Crises of Lethargic Encephalitis.* Nerv. Ment. Dis. Publ. Co., New York and Washington.

JOHNSON T.N. & CLEMENTE C.D. (1959) An experimental study of the fiber connections between the putamen, globus pallidus, ventral thalamus and midbrain tegmentum in the cat. *J. comp. Neurol.* **113**, 83–102.

KINSTON W.J., VADAS M.A. & BISHOP P.O. (1969) Multiple projection of the visual field to the medical portion of the dorsal lateral geniculate mucleus and the adjacent nuclei of the thalamus of the cat. *J. comp. Neurol.* **136**, 295–316.

KUHLENBECK H. & MILLER R.N. (1949) The pretectal region of the human brain. *J. comp. Neurol.* **91**, 369–408.

LHERMITTE J. DE MASSARY & KYRIACO (1928) Syndrome de Parinaud, crises oculogyres, rire spasmodique, narcolepsie en apparence essentielle, dans l'encéphalite prolongée. *Revue neurol.* **44**, 154–7.

MAGOUN H.W., ATLAS D., HARE W.K. & RANSON S.W. (1936) The afferent pathways of the pupillary light reflex in the monkey. *Brain* **59**, 234–49.

MATHERS L.H. & RAPISARDI S.C. (1973) Visual and somatosensory receptor fields of neurons in squirrel monkey pulvinar. *Brain Res.* **64**, 65–83.

McCOWAN P.K. & COOK L.C. (1928) Oculogyric crises in chronic epidemic encephalitis. *Brain* **51**, 285–309.

MORAX P-V. (1937) *Les Paralysies des Mouvements Associés des Yeux.* Thèse de Paris.

NAUTA W.J.H. & MEHLER W.R. (1966) Projections of the lentiform nucleus of the monkey. *Brain Res.* **1**, 3–42.

ORZECHOWSKI C. (1927) De l'ataxie dysmétrique des yeux. *J. Psychol. Neurol., Lpz.* **35**, 1–18.

PASIK P. & PASIK T. (1973) Extrageniculate vision in the monkey. V. Role of the accessory optic system. *J. Neurophysiol.* **36**, 450–7.

ROTH W.C. (1901) Demonstration von Kranken mit Ophthalmoplegie. *Neurol. Zentbl.* **20**, 921–3.

ROUX J. (1910) Hémiplégie oculaire double, abolition de tous les mouvements volontaires avec conservation des mouvements sensorio-réflexes. *Revue neurol.* **18**, 57–61.

SCHUSTER P. (1936) Beitrage zur Pathologie des Thalamus opticus. *Arch. Psychiat. NervKrankh.* **105**, 358–432, 550–622; **106**, 201–33.

SEGARRA J. (1970) Cerebral vascular disease and behavior. I. The syndrome of the mesencephalic artery. *Archs Neurol.* (Chicago) **22**, 408–18.

SNIDER R.S. & LEE J.C. (1961) *A Stereotaxic Atlas of The Monkey Brain* (Macaca mulatta). University of Chicago Press, Chicago.

STRASCHILL M. & HOFFMAN K.P. (1969) Response characteristics of movement-detecting neurons in the cat's pretectal region. *Expl Neurol.* **25**, 165–76.

STEINERT H. & BIELSCHOWSKY A. (1906) Ein Beitrag zur Physiologie und Pathologie der vertikalen Blickbewegung. *Münch med. Wschr.* **53**, 1613–16, 1664–8.

TER BRAAK J.W.G. (1936) Untersuchungen ueber optokinetischen Nystagmus. *Archs néerl. Physiol.* **21**, 309–76.

TILING Th. (1873–4) Beitrag zur Diagnostik der Heerderkrankungen in den Groshirnhemisphären. *Sankt Petersb. med. Z.* **4**, 251–9.

TOURNIER C. (1898) Double hemiplégie, trismus persistent, syndrome de paralysie glosso-labio-faciale pseudobulbaire d'origin cérébrale, ophthalmoplégie ne portant que sur les mouvements volontaires avec conservation des mouvements réflexes. *Revue Méd.* **18**, 671–9.

TREVARTHEN C.B. (1968) Two mechanisms of vision in primates. *Psychol. Forsch.* **31**, 299–337.

TROJANOWSKI J.Q. & JACOBSON S. (1975) Peroxidase labeled subcortical afferents to pulvinar in rhesus monkey. *Brain Res.* **97**, 144–50.

VAN BOGAERT L. (1928) Sur des modalités exceptionelles des crises oculogyres. *J. Neurol. Psychiat., Brux.* **28**, 379–86.

WALD G. & BURIAN H.M. (1944) The dissociation of form vision and light perception in strabismic amblyopia. *Am. J. Opthal.* **27**, 950–63.

WILSON S.A. KINNIER (1940) published posthumously by his son-in-law. In: Bruce A.N. (Ed.) *Neurology*, p. 798. Arnold, London.

DYSFUNCTION IN THE VISUAL PERCEPTION
OF SPACE AND MOTION

MORRIS B. BENDER

Introduction

Among the disciplines of medicine, neurology now stands sovereign. Its primacy was secured in the century between 1850 and 1950 by such gifted physicians as Sir Gordon Holmes. Their painstaking and often brilliant clinical observations, recorded in the European and American literature of their times, continue to deserve our respectful attention. Sir Gordon wrote his first article in 1901, and an impressive series of papers thereafter on the behavioural aspects of cerebral dysfunction, emphasizing disorders of visual perception (Head & Holmes 1910; Holmes 1916, 1917). Many of his descriptions and those of his contemporaries provoked more rigorous physiological and psychophysical investigations which, in general, did little more than corroborate the clinical findings. Laboratory scientists generated long lists of numbers—often at great cost per digit—that failed to yield much additional insight into cerebral processes or the mechanisms of perceptual disorders. Had we to depend entirely on the laboratories, neurology would now be a thrall among the clinical sciences and not their Queen.

The history and clinical aspects of disorders in perception have been compiled by Critchley in a masterful volume on the parietal lobes (1953). Many of the descriptions contained therein are based on his own observations of phenomena to which I will refer. The lesions which underlie perceptual distortions of a given type may be localized in either the central or peripheral portion of any of the various sensory systems. In defective visual perception, focal lesions may be found to involve the visual, oculomotor, vestibular, or cerebellar systems, either singly or in combination with one another.

Disorders in perception of visual space

The characteristic finding in cases of localized cerebral lesions involving the visual system is an impairment of function in restricted homonymous regions of the visual fields. Even when the spontaneous report of perceptual difficulty suggested a symmetrical disturbance of function over the whole field of vision, further testing most often shows a disparate regional involvement. For example, a patient, D.G., who complained about general disturbances in visual perception of depth, was found to experience micropsia and macropsia in the left homonymous half field. These distortions corresponded respectively to the illusion of teleopsia and pelopsia which the patient reported on simple confrontation testing. Careful perimetric examination revealed the additional findings of homonymous bilateral relative scotomata in three quadrants of the visual field (Bender *et al* 1957). In our experience, this finding is not uncommon among patients who complain of visual defects; i.e. there is some loss of 'simple' visual sensations in distinct regions of the field, frequently accompanied by complex perceptual aberrations (Bender & Diamond 1970). But whether the defect in the field may be as phenomenologically simple as a spatially localized loss of acuity, or whether it is a complex alteration in spatial or temporal interactions, the basic correlate of all defects in visual perception of space has been involvement of restricted regions of the entire visual sensory field.

Our knowledge of visual disorientation in three-dimensional space may be traced to the systematic work of Holmes (1918a, b, c; 1919a, b) carried out in 1918 during the First World War and thereafter, often on patients with bilateral injuries of the brain. According to Holmes and Horax (1919), the important features of visual disorientation comprise some or all of the following: (1) An error of absolute localization of objects seen in space, (2) errors in relative localizations in depth, (3) an inability to compare the dimensions of two or more objects, (4) difficulty in avoiding objects when walking and in finding one's way about; this may be coupled with impairment of topographical memory, (5) difficulty in counting objects in visual space, (6) inability to recognize movement in the sagittal plane, (7) impairment of visual attention, (8) disturbed ocular movements, including the so-called fixation of gaze, and (9) at times loss of stereoscopic vision.

During the Second World War we observed patients who mislocalized objects presented anywhere in the visual field, regardless of the nature and extent of the visual defect, while in other cases the errors in localization were more or less confined to amblyopic areas. These areas varied in shape and size, often comprising an entire half field, but at times occupying only a quadrant or a sector. A surprising finding in some patients with complete homonymous hemianopias was that they failed to localize correctly targets displayed in the remaining, perimetrically intact, visual half field. The localization errors were encountered in every part of these 'normal' fields. More detailed testing demonstrated that there were other functional deficits in the supposedly preserved areas, including alteration in flicker fusion frequency, visual thresholds for stroboscopic motion, velocity judgements, and visual after-imagery (Bender & Teuber 1948, 1949). Other patients with brain injuries sustained in battle showed a change in the subjective coordinates of the field of vision, with a shift away from the patient in depth, and again, a lateral shift into the preserved field (Bender & Teuber 1948, 1949). The mislocalization occurred for targets within amblyopic areas and the pointing error was toward the intact field. In attempting to bisect lines, these patients marked the division further toward the visually good side of geometric centre.

The phenomenon of mislocalization of visual targets at the boundary of homonymous hemianopia in the so-called intact portions of the field of vision has also been observed (Corin & Bender 1972). The most common error was mislocalization toward the intact visual field.

Holmes described examples of visual disorientation and inattention, as well as teleopsia and loss of stereopsis in patients with acute lesions localized to one of the occipital lobes. However, it must be emphasized that there have been many instances of such visual disturbances in which both cerebral hemispheres were involved by oedema or other secondary factors. Although Riddoch (1935) claimed that disorientation in visual space was due to a localized lesion of the brain, visual mislocalization in three-dimensional space is almost always due to bilateral involvement, as noted by Holmes (1945). To illustrate this important point, consider the patient H.P., a 52-year-old man, with two metastatic lesions in the right cerebrum as was demonstrated by angiography in September 1975. At that time he was lethargic and had left-sided hemimotor, hemisensory and hemivisual defects, especially during double simultaneous stimulation. There also developed a loss of optokinetic nystagmus (OKN) to stripes moving from left to right followed by a complete disregard of personal and extrapersonal space on the left. He was treated with steroid medication and within three days his organic mental status improved. The phenomena of sensory and visual extinction as well as unilateral OKN deficit disappeared and he could correctly localize objects in his defective left visual field. Yet, computerized tomography scan performed two months later while he was in this improved state demonstrated no essential change in the size or distribution of the two focal metastatic lesions. It must be concluded that the rapid reversal of his hemispatial disorientation and the disappearance of the associated abnormal perceptual interactions were determined by rapid decrease in oedema or other factors which usually affect the function of both cerebral hemispheres. We have recorded many such instances of this dramatic response to steroids and have often observed the phasic appearance of complex hemispatial defects synchronous with fluctuating deficits in mental status (Bender & Diamond 1965). In several cases, when spatial orientation has been restored, we have seen it redeveloped when steroids were discontinued.

Extravisual influences on perception of visual space

It is a well-known but often neglected fact that visual perception of space entails more than a sensing of objects in the visual field through a fixed set of receptor actions and neural transformations (Diamond 1964). Spatial vision depends upon interaction effects in whole regions of the eye and brain and not simply upon point-to-point projection from an external target via retina to brain. The extensive interrelationships between vision and other sensorimotor and cognitive functions that operate in normal perceptual processes are very apparent in the evolution of disordered perception of space and motion. For this reason, many abnormal perceptual phenomena in vision occur only when the influences of body, head, and eye movements are brought into play or when the patient is simultaneously stimulated through another sense modality (Bender 1970).

Various sensory inputs may strongly influence visual perception. Profound abnormal heteromodal interaction effects on vision may be noted in patients who offer no specific visual complaints and who show little, if any, field defects for perception of light, motion, form or colour on standard perimetry. The phenomenon of unilateral visual extinction, an example of interaction within a single modality, such as occurs between a pair of visual stimuli on the left and right sides, was noted by Sir Gordon in 1911. A target exposed in one region of the visual field may become effectively invisible as soon as another target is introduced into the opposite or less affected portion of the field of vision (Bender & Furlow 1945). Auditory or somatosensory stimuli may also interfere with visual perception in different ways. Crossed modal or abnormal interaction effects may result in distortion in the form of a visual percept, a bleaching of its colour, and obscuration or complete extinction of the visual image. Transmodal displacement or spatial transposition of a visual percept in one half field of vision may occur when an optical stimulus is presented concurrently with a tactile, thermal, acoustic, or other extravisual stimulus (Bender 1952, Diamond & Bender 1965).

It is also significant that there are reciprocal influences of vision upon other sensory functions. This was illustrated by many patients we encountered in whom a visual stimulus caused an alteration of a haptic percept and vice versa. For example, a patient might, under simple conditions of testing, correctly perceive that he had been touched on either hand. Yet if the right hand of this same patient were touched while he watched an examiner rub one side of his own face the patient reported either that he felt nothing at all or else that he felt a touch on the cheek. The same type of extinction of a tactile stimulus on the hand occurs when the examiner waves a hand vigorously in the patient's field of vision.

The foregoing class of perceptual abnormalities, especially those which reflect crossed modality interaction effects, are most often observed as part of a highly organized syndrome of unilateral disorientation in visual space or hemispatial inattention. Hemispatial 'inattention', as described by Holmes in 1919a, b, is a syndrome consisting of a neglect of, or inattention to, one-half of extrapersonal space, especially of the periphery and much less neglect in the centre. Patients with this disorder omit material on one side in reading or drawing and even manifest unilateral asymmetries of response when dressing themselves. On the basis of such observations it has been suggested that the right parietal lobe has 'special function in relation to visual-spatial condition'. However, in an analysis of our own series of cases it was shown that parietal lesions in either hemisphere is neither a necessary nor a sufficient condition for obtaining asymmetrical responses to spatial stimuli (Battersby *et al* 1956). Visual field deficits and unilateral somatosensory signs in combination with mental changes appear to be more directly related to the occurrence of spatial inattention than the location of a lesion in the brain, as suggested by others (Hecaen 1962, McFie *et al* 1950, Patterson & Zangwill 1944). Unilateral visual-spatial inattention or imperception is due to defective sensory functions, primarily visual, superimposed upon a background of altered mental function which shifts the normal lateral perceptual bias away from the defective half space (Diamond *et al* 1966). It is not a hemispatial agnosia in the traditional sense of the term.

When the syndrome of hemispatial imperception is full-blown, the defects extend beyond a single sensory field to include other sense modalities, as well as movements of the eyes, head and body on the affected side, and especially to involve general mental functions. An example of this was found in a patient (E.K.) with a large metastatic tumour in the right hemisphere and another smaller tumour in the left hemisphere. She was able to enlarge her field of search from the midline to the right side by appropriate rotation of eyes, head and trunk. She could also make assumptions about the remainder of the unseen portion of the right-hand space behind her, but she did not turn or scan to the left of the midline nor was she able to imagine any content in the left half of space. Other such patients, if they hear a sound, like the sudden clatter of a typewriter originating in the defective field, will turn away from the sound to search for its source in the opposite intact field (Diamond & Bender 1965).

As previously stated, the spatially asymmetrical distribution of disturbances in visual perception, which is recognized as a cardinal feature of illusions developing out of localized cerebral pathology, does not imply that the other regions of the visual field, even the half field on the same side as the lesion, are free from sensory loss or perceptual defects. Spatial and temporal induction effects occur across the fixation point so that illusory phenomena can be expected and in fact are observed in the 'intact field'. Here again, careful plotting of colour fields or measurement of critical flicker frequency will frequently demonstrate an abnormality so that there will be some impairment of visual function in all four quadrants, although the principal losses will be in the expected visual half field.

Disturbances in visual perception of space and its coordinates may also be found in patients who have lesions of the vestibular, kinaesthetic, oculomotor, or cerebellar systems. Accurate visual estimation of distance and size, the comparison of different areas, and the localization of objects in visual space require fine coordinating movements of the eyes and occasionally of the head and body. Mislocalization of objects in visual space is common in patients with brainstem pathology and resultant conjugate gaze paralysis. In cases of isolated abducens palsy the patient frequently mislocalizes to the side opposite the palsy when only the affected eye is tested. Patients with lateral medullary lesions may report alteration in the coordinates of their visual space so that the entire visual field is skewed or even inverted. Such patients may see a piece of furniture on the ceiling, while erect objects may appear to be severely tilted. Disturbances in conjugate gaze may interfere with awareness of unilateral visual space and give the appearance of visuo-spatial neglect. Judgement of verticality in visual space may also be impaired in patients with lesions of the cerebellum (Halpern 1951, 1963).

Spatial and temporal factors in disturbances of perception of visual space

In plotting a suspected defect in homonymous quadrant or hemianopic field of vision the greatest impairment will be found in the periphery and least in the centre. In tests for perception of different colours and size of targets in the normal subject the acuity is found to be best in the centre. In patients with a unilateral lesion of the optic radiation an advancing quadratic or hemianopic defect develops as a progressive constriction of the contralateral field. During recovery the visual field enlarges from the centre to the periphery (Bender & Kanzer 1939, Bender 1963). In most patients the lesion is seldom discrete and free of surrounding oedema or vascular reaction.

Numerous abnormal spatial or temporal interaction effects will occur in association with lesions of the cerebrum. However, most of these are discovered only by detailed qualitative testing of the patients because the illusory percepts do not exist independently of the visual space. Thus, visual space, although it normally has certain potential for development, has no independent existence apart from the external events that occupy it. Many patients, who may report no alteration in the perceived shape of objects, when tested under appropriate conditions, will report various topographic visual aberrations, such as crowding of objects, or the bending, rotation, curving or stretching of contours in the periphery of a visual half field, and little if at all in the centre of the affected field.

This is also true of the defects involving temporal factors in perception which we have observed in patients with cerebral lesions. Such defects include rapid visual adaptation time to fixed or intermittent stimuli, abnormal persistence of visual percepts in time, 'palinopsia', and discontinuities in perception, such as flickering vision or decomposition of movement with multiple image formation. Disturbances in visual perception of motion occur for specific time rates of change and may involve a restricted region of the field of vision. Again, significant changes in visual perception based on temporal factors may be completely overlooked unless suitable testing is conducted.

Disorders in visual perception of motion

It is well known that a normal observer can be tricked into thinking he sees continuous motion when he is actually viewing a discrete sequence of pictures, alternating with periods of darkness at a rate of only 15 frames per second. A necessary condition for the visual perception of movement is successive stimulation of adjacent retinal loci. Perception of real movement is always complicated by the existence of the phenomena of apparent movement including the well known phi (φ) effect. In the case of fine movement, the appearance of continuous movement may be produced simply by increasing the successive light stimulation of discrete retinal loci to a critical frequency, and the absence of continual displacement of the stimulus on the retina. In the phenomenon of real movement, there is experiential correlation of object displacement projected over the retina. The perceived path of movement can be determined by the specific direction of the objectively moving surround. The speed of movement should also be considered. The perception of moving contour is held to be dependent upon the summation of neural excitation in the visual cortex on the two phases of the stimulation sequence. A fixed luminous source and a non-articulated surround, such as darkness or ganzfeld, one which reduces to a minimum any frames of reference instability, may be seen as moving in an erratic, unpredictable fashion. Darkness has proved to be the most efficient contour-free situation for the production of illusory autokinetic movement.

Cerebral lesions and defects in visual perception of motion

Abnormalities in the visual perception of motion may be found in cases of a localized lesion of the brain (Riddoch 1917). One example of defect in perception of motion is known as palinopsia, observed by Holmes in 1931 and reviewed by Critchley (1951, 1953). In the phenomenon of palinopsia, movement of a target along a given path within a defective field of vision (rendered so by a traumatic or neoplastic lesion in the opposite posterior half of the cerebrum) will evoke a visual sensation of a series of separate images of the single target situated along the path of motion. As soon as the target crosses the midvertical and moves through the affected into the normal half field, the series of perseverated images disappear and a single, true image, moves smoothly (Bender & Teuber 1949, Bender *et al* 1968). The appearance of a series of separate still images in the defective field along the path of motion may be due to interference by the brain lesion with the normal φ phenomenon. This conclusion is based on the hypothesis that the φ phenomenon may be the basis both for the perception of real as well as apparent motion (Kolers 1968, Spigel 1968).

Experience in human patients with cerebral lesions provides some significant insight into the function of neocortex with respect to the perception of real and apparent movement (Bender & Teuber 1949, Teuber *et al* 1960). In a study of Naval casualties with penetrating head injuries during the Second World War, it was found that disorders in the visual perception of motion frequently occurred as a prominent though never as an isolated symptom of disorganization in vision. Moreover, the disturbance was found to involve not the entire field of vision but homonymous halves or quadrants. Such cases afforded a singular opportunity for the study of alterations in perception of movement because the patient could often describe directly what was seen in the affected part of the field and compare these impressions with those in other, less impaired, regions of the field of vision. The phenomena observed in this fashion have obvious significance for understanding of the physiological basis of visual perception of motion in the normal. The following visual dysfunctions were noted: (1) illusory motion of stationary objects ('drifting' of images), (2) distortions in the perceived path of actually moving objects, e.g. an object moving in a straight line seemed to the patient to follow a curved path in the impaired sector of the field, (3) alterations in the apparent speed of actually moving objects. To the patients the test objects appeared to 'slow down' or 'speed up' upon traversing the most impaired homonymous quadrants of the plotted field of vision, (4) apparent multiplication of single, actually moving objects, resulting in monocular diplopia or polyopia.

The occurrence of these perceptual disturbances depended upon the mode of stimulation. Testing conditions were controlled with regard to the actual speed of the moving stimuli in the patient's field. Results of these tests can be described as follows:

(a) Spatial factors played a role in the production of distortions in the path of seen movement. The distortions occurred consistently in certain directions. Thus, the path of objects moving through a lower quadrant of the field of vision was distorted toward the fixation point or towards the midvertical meridian. The apparent 'drifts' of actually stationary objects in the affected quadrants of the field of vision occurred in the same directions.

(b) Similarly, temporal aspects of stimulation influenced these visual phenomena in a systematic fashion. The visual perception of true motion varied with the speed of the presented moving object. Slow motion, below 5 degrees per second, produced the impression of a single stationary object. More rapid motion produced an apparent elongation or duplication of the image (monocular diplopia). As the rate was increased beyond 20 degrees per second, the patient complained of formation of multiple images or seeing a 'string' of objects spread out along the path of the actual movement of the single object. In the affected fields the patients also had difficulties in assessing actual speeds. Whenever movement of an object was perceived, they either underestimated or overestimated the true rate. They underestimated slow speeds and overestimated moderately rapid speeds.

(c) Although the symptoms thus far described were limited to homonymous quadrants, there were indications of interaction across the midline of the field of vision. Thus, an object seen to be moving into one field of vision may lead to an optic illusion of motion in the opposite defective field. Associated with this there was polyopia for an object exposed in the defective half field.

(d) Disturbances of visual perception of true motion were invariably accompanied by corresponding changes in the perception of stroboscopic movement, i.e. the apparent movement produced by alternating exposures of two spatially separate, stationary stimuli. Moreover, these patients showed marked fluctuation in all visual thresholds in the impaired sectors of the field, such as 'extinction' on bilateral simultaneous stimulation and a reduction of fusion frequencies of visual flicker and in visual adaptation time.

A most significant finding involved the occasional replacement of the continuous vision of a moving object by the appearance of successive stationary objects. At times the path of a target moving with constant velocity was seen by some patients with cerebral lesions as curved rather than straight (Teuber & Bender 1949).

Tests made under controlled conditions indicated that perception of actual motion was changed concomitantly with that of stroboscopic motion and flicker, suggesting that these three functions have a common physiologic basis. Multiplication of visual images may also depend on the abnormal intermittence of neural activity subserving vision. Similar intermittence, but with different temporal characteristics, may exist in normal vision. The visual perception of multiple images of a moving object is experienced by the normal observer when an object is about to reach the critical speed and assumes the appearance of a streak. One might suppose that the critical flicker speed was lower for patients with brain injury, just as thresholds for other visual functions were changed in these cases. The assumption of continual intermittence of cerebral process in vision is useful in understanding physiology of vision and some disorders in vision.

Disorders of visual perception of space in diffuse bilateral disease of the brain

Examples of disorder of visual perception in space and in optic illusions of motion may be found in patients with diffuse bilateral involvement of the brain, e.g. due to drug intoxications, delirium associated with systemic infection or metabolic disorders and in degenerative or arteriolar disease.

Although there may be some asymmetry with respect to the portion of visual space in which the illusory phenomena become manifest, the characteristic feature of the perceptual disorders associated with diffuse cerebral disease is the general constriction of visual space. In unilateral hemispatial disorders there is an asymmetrical or unilateral constriction of visual function, whereas in diffuse cerebral disease there is a bilateral constriction of vision. There is a marked reduction in the use of information from the peripheral field of vision and a disregard of visual background leading to constricted fields. The patient may be unable to perceive relationships between adjacent spots in a defective visual field so that the φ phenomenon, for example, appears to be absent. An illustration of this is the failure to perceive a figure whose contour is discontinuous but clearly defined by a number of smaller figures. For example, when presented with a figure composed of repeated small numerals arranged to outline the pattern of a larger figure, the patient with severe bilateral encephalopathy, such as Alzheimer's disease, may report that only the small individual numbers of which the larger pattern is constructed were seen. When this occurs, he may still fail to perceive the main figure, even when it is suggested to him or outlined for him. A large '3' drawn of little '2's' is recognized only as the cipher '2' or a number of '2's'. Again, if the large '3' is outlined in heavy dots, the patient reports seeing dots. However, if the '2's' or the dots are connected with lines so that the outline of the large '3' appears to be continuous, the patient sees the '3'. When too much information is presented, the useful field contracts to a small region around the fixation point. This is a response to an overload of the defective visual system (Bender & Diamond 1975). Extraneous visual stimuli destroy peripheral recognition because the whole stimulus pattern is complex. Such patients see the small '2' as a whole central figure but they miss the figures outside of the central field which normal subjects would scan, integrate and thus identify the pattern of the figure '3'.

Other perceptual disorders show the relatively greater involvement or impairment of the peripheral fields in diffuse encephalopathies, such as the illusion of panoramic perspective or the common failure to perceive objects or motion outside the central field, particularly when the patient is fixating. Hallucinations may occur in these cases and, like the illusory phenomena, are usually marked by their spatial asymmetry. They frequently develop in the central field and may, in fact, evolve from a simple illusion through a sequence of changes. For example, a patient with toxic encephalopathy may fix his gaze on a small, dark speck observing that it appears to enlarge, to change its position and its colour and, finally, to assume the appearance of a moving insect which may become multiple (visual hallucination of motion or zoopsia).

Frequent visual illusions of motion are common in these cases. They may be related, in part, to the fact that apparent movement of an object in space depends not only on the relative motion of the image and eyes, as noted above, but also on the relative movement of the object and the background field, effects of autokinesis and the φ phenomenon. When the background is neglected, as in darkness, the position of a fixated object will tend to become unstable, producing an illusion of motion in the same way that an absence of background gives rise to autokinetic phenomena in the normal person. Lesions within the cerebellum, vestibular or oculomotor system are known to produce optic illusions of movement of a luminous target in a darkened room or ganzfeld. The illusory motion reported by patients in this category most often consists of a slow, steady drift of a single figure or of identical figures arranged in a regular pattern. The space of the apparent movement is usually confined to the paracentral region of the field if the cerebral dysfunction is symmetrical. If there is accentuated unilateral involvement of the visual system, the illusion will most frequently consist of movement away from the side of the lesion toward the centre of the visual field.

Disturbances in visual perception of motion due to lesions of the vestibular or oculomotor systems

Many of the perceptual distortions of movement in man, especially illusory motion, may be seen in association with disease of the oculomotor and vestibular systems (Holmes 1936, 1938, Bender 1965). It will be remembered that an object and its surroundings usually appear stationary when the eyes and the retinal images are fixed or, if the eyes are moving, when the angular velocity of the image across the retina is equal and opposite in direction to the angular velocity of the moving eye. In most other cases, the object is seen to move in the field of vision. Thus, a target is perceived to be in motion when its image either traverses the receptor field of a stationary eye or moves on the retina at some angular speed other than that of the moving eye, or else moves in a direction which is not opposite to the eye movement.

Examples of altered visual perception of motion may be found in patients with brainstem disease and difficulties in maintaining a perceived visual image stable during head turning. They may report seeing horizontal movement of an entire visual environment. Thus a woman with a unilateral lesion within the vestibular nucleus complained that every time she turned her head quickly to the left all objects moved to the right. Another woman with a metastatic lesion to the brainstem and defects in eye movement stated that when she moved her head horizontally, side to side, viewed objects moved up and down. The same patient complained that vertical oscillations of the head induced the optic illusion of horizontal motion (Bender & Feldman 1967). Patients with nystagmus may have oscillopsia in the plane of nystagmus on direct forward gaze. Vertical oscillopsia can also be seen in vertical nystagmus due to bilateral brainstem disease. At times vertical oscillopsia may be found without grossly visible nystagmus. However, such patients have vertical motions of retinal vessels on funduscopy or 'retinal nystagmus'. Oscillating vision in rotary or oblique planes has also been observed. A rare form of disorder in visual perception of motion is oscillations in depth. This occurs in patients with asymmetrical and unequal nystagmus in the two eyes (Bender 1965).

Summary

In summary, some observations on diverse disorders of visual perception are reviewed; these observations have led to a number of general propositions that are both testable and predictive.

Focal involvement of the nervous system will usually result in asymmetrical disturbances in perceptual functions. If a disease process primarily affects one cerebral hemisphere, the principal changes in perception will arise in a portion of the sensory field opposite the site of the lesion. There is no distinct area of the cortex which if destroyed will cause a disturbance in the organization of a sensory space. Any visuo-spatial disorientation or spatial agnosia is due to a general disturbance in brain function, superimposed on a predominately unilateral neural sensory deficit including vision.

No specific type of perceptual illusion taken in isolation can localize pathology in the cerebrum. Correlation between alteration in function and site of lesion must be based on larger patterns of neurological deficits. Extensive interrelationships among the various sensory and motor systems that characterize normal perceptual function are reflected in the wide variations of perceptual illusions caused by lesions in the nervous system.

Vestibular, oculomotor, kinaesthetic and cerebellar systems have a profound influence upon visual function, through reciprocal interactions with the visual projection system itself and with the subject's state of alertness or mental state.

Diffuse bilateral cerebral disorders without significant focal accentuation produce generally symmetrically distributed perceptual deficits. The principal manifestation of these deficits is a constriction of visual or other sensory space from the periphery towards the centre. The degree of constriction appears to be directly related to the information content of stimulus patterns in the sensory field.

The fact that perception of flicker, apparent motion, and real motion are simultaneously altered in disease, suggests that there is a unitary physiological factor underlying these three functions. The multiplication of images, in particular, indicates that the common mechanism might be an abnormal intermittence of cerebral activities subserving vision. A similar intermittence, though with different time characteristics, may exist in the process of normal vision. The perception of multiple images of a flickering light is experienced by the normal observer when the rate of flicker is about to reach the critical value at which it assumes the appearance of a steady source. One might suppose that this critical rate is lowered in patients with brain injury.

Lesions of the vestibular or oculomotor systems will also affect visual perception of motion, as well as the stabilization of visual images in space during eye-head-body motions. It appears that the phenomena observed in patients with brain lesions are not essentially different from those which play a role in normal perceptual activity.

References

BATTERSBY W.S., BENDER M.B., POLLACK M. & KAHN R.L. (1956) Unilateral 'spatial agnosia' ('Inattention'). *Brain* **79**, 68–93.

BENDER M.B. (1945) Polyopia and monocular diplopia of cerebral origin. *Arch. Neurol. psychiat.* **54**, 323–38.

BENDER M.B. (1952) Disorders in perception. In: Aring C.D. (Ed.) *American Lectures in Neurology*, No. 120. Charles C. Thomas, Springfield, Illinois.

BENDER M.B. (1963) Disorders in visual perception. In: Halpern R. (Ed.) *Problems of Dynamic Neurology*, pp. 319–75. Grune & Stratton, New York.

BENDER M.B. (1965) Oscillopsia. *Archs. Neurol.* **13**, 205–13.

BENDER M.B. (1970) Perceptual interactions. In: Williams D. (Ed.) *Modern Trends in Neurology*, pp. 1–28. Butterworth, London.

BENDER M.B. & DIAMOND S.P. (1965) An analysis of auditory perceptual defects. *Brain* **88**, 675–86.

BENDER M.B. & DIAMOND S.P. (1970) Perception and its disorders. *Res. Publ. Assoc. Nerv. Ment. Dis.* **48**, 176.

BENDER M.B. & DIAMOND S.P. (1975) Sensory interaction effects and their relation to the organization of perceptual space. In: Tower D.B. (Ed.) *The Nervous System*, Vol. 3, *Human Communication and its Disorders*, pp. 393–402. Raven

Press, New York.

BENDER M.B. & FELDMAN M. (1967) Visual illusions during head movement in lesions of the brainstem. *Archs. Neurol.* **17**, 354–64.

BENDER M.B., FELDMAN M. & SOBIN A.J. (1968) Palinopsia. *Brain* **91**, 321–38.

BENDER M.B. & FURLOW L.T. (1945) Phenomenon of visual extinction in homonymous fields and psychological principles involved. *Arch. Neurol. & Psychiat.* **53**, 29–33.

BENDER M.B. & KANZER M. (1939) Dynamics of homonymous hemianopias and preservation of central vision. *Brain* **62**, 404–21.

BENDER M.B., POSTEL D.M. & KRIEGER H.P. (1957) Disorders in oculomotor function in lesions of the occipital lobe. *J. Neurol. Neurosurg. Psychiat.* **20**, 139–47.

BENDER M.B. & TEUBER H.L. (1946) Phenomena of fluctuation, extinction and completion in visual perception. *Arch. Neurol. Psychiat.* **55**, 627–58.

BENDER M.B. & TEUBER H.L. (1947–8) Spatial organization of visual perception following injury to the brain. *Arch. Neurol. Psychiat.* **58**, 721–39 and **59**, 39–62.

BENDER M.B. & TEUBER H.L. (1948) Disorders in the visual perception of motion. *Trans. Amer. Neurol. Assoc.* **73**, 191–3.

BENDER M.B. & TEUBER H.L. (1949) Disturbances in visual perception following cerebral lesions. *J. Psychol.* **28**, 223–33.

CORIN M. & BENDER M.B. (1972) Mislocalization in visual space with reference to the midline at the boundary of a homonymous hemianopia. *Archs. Neurol.* **27**, 252–62.

CRITCHLEY M. (1951) Types of visual perseveration; 'Palinopsia' and illusory visual spread. *Brain* **74**, 267–99.

CRITCHLEY M. (1953) *The Parietal Lobes.* Edward Arnold, London.

DIAMOND S.P. (1964) Input–output relations. *Ann. New York Acad. Sci.* **112**, (Part 1) 160–71.

DIAMOND S.P. & BENDER M.B. (1965) On auditory extinction and alloacousis. *Trans. Amer. Neurol. Assoc.* **90**, 154–7.

DIAMOND S.P., RUTSCHMANN R. & BENDER M.B. (1966) Spatial bias and asymmetries in psycho-physical judgments. *Trans. Amer. Neurol. Assoc.* **91**, 145–51.

HALPERN L. (1951) Syndrome of sensori-motor induction in combined cerebellar and labyrinthian injury. *J. Nerv. & Ment. Dis.* **114**, 137.

HALPERN L. (1963) Problem of dynamic neurology. In: Halpern L. (Ed.) *Studies on the Neurobiological effects of Colours in Problems of Dynamic Neurology*, pp. 399–422. Grune & Stratton, New York.

HEAD H. & HOLMES G. (1911) Sensory disturbances from cerebral lesions. *Brain* **34**, 102–254.

HECAEN H. (1962) Clinical symptomatology in right and left hemispheric lesions. In: Mountcastle V.B. (Ed.) *Interhemispheric Relations and Cerebral Dominance*, pp. 215–44. Johns Hopkins Press, Baltimore.

HOLMES G. & LISTER W.T. (1916) Disturbances of vision from cerebral lesions. *Brain* **39**, 34.

HOLMES G. (1917) Visual localization and orientation. *Brit. med. J.* **2**, 826.

HOLMES G. (1918a) Disturbances of vision by cerebral lesions *Amer. J. Ophthalm.* (Sect. 3) **1**, 270.

HOLMES G. (1918b) Disturbances of vision by cerebral lesions *Brit. J. Ophthalm.* **2**, 353.

HOLMES G. (1918c) Disturbances of visual orientation. *Brit. J. Ophthalm.* **2**, 506.

HOLMES G. (1919a) The cortical localization of vision (Montgomery lectures I). *Brit. med. J.* **2**, 193.

HOLMES G. (1919b) Disturbances of visual space perception (Montgomery lectures II). *Brit. med. J.* **2**, 230.

HOLMES G. (1931) Contribution to the cortical representation of vision. *Brain* **56**, 470–9.

HOLMES G. (1936) Looking and seeing; movements and fixation of eyes (John Mallet Purser lecture). *Irish J. med. Sci.*, p. 565.

HOLMES G. (1938) The cerebral integration of the ocular movements (Victor Horsley memorial lecture). *Brit. med. J.* **2**, 107.

HOLMES G. (1945) The organization of the visual cortex in man (Ferrier lecture). *Proc. Roy. Soc.* **132**, 348–61.

HOLMES G. & HORAX G. (1919) Disturbances of spatial orientation and visual attention with loss of stereoscopic vision. *Arch. Neurol. Psychiat.* **1**, 385–407.

KOLERS P.A. (1968) Some differences between real and apparent visual movement. In: Haber R.N. (Ed.) *Contemporary Theory and Research in Visual Perception*, pp. 122–36. Holt, Rinehart & Winston, New York.

MCFIE J., PIERCY M.F. & ZANGWILL O.L. (1950) Visual spatial agnosia associated with lesions in the right cerebral hemisphere. *Brain* **73**, 167–90.

PATTERSON A. & ZANGWILL O.L. (1944) Disorders in visual space perception associated with lesions of right cerebral hemisphere. *Brain* **67**, 331–58.

RIDDOCH G. (1917) Dissociation of visual perception due to occipital injuries, with especial reference to appreciation of movement. *Brain* **40**, 15.

RIDDOCH G. (1935) Visual disorientation in homonymous half fields. *Brain* **58**, 376.

SPIGEL I.M. (1968) Problems in the study of visually perceived movement. An introduction. In: Haber R.N. (Ed.) *Contemporary Theory and Research in Visual Perception*, pp. 103–21. Holt, Rinehart & Winston, New York.

TEUBER H.L. & BENDER M.B. (1949) Alterations in pattern vision following trauma of occipital lobes in man. *J. Gen. Psychol.*, **40**, 37–57.

TEUBER H.L., BATTERSBY W.S. & BENDER M.B. (1960) *Visual Field Defects After Penetrating Missile Wounds of the Brain.* Harvard University Press, Cambridge, Massachusetts.

PARIETAL CORTEX IN VISUAL ORIENTATION

G. ETTLINGER

In 1918 Gordon Holmes described 6 patients having 'disturbances of visual orientation'. He defined disturbances of visual orientation as '. . . an affection of the power of localizing the position in space and the distance of objects by sight alone . . .' and in particular, '. . . the patient was unable to touch accurately any object within his reach and vision, though the movements of one or both arms were intact; in walking he collided with easily visible objects and had difficulty in finding his way around them, and frequently he could not recognize the relative positions of two similar objects in space. In attempting to touch an object he made mistakes in all three planes of space, that is in judging its lateral and vertical position as well as its distance, though the errors were always greater in the estimation of distance.'

Holmes referred to 5 single case-reports of this syndrome in the earlier literature, and subsequently with Horrax (1919) described one additional case. In 9 of these 12 cases the parietal lobes were known (or likely) to have been injured by perforating missiles; in the remaining 3 parietal lesions were due to vascular disease and the medial surfaces of the hemispheres were free from gross damage. Therefore Holmes regarded destruction of the lateral parietal cortex (in particular, of the angular and marginal gyri) as the essential lesion.

Holmes (1918) also noted that similar disturbances had been described by various authors in monkeys after removals of lateral parietal cortex from both hemispheres. For instance, Ferrier (1886) wrote of a monkey with bilateral removals of the region thought to be equivalent to the angular gyrus: 'On the fourth day (after operation) some indications of returning vision were observed, but the animal never during the whole period of its survival—over two months—regained perfect vision, but always exhibited some uncertainty or want of precision in its endeavours to seize things offered it, or to pick up minute articles of food from the floor, such as currants or grains of corn'.

The clinical syndrome described by Holmes was subsequently termed 'Visual Disorientation'. Its place in the wider constellation of disorders of spatial orientation has been reviewed by Benton (1969). Progress since Holmes has been made in 3 ways: (i) fractionation of the syndrome into independent clinical elements; (ii) quantitative analysis of certain elements in unselected series of patients; and (iii) comparative studies, both behavioural and electrophysiological, with monkeys.

(i) Fractionation of visual disorientation into clinically independent elements

Little further work was done until the Second World War, when intensive investigations of parietal syndromes began in this country, in France and the U.S.A. In consequence, particularly of the study of unilateral parietal syndromes, it is now widely accepted that : (a) defective visual localization; (b) topographical disturbances (of orientation and/or memory); (c) disorders of visual fixation (termed by Holmes 'Ocular symptoms'); and (d) certain other elements (e.g. visual inattention; loss of stereoscopic vision) can each occur as a clinical condition independently of the others. However, each element is frequently but not always associated with yet a further complex disturbance now variously termed 'Constructional Apraxia' or 'Visual-spatial Agnosia'. An example of such clinical dissociation of elements is the case of Godwin-Austen (1965).

The cardinal element (i.e. that necessary and sufficient to distinguish 'Visual Disorientation' from, for instance, 'Constructional Apraxia' or 'Visual-spatial Agnosia') is defective visual localization of objects in extra-personal space. This is evident from cases like those described by Riddoch (1935), Brain (1941) and by several others in which defective localization is confined to homonymous contralateral half-fields in association with a unilateral parietal lesion. Holmes (1952) was aware of this when he wrote: 'Unilateral loss of orientation produces less obvious symptoms and is usually not recognized by the subject, but he is unable to point to, or otherwise indicate, the position of an object in the affected homonymous halves of the field of vision'.

(ii) Quantitative analyses in unselected series of patients

(a) Defective visual localization. Ratcliff and Davies-Jones (1972) assessed the accuracy of reaching for a white visual target (5 mm at 33 cm) in 49 subjects with chronic missile wounds of the brain, and in 22 control subjects. The lesions were 'posterior' (i.e. post-Rolandic) in 40 (in 13 left-sided, 16 right-sided and 11 bilateral). Each half-field was tested individually with each hand (e.g. the right half-field with the right- and separately with the left-hand).

A significant association between defective localization and a posterior cerebral lesion was found—no subject with an anterior lesion was defective in any quadrant, whereas 90% of those with posterior lesions were defective in at least one quadrant. Localization was not related to the laterality of the lesion nor to the hand used in reaching. Grossly defective localization in at least one quadrant was not associated with visual field defect, but was associated with cortical sensory defect.

Three of the 29 patients with unilateral lesions were hemianopic. Thirteen of the remaining 26 patients were grossly defective in the contralateral fields (in at least one quadrant), 11 were mildly defective and 2 localized normally. Gross defect was never observed in one quadrant without some impairment of localization in the other quadrant of the same half-field, but there was no correlation between the degree of impairment in the 2 half-fields. (However, in 2 of the 11 patients with *bilateral* posterior lesions localization was grossly defective in all remaining quadrants; and in 3 other men of this group there was mild impairment throughout the visual field.) Ten subjects with unilateral injuries were impaired (but mildly) in quadrants ipsilateral to the lesions. No patient showed the full syndrome originally described by Holmes in 1918.

In summary: the majority of patients with posterior wounds localized inaccurately; the hand used was not relevant; the side of lesion was not relevant but the defect was more severe in the quadrants contralateral to a unilateral lesion than in the ipsilateral quadrants; in patients with unilateral wounds a similar degree of impairment was found within the half-fields but not between the 2 half-fields; and severe inaccuracies were associated with defective tactile sensitivity but not with field defect.

(b) Topographical disorientation. Semmes *et al* (1955) and Weinstein *et al* (1956) studied 62 patients with traumatic injury and 17 control subjects on a task of topographical orientation. The subjects were required to follow by locomotion routes represented on maps. Five of the path-diagrams were perceived visually; 5 were perceived by touch alone with the hand contralateral to the injury; and 5 with the ipsilateral hand. Subjects with lesions that extended beyond one lobe were included in more than one grouping. There were 43 patients with unilateral lesions (with involvement of the frontal lobes in 17; parietal, 15; temporal, 13; and occipital, 14); and in addition to the 11 left- and 22 right-sided cases, there were 19 cases of bilateral lesion (with frontal involvement in 15; parietal, 8; temporal, 6; and occipital, 5).

A significant association between topographical disorientation and a parietal lesion was found but no other differences were significant, for instance between any other lesion group and controls, or between groups with left- or right-sided lesions; or between unilateral or bilateral lesions; or between modes of presenting the path-diagrams. However, the subsequent analysis of the same observations by Weinstein *et al* (1956) indicated that topographical disorientation, for both the visual and tactile path diagrams, was associated with severe sensory defect, but not with field defect or epilepsy. Although aphasic patients were significantly impaired in comparison with non-aphasics, this difference could be wholly ascribed to differences in intelligence; but these differences in intelligence could not account for the differences in topographic orientation between groups with and without sensory defect. Later, Semmes *et al* (1963) found a significant but not strong association between topographical orientation (in 'extra-personal' space) and performance on a (visual) test of orientation on the patient's own body ('personal space').

In summary: topographic disorientation was associated with parietal injury and with sensory defect; all other possible contributing factors such as the modality of the task, the use of the ipsilateral or contralateral hand, a unilateral or bilateral injury, a left- or right-sided injury, the presence of a field-defect, or aphasia or epilepsy were found to be of no importance except in so far as any factor was related to lowered intelligence.

(c) Other elements. Quantitative analyses of certain other elements have been reported for unselected series of cases. For example, Carmon and Bechtoldt (1969) and Benton and Hécaen (1970) have found defective stereopsis to be associated with right-sided lesions—but no other groupings by site of injury or associated defects were made. Bender and Jung (1948) and Teuber and Mishkin (1954) have investigated the patient's ability to align a rod with the vertical. Semmes (1965) has found that impaired tactual shape discrimination is associated with sensory defect and, independently, with impaired topographical orientation, even when the paths were presented visually. None of these investigations is contributory to the present theme.

(iii) Comparative studies in monkeys

(a) Behavioural. 1. Reaching may be severely inaccurate for weeks or months after unilateral parietal ablations restricted to Brodmann's areas 5 and 7, as in the reports of Hartje and Ettlinger (1973) and Mountcastle (1975). Irrespective of the position of the target to the side ipsilateral or contralateral to the ablation, reaching with the contralateral arm is inaccurate (and more so in the dark than in the light), whereas with the ipsilateral arm the monkey reaches accurately (although in the dark it may be somewhat inaccurate, probably due to an additional wider spatial disorientation). Reaching for the mouth is accurate except in rare instances of short duration after larger bilateral removals. Ettlinger and Kalsbeck (1962) reported an insignificant but suggestive trend for a correlation between the anterior extent of the posterior parietal ablation and the inaccuracy of reaching; and also evidence of contralateral neglect in the dark. The observations of Haaxma and Kuypers (1975) suggest that area 7 is more important than area 5; and that occipito-frontal fibre tracts may form part of a system, independent of parietal cortex, for the guidance of finger-movements in retrieval of reward.

2. Gross alterations of behaviour resembling topographical disorientation follow *bilateral* removals of posterior parietal and pre-occipital cortex, and are illustrated in the unpublished film recorded with Miss R. M. Ridley. As

noted by Bates and Ettlinger (1960) there may be only slight degeneration in the lateral geniculate nuclei of such monkeys; their performance on tasks of visual shape discrimination may be unimpaired; and only posture, spontaneous movements, reaching and placing may be abnormal on neurological examination. These alterations last for up to a few months.

3. The same bilateral cortical removals may in some, but not all, animals be associated with subtle disturbances of spatial discrimination both in the light and dark, evident when there is separation between test-objects and the site of response (e.g. Bates & Ettlinger 1960).

(b) Electrophysiological. Hyvärinen and Poranen (1974) have shown that cells in area 7 are activated during reaching and visual fixation. Mountcastle *et al* (1975) have studied a larger population of cells and compared the functions of areas 5 and 7. Many cells respond at much higher rates during active movements initiated by the animal than during similar passive movements imposed by the investigators—for example rotation of one or more joints. Other cells are yet more specific, in that the active movement—projection of the arm and manipulation with the hand—must be towards a particular target known from previous experience to be desirable. The discharge patterns then hardly differ when the projected movements differ greatly (e.g. by 60° in space; or after occlusion of fixation; or whether the movement is towards a visual or tactile target). Curiously, such cells if situated in area 7 are 5 times more likely than if in area 5 to be active during projection of both contra- and ipsi-lateral arms.

In summary: the evidence from behavioural investigations in the monkey indicates that parietal removals produce defects possibly related to visual disorientation in man. However, there are clear differences: in man the defect relates to the contralateral fields but the arm is irrelevant; in the monkey the defect relates to the contralateral arm but the field is irrelevant. Moreover, the electrophysiological evidence from the monkey also supports an organization with emphasis on arm rather than field (although certain cells respond only to stimulation by visual targets).

Current problems

(a) The clustering of elements. As already noted, the cardinal element of Holmes' 'Visual Disorientation' is defective visual localization. In individual cases defective localization has been reported in the absence of the other elements (assessed clinically, not quantitatively). However, in no unselected series of patients has performance on localization, topographical orientation, topographical memory and visual attention been evaluated quantitatively and correlated. Elements which clinically (i.e. considering only severe grades of defect in individual cases) appear independent could still statistically (i.e. considering all grades of defect in unselected series) be found to be inter-

dependent. Moreover, any element of visual disorientation might also be significantly correlated with a parietal disorder (such as defective construction, with blocks or matches, or such as defective spatial analysis, on Raven's Matrices or on Cube Analysis) which has not traditionally formed part of the constellation of elements termed 'Visual Disorientation'. Information in respect of clustering should have diagnostic value; it might also have explanatory value; but significant correlations might merely reflect anatomical overlap or proximity of functionally independent systems.

(b) The nature of defective visual localization. So far it has been established that the disturbance is unrelated to paresis of an arm, crossing the midline with an arm, amblyopia or field defect, defective fixation or any general mental deterioration (dementia or confusion). The association with sensory defect reported by Ratcliff and Davies-Jones (1972) is almost certainly anatomical and not functional (as is the association between topographical disorientation and sensory loss reported by Weinstein *et al* 1956). Nonetheless, it is curious that no investigation has been undertaken of the relationship between visual and non-visual localization in parietal and other cases. (Non-visual localization could require reaching for a target previously but no longer seen; or for a target previously felt.) Indeed, there are suggestions that 'Visual Disorientation' is not always exclusively visual: case 1 of Holmes (1918) had difficulty in moving round an obstacle into which he had run; case 5 did not localize sounds accurately; a patient of Brain (1941) was more severely disorientated in the dark than light; a patient of Paterson and Zangwill (1944) reached inaccurately with the eyes closed but not with the eyes open; and, in another element, the comparable failure on visual and tactual path diagrams of the patients of Semmes *et al* (1955).

Also, no attempt has been made to account for the systematic errors of localization in individual patients in terms of the exact locus or depth of the lesion. If, on an admittedly naïve view, the errors were due to systematic deformation of a visual coordinate system onto which targets for reaching were mapped, then compression of certain parietal sites might be expected to lead to one kind of error, whereas expansion (due to necrosis of adjacent tissue) to errors of opposite sign.

And yet other kinds of investigation remain untried: would an oscillating (i.e. moving) or flickering target be localized more accurately than a static one in the belief that separate coordinates might underlie separate detection systems? How do errors vary with the distance of the target? Do verbal reports of position correspond with attempts to touch?

(c) Differences between man and monkey. In both man and monkey the responsible lesion seems to be lateral parietal, caudal to sensory projection cortex; and yet the organization is different. The reason for the difference may relate to the arboreal habitat of the typical simian species, in which much of the external environment is generally within arm's reach. In contrast,

man's world is more remote and pointing at targets within an arm's reach may represent untypical usage of a human system that normally operates at greater distances. When we close our eyes we still 'visualize' the space around us; and even in the dark our targets may be mapped through somatosensory inflow onto the visual coordinate system(s). Conversely, the monkey may 'tactualize' the world so that even with its eyes open, targets are signalled through visual inflow into the somatosensory reaching system(s). Hyvärinen and Poranen (1974) wrote: 'In visually activated cells . . . often only stimuli presented close to the animal, within its reach, activated the cells' (p. 679). Mountcastle *et al* (1975) wrote of visual fixation cells in area 7: 'The discharge rates . . . increase when the animal fixates certain objects . . . The effect of such an object is maximal if it is located within arm's reach . . .' (p. 886).

According to this view, a unilateral parietal injury in a patient blind from birth might give rise to inaccurate reading with the contralateral arm irrespective of the position of the target. Also, apes could show an intermediate organization. Such a view would, in evolutionary terms, be compatible with the observation that visual disorientation in man is associated with sensory defect (not with field defects), and yet affects the fields and not the arms. It is also compatible with evidence, for example from Hamilton (1964, 1967), that both in man and monkey there exists a system, related in both species to arm but not to field, which is responsible for adaptation under certain conditions to the displacements of the visual world when the subject wears prisms. Hamilton (1967) suggests that this system may be subcortical. Perhaps this system mediated reaching in all primates at an earlier evolutionary stage: divergence between the ancestors of man and monkey may then have occurred when the cortex assumed control of the simple reaching response. In present-day man, on account of his pre-eminently visual environment, integration of vision and limb position takes place in a mapping system more closely linked to visual than kinaesthetic afferents, perhaps in the angular and marginal gyri.* However, in the present-day monkey there may, as suggested by Mountcastle *et al* (1975), be little 'integration' or 'association' between afferents of separate senses. Instead, commands to move the limb may originate in areas 5 and 7, the direction of limb movement being determined by an efferent system directly responsive to inflow from different sense-modalities.

Acknowledgments

I am grateful to various colleagues for helpful comments on this paper.

* An attempt has been made to reconcile the existence in man of a visual system with the existence in the monkey of a somatosensory system for reaching. There is some evidence from within man of separate neural systems for targets within 'walking distance' and 'grasping distance' from Brain (1941, p. 255) and Paterson and Zangwill (1944, p. 338).

References

BATES J.A.V. & ETTLINGER G. (1960) Posterior biparietal ablations in the monkey: changes to neurological and behavioral testing. *Arch. Neurol.* (Chicago) **3**, 177–92.

BENDER M. & JUNG R. (1948) Abweichung der subjectiven optischen Vertikalen und Horizontalen bei Gesunden und Hirnverletzen. *Ach. f. Psychiatr. u. Z. Neurol.* **181**, 193–212.

BENTON A.L. (1969) Disorders of spatial orientation. In Vinken P.J. & Bruyn G.W. (Eds) *Handbook of Clinical Neurology*, Vol. 3, 212–28.

BENTON A.L. & HÉCAEN H. (1970) Stereoscopic vision in patients with unilateral cerebral disease. *Neurology* **20**, 1084–8.

BRAIN W.R. (1941) Visual disorientation with special reference to lesions of the right cerebral hemisphere. *Brain* **64**, 244–72.

CARMON A. & BECHTOLDT H.P. (1969) Dominance of the right cerebral hemisphere for stereopsis. *Neuropsychologia* **7**, 29–39.

ETTLINGER G. & KALSBECK J.E. (1962) Changes in tactile discrimination and in visual reaching after successive and simultaneous bilateral posterior parietal ablations in the monkey. *J. Neurol. Neuros. Psychiat.* **25**, 256–68.

FERRIER D. (1886) *The Functions of the Brain*, 2nd edn. Smith, Elder & Co., London.

GODWIN-AUSTEN R.B. (1965) A case of visual disorientation. *J. Neurol. Neuros. Psychiat.* **28**, 453–8.

HAAXMA R. & KUYPERS H.G.J.M. (1975) Intrahemispheric cortical connexions and visual guidance of hand and finger movements in the rhesus monkey. *Brain* **98**, 239–60.

HAMILTON C.R. (1964) Intermanual transfer of adaptation to prisms. *Am. J. Psychol.* **77**, 457–62.

HAMILTON C.R. (1967) Effects of brain bisection on eye–hand coordination in monkeys wearing prisms. *J. Comp. Physiol. Psychol.* **64**, 434–43.

HARTJE W. & ETTLINGER G. (1973) Reaching in light and dark after unilateral posterior parietal ablations in the monkey. *Cortex* **9**, 344–52.

HOLMES G. (1918) Disturbances of visual orientation. *Br. J. Ophthal.* **2**, 449–68 and 506–16.

HOLMES G. (1952) *Introduction to Clinical Neurology*, 2nd edn. E. & S. Livingstone Ltd, Edinburgh.

HOLMES G. & HORRAX G. (1919) Disturbances of spatial orientation and visual attention, with loss of stereoscopic vision. *Arch. Neurol. Psychiat.* (Chicago) **1**, 385–407.

HYVÄRINEN J. & PORANEN A. (1974) Function of the parietal association area 7 as revealed from cellular discharges in alert monkeys. *Brain* **97**, 673–92.

MOUNTCASTLE V.B. (1975) The view from within: pathways to the study of perception. *Johns Hopkins Med. J.* **136**, 109–31.

MOUNTCASTLE V.B., LYNCH J.C., GEORGOPOULOS A., SAKATA H. & ACUNA C. (1975) The posterior parietal association cortex of the monkey: command functions for operations within extrapersonal space. *J. Neurophysiol.* **38**, 871–908.

PATERSON A. & ZANGWILL O.L. (1944) Disorders of visual space perception associated with lesions of the right cerebral hemisphere. *Brain* **67**, 331–58.

RATCLIFF G. & DAVIES-JONES G.A.B. (1972) Defective visual localization in focal brain wounds. *Brain* **95**, 49–60.

RIDDOCH G. (1935) Visual disorientation in homonymous half-fields. *Brain* **58**, 376–82.

SEMMES J. (1965) A non-tactual factor in astereognosis. *Neuropsychologia* **3**, 295–315.

SEMMES J., WEINSTEIN S., GHENT L. & TEUBER H.L. (1955) Spatial orientation in man after cerebral injury: I. Analyses by locus of lesion. *J. Psychol.* **39**, 227–44.

SEMMES J., WEINSTEIN S., GHENT L. & TEUBER H.L. (1963) Correlates of impaired orientation in personal and extrapersonal space. *Brain* **86**, 747–72.

TEUBER H.L. & MISHKIN M. (1954) Judgment of visual and postural vertical after brain injury. *J. Psychol.* **38**, 161–75.

WEINSTEIN S., SEMMES J., GHENT L. & TEUBER H.L. (1956) Spatial orientation in man after cerebral injury: II. Analysis according to concomitant defects. *J. Psychol.* **42**, 249–63.

VISUAL LOCALIZATION AND VASCULAR DISEASE

DR R. W. ROSS RUSSELL

Gordon Holmes, while serving as a Medical Officer in the B.E.F. in France in the First World War, saw a number of brain-damaged soldiers who presented an unusual clinical syndrome combining both a visual and oculomotor disturbance. The visual defect included disorientation and defective visual localization in space, an inability to estimate absolute and relative distance and a failure to recognize relative lengths and sizes. A further feature was a restriction of visual attention so that patients failed to take notice of images falling on different parts of the retina, though retinal sensibility was intact. The disorder of eye movement comprised a difficulty in visual fixation and pursuit, a failure to converge and accommodate on near objects and absence of reflex blinking to menace (Holmes 1918, Holmes & Horrax 1919). Holmes was at pains to point out that these defects were not due to a disturbance of elementary visual perception since central visual acuity in most cases was unaffected. Although all his patients had visual field defects on conventional testing, usually involving the lower quadrants and usually bilateral, he showed that equivalent field defects produced by wounds of the striate cortex or of the anterior visual pathways did not produce the syndrome. Furthermore defective localization was not itself due to oculomotor disorder since it persisted even when fixation was accurately achieved and could not be demonstrated in patients with total ophthalmoplegia from other causes. As in normal patients, however, localizing errors were smaller when the images fell on macular, rather than extramacular, portions of the retina.

The site of the responsible lesion in the brain was determined at autopsy in two patients and in the remainder deduced by careful craniometric measurements. All patients showed bilateral damage. On the lateral surface of the hemisphere the damaged regions centred on the supramarginal and angular gyri extending to a variable extent into the adjoining occipital, temporal and parietal convolutions involving the upper fibres of the radiation. On the medial surface the splenium was constantly involved.

Holmes' original patients all had high velocity penetrating head injuries and in his experience of many hundreds of brain-damaged soldiers he recognized the syndrome in only a few. He was aware that similar cases had been described before in the German literature but surmised that such patients would rarely be seen in civilian practice, where focal brain lesions due to tumour or vascular disease tend to affect only one hemisphere. Further observations on traumatic lesions were published during the Second World War, but otherwise the syndrome has attracted little attention.

It may be remarked that fragments of what Holmes described are part of every-day neurological experience, for example many patients with unilateral parietal lesions show the phenomenon of visual inattention or defective localization in the affected half field especially when this is on the left side and when the condition is evolving or recovering. In other patients with widespread cerebral vascular disease, visual disorientation may co-exist with other defects of an apraxic or aphasic kind and with a generalized dementia.

In recent years, a striking clinical syndrome having much in common with that so clearly described by Holmes, has been observed in patients following an acute reduction in overall cerebral perfusion. It is true that the patients often show defects outside the visual sphere but their principal symptoms are visual disorientation and impairment of movement under visual guidance and the brunt of the damage falls on the posterior parts of the hemispheres. Reference will be made briefly to five of these patients studied personally to offer some speculations on the underlying vascular disturbance.

Of the five patients, two showed only a temporary defect which recovered completely and the following description applies mainly to the remainder who had more lasting deficits and who were studied at various times after acute ischaemia from three days to three years. Although difficult to test in the early stages, central visual acuity eventually became normal in all patients once correct fixation had been achieved. Visual fields to formal testing showed a lower altitudinal hemianopia in two patients; the third patient had full visual fields but visual inattention in the right half field (Fig. 7.1). Colours were correctly perceived.

The most disabling symptom in all three patients was in the location and orientation of visual stimuli both relative to the patient and relative to each other. All patients had great difficulty in negotiating articles of furniture and moving around due to an inability to perceive their surroundings in three dimensions. They tended to walk into walls and doors which they could see clearly but in altered perspective. This loss of depth perception leads to a cautious approach to the environment which is easily mistaken for hysteria.

Defective localization of visual stimuli in all three dimensions of space was the most striking common characteristic. Small finger movements were quickly perceived except when movement was towards or away from the patient. The reaction to menace was usually absent though the patient blinked when his own hand approached his eyes. All three patients had difficulty in selecting the nearest or furthest away of a group of objects or in judging the relative size or length, sometimes thickness, in the absence of tactile clues. Common objects were readily identified but were handled

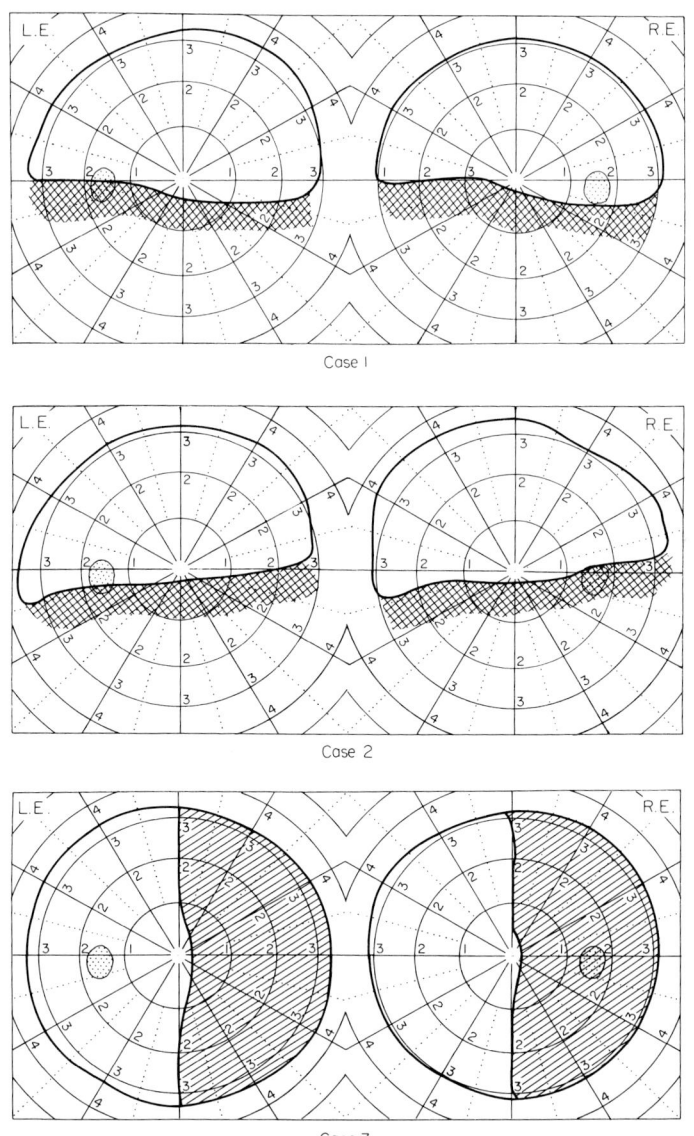

Fig. 7.1 *Primary visual defect.* Case 1. T.D. M. 36 yrs. Visual Acuity 6/5 R. and L. Congruous lower altitudinal hemianopia. Case 2. G.A. F. 56 yrs. Visual Acuity 6/9 R. and L. Lower altitudinal hemianopia Formed hallucinations (moving patterns). Case 3. C.W. F. 36 years. Amaurosis fugax on standing. Visual Acuity 6/6 R. and L. Fields full to confrontation. In attention R. half field.

confidently only when their position could be appreciated by tactile means; tasks involving accurate visuo-spatial localization such as pouring out liquid from a jug or putting an object on a shelf were performed with extreme difficulty. Two patients showed restricted visual attention and had difficulty in appreciating a group of objects, although each individual object could be correctly perceived. This gave rise to difficulty in reading and copying words (though not individual letters) and in counting, although the patients had no difficulty when allowed to touch the objects with their fingers.

Intimately associated with the visual defect and probably resulting from it are the disturbances of ocular movement and fixation. Two of the three patients had difficulty in fixing their gaze on static or moving objects within the field of vision. When spoken to or asked to look at an object the patient would stare in the wrong direction, roll his eyes around awkwardly until finding by chance the point he sought. Willed voluntary eye movement appeared normal as were the oculocephalic reflexes. The optokinetic drum elicted no response, either fast or slow. Convergence and accommodation were particularly difficult. The third patient showed no abnormality of eye movement.

It must be emphasized that the three severely affected patients showed some defects outside the purely visual sphere. Case one had a left hemiparesis which rapidly recovered and also dyscalculia and right/left disorientation; he also was unable to write or read fluently. Case two had no hemiparesis or sensory loss; she had a mild intellectual impairment and marked motor apraxia of the upper limbs and gait. She also showed dysgraphia and dyscalculia and some visuo-spatial perceptual loss indicated by slowness in interpretation of complex pictures. Case three had no motor signs but mild sensory loss of cortical type with tactile inattention of the right side as well as dysgraphia, dyscalculia and right/left disorientation. She could not copy simple geometric figures and was poor at picture interpretation.

Localization of the responsible lesions was aided by scintiscan and computerized axial scanning in those patients with permanent defects. Scintiscan showed in one patient a left parietal lesion with a probable lesion on the other side also, while in the other two patients axial scanning showed bilateral lesions in the occipital and occipito-parietal regions extending forward on both sides of the midline to the frontal areas (Figs. 7.2 and 7.3a, b). The medial surface of the hemisphere was involved only at the posterior pole and no lesion was visible in the corpus callosum.

Holmes favoured the view that the defect in visual orientation resulted not from involvement of a particular centre for visual localization but from a failure of integration. As he put it 'Abnormal functions are not purely sensational but are the result of mental synthesis of more elementary visual perception. They should be interpreted as the effects of an injury of association pathways between those portions of the occipital cortex which

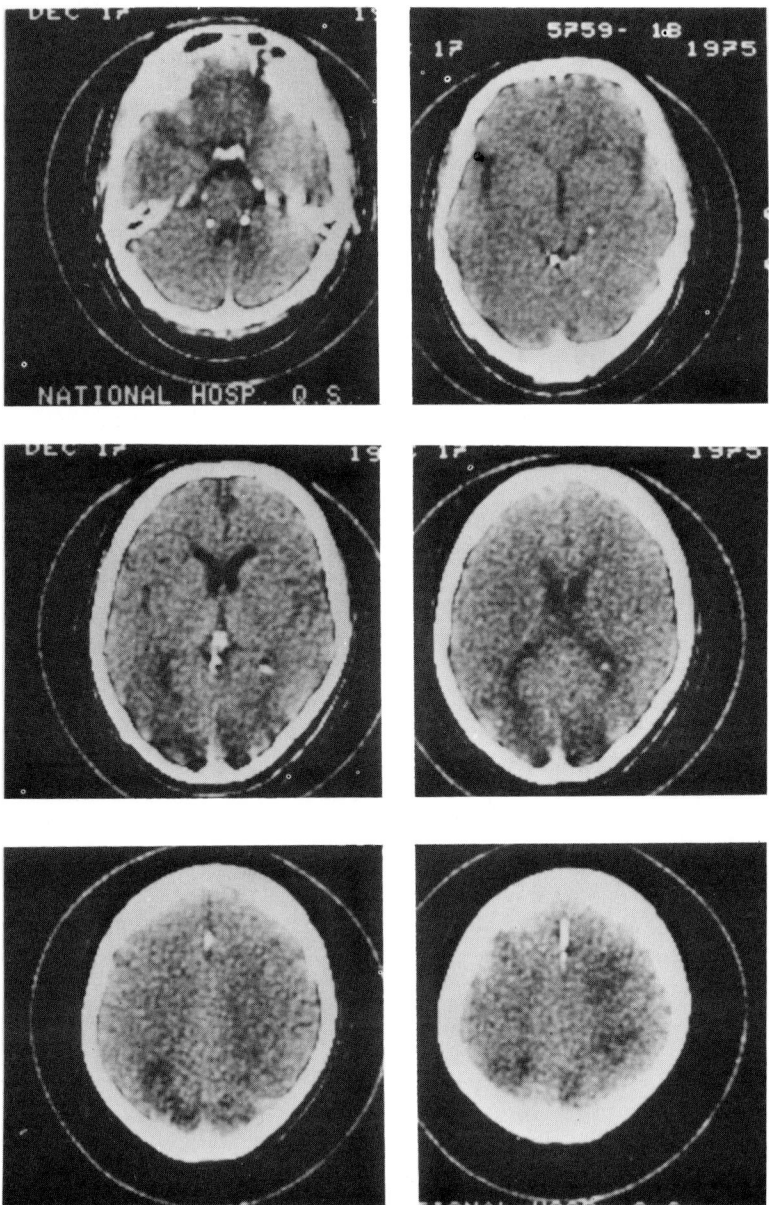

Fig. 7.2 Computerized Axial Scan (Case 1) showing bilateral occipito-parietal infarction with forward extension into the frontal region on the right side.

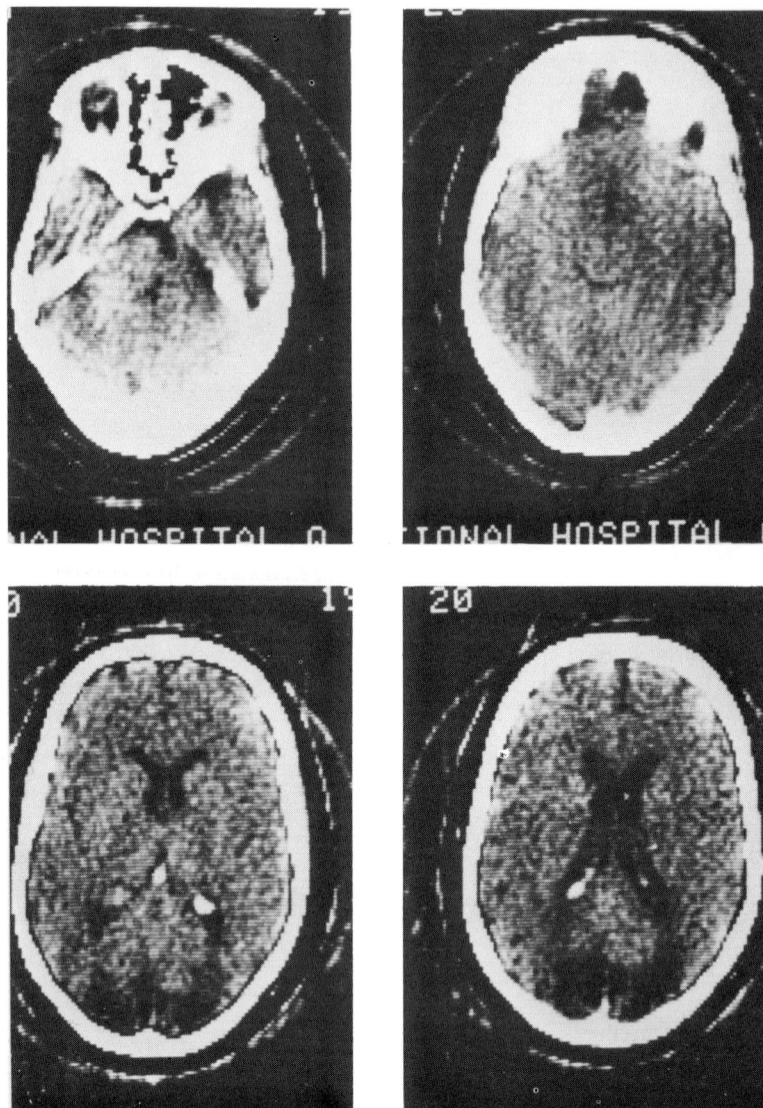

Fig. 7.3a, b   Computerized Axial Scan (Case 2) showing extensive bilateral occipito-parietal infarction extending forward on both sides in the watershed distribution.

are concerned in visual perception and the rest of the brain'. In the present series the lesions were more extensive and the radiological changes are not sufficiently exact to determine which association tracts were interrupted and whether the cortex as well as the white matter was involved, although damage to both is likely. The location of the lesions suggests that they may interrupt

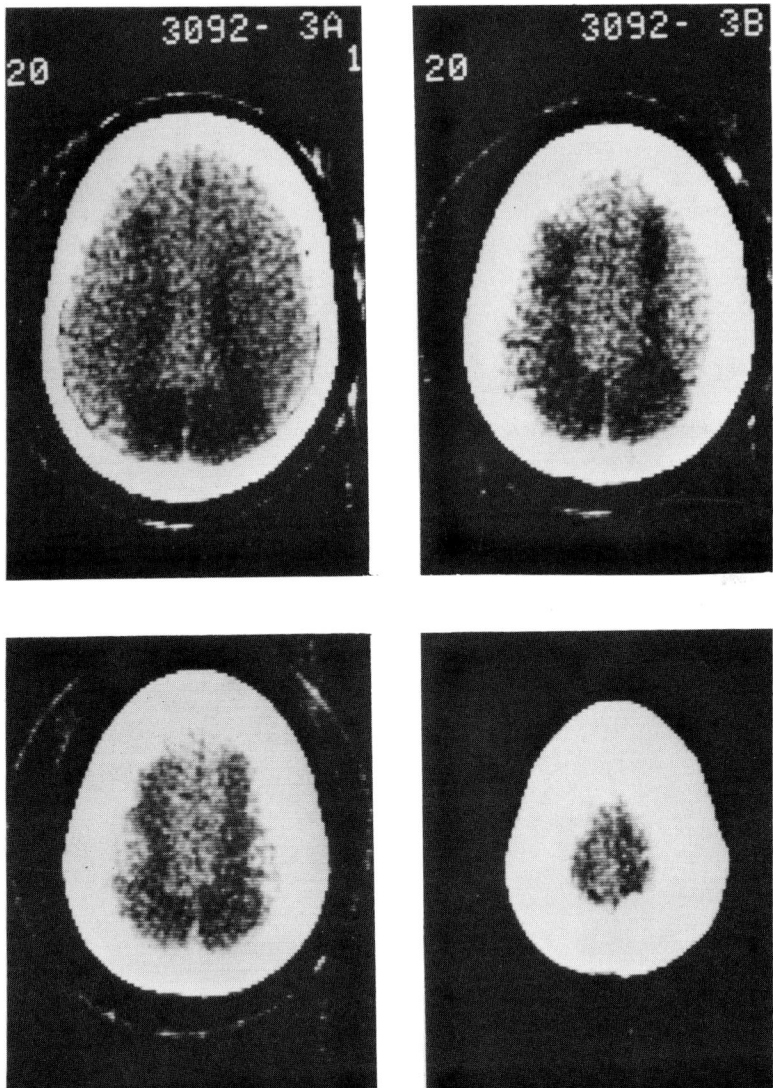

Fig. 7.3b

association tracts linking the visual association area with parietal and frontal lobes. The present small series shows that the four main features Holmes described, namely visual disorientation, visual field defect, visual inattention and oculomotor disorder are not necessarily linked, the oculomotor disorder tending to recover first. In case two, for instance, visual disorientation persisted in association with elements of the Gerstmann Syndrome but without Holmes' other three components.

Four of the five patients had episodes of cardiac dysrhythmia, either spontaneous in the course of myocardial infarction or related to anaesthesia or surgery, and in three patients periods of hypotension lasting three, twelve and forty-eight hours were documented. One patient had mild systemic hypertension and extensive extracranial arterial disease. She suffered many syncopal attacks while walking or standing (Table 7.1). The circulatory factor common to these patients is generalized cerebral hypotension, a severe but temporary global reduction in blood flow from insufficient perfusion pressure followed in most instances by re-establishment of the circulation. The degree of ischaemia must be critical, for we already know that if it is too prolonged the whole brain or the cerebral and cerebellar cortex may be diffusely damaged resulting either in death or in an apallic state. If the ischaemia is insufficient to cause infarction, the patient may exhibit a

Table 7.1   Underlying circulatory disorder in five patients showing visual disorientation

Case 1	T.D. M, 36 yrs	Myocardial infarction: coronary artery stenosis Bypass graft L. and R. coronary arteries ? Short period of cardiac dysrhythymia post operative (10 mins). Normal B.P. thereafter	Single episode Severe cerebral hypotension
Case 2	G.A. F, 56 yrs	Ascending polyneuritis. Anoxia (pO₂40) Assisted respiration Loss of consciousness Systemic hypotension (intermittent) 2 days (60 mm Hg)	Single episode severe cerebral hypotension Mild hypotension 2 days
Case 3	C.W. F, 36 yrs	Bilateral carotico-vertebral occlusion Premature atherosclerosis Bilateral low pressure retinopathy Recurrent syncope and amaurosis fugax	Chronic cerebral hypotension Small postural variations
Case 4	R.G. M, 60 yrs	Myocardial infarction. Asystole 2 mins Hypotension 3 hours. Normotensive thereafter	Transient circulatory arrest Short lived cerebral hypotension
Case 5	P.M. M, 47 yrs	Tuberculous pericarditis. Pericardectomy Hypotension variable. 12 hours (50 mm Hg)	12 hours cerebral hypotension

I am indebted to Dr C.J. Earl for permission to refer to Case 2.

transient visual disturbance, seldom well documented, during his recovery. In only a few patients does the condition persist.

The reason why a generalized hypotension should cause localized hemisphere defects was obscure until the concept of border zone or watershed infarct was introduced by Zülch in 1955. He suggested that, during a period of hypotension, focal regions in the most distal portions of the arterial tree at the junction of adjacent vascular territories are the regions with the lowest perfusion pressure; this might be too low for the autoregulatory capacity of the cerebral circulation, producing localized border zone infarcts while other regions escaped. This concept has been expanded by Meyer (1958) and later by Romanul and Abramowitz (1964) who showed the importance of extracerebral arterial occlusion in predisposing to a low cerebral perfusion pressure and in determining the location of the infarct. They also studied the changes, previously thought to be due to endarteritis obliterans, in pial arteries overlying the border zones, attributing these instead to the effects of reduced blood flow. Finally Brierley and Excell succeeded in producing posterior parieto-occipital lesions in monkeys with intact extracerebral arteries by subjecting them to a series of acute hypotensive episodes. In clinical cases, Adams *et al* (1966) and Gilman (1965) have shown that localized infarction is usually associated with repeated severe falls in blood pressure rather than with sustained hypotension.

The importance of the border zones in the context of visual disturbance is that the ACA/MCA and MCA/PCA zone runs in a sickle-shaped fashion on the lateral surface of the hemisphere and that the regions most constantly involved are the parieto-occipital area and the occipital poles (Russell 1973). It is true that certain embolic lesions such as that produced by air or foam also have a predilection for border zones and this could possibly explain those patients showing visual defects after open heart surgery. Low perfusion pressure, however, seems a likelier explanation since it is a factor common to all the patients presented here.

It is clear from the natural history of these patients that considerable recovery may occur in the weeks following vascular damage. One of the five patients reported here who showed marked visual disorientation and who made a complete clinical recovery later died of unrelated causes; no cerebral lesions were found at autopsy. In this case, watershed ischaemia rather than infarction must have occurred.

There are obvious practical lessons to be learnt, notably the importance of correcting systemic hypotension from cardiac causes and the realization that patients with occlusive cerebral arterial disease are particularly at risk. We must hope that further clinical observations on these patients, who must inevitably be seen in increasing numbers, combined with the marvellous potential for cerebral localization offered by the computerized axial scan will take us further along the path so clearly signposted by Gordon Holmes.

References

ADAMS J.H., BRIERLEY J.B., CONNOR R.C.R. & TREIP C.H.S. (1966) The effects of systemic hypotension upon the human brain. *Brain* **89,** 235–68.

BRIERLEY J.B. (1963) Neuropathological findings in patients dying after open heart surgery. *Thorax* **18,** 291–304.

BRIERLEY J.B. & EXCELL B.J. (1966) The effects of profound systemic hypotension upon the brain of *Macacus rhesus*: physiological and pathological observations. *Brain* **89,** 269–98.

GILMAN S. (1965) Cerebral disorders after open heart operations. *New England Journal of Medicine* 489–98.

HOLMES G. (1918) Disturbance of visual orientation. *British Journal of Ophthalmology* **2,** 449–506.

HOLMES G. & HORRAX G. (1919) Disturbance of spatial orientation and visual attention. *Archives of Neurology and Psychiatry* (Chicago) **1,** 385.

MEYER J.E. (1958) Zur Lokalisation arteriosklerotischer Erwreichungsherde in arteriellen Grenzgebieten des Gelhirns. *Arch. Psychiat. Nervenk* **196,** 421–32.

ROMANUL F.C.A. & ABRAMOWICZ A. (1964) Changes in brain and pial vessels in Arterial border zones. *Archives of Neurology* **11,** 40–65.

ROSS RUSSELL R.W. (1973) The posterior cerebral circulation. *Journal of the Royal College of Physicians of London* **7,** 24–46.

ZÜLCH K.J. (1955) On circulatory disturbances in borderline zones of cerebral and spinal vessels. Proceedings of 2nd International Congress of Neurology, London. (abst) *Excerpta Medica* **8,** 894–5.

NEURONAL MECHANISMS
OF THE MIGRAINOUS VISUAL AURA

G. BAUMGARTNER

The transient focal neurological symptoms preceding classical migraine (ophthalmic migraine, migraine accompagnée) have rather similar characteristics in different individuals. For this reason, Airy as early as 1870 assumed that they may indicate pathological neuronal processing, in which fragments of the functional neuronal organization of the cortex may be reflected. Following similar ideas, we have tried to correlate the focal symptoms at the beginning of classical migraine with neuronal data from animal experiments, both in normal and pathological conditions. The underlying basic assumption is that the prodrome of classical migraine is initiated by local cortical hypoxia.

Material

Prerequisites for such a correlation are clear descriptions of the subjective phenomena. To obtain these descriptions we have re-examined 200 migraine patients. In 87, the diagnosis of classical migraine (46 ophthalmic migraines, 41 migraine accompagnée) was confirmed and these patients were asked for a detailed description of the evolution of the focal symptoms. The details of these examinations are reported elsewhere (Bücking & Baumgartner, 1974) but they are summarized as follows.

(a) Visual symptoms

Since the symptoms may vary from attack to attack in the same individual, the assumption of a relatively stable characteristic of their development may be questioned. If the different descriptions are accumulated, a typical sequence of the visual disturbance at the onset of the attack can usually be established. Of 84 patients with disturbances of vision in connection with the headaches, 52 reported as a first sign only 'defective vision'. No one was able to describe clearly the kind of defect, or to relate it to one eye or to one half of the visual field. 'Something is different with my eyes, I can't tell you what, but

111

I know I shall have another migraine in a few minutes'. Following these changes, or without this preceding warning, 48 patients reported scintillations in the entire visual field, sometimes with a preponderance in one half. These scintillations often were compared with the interference on a television screen. During these phases, no real deterioration of vision was observed. In 23 patients the scintillation was followed by dysopias, i.e. perceptions of translucent, sometimes moving spots, mostly in one half or one quarter of the visual field. Scintillating scotomas were reported following the entoptic scintillations and spot perceptions in 26 cases; the scotomas were always binocular and corresponded to the characteristic fortification spectra of the literature (Fig. 8.1). Bright zig-zag line elements were commonly described, consisting of either one or two stripes slowly spreading across the field. The single line elements were magnified when the fortification band was propagating to the periphery of the visual field. At the same time, the speed of the spread seemed to accelerate. The fortification lines were

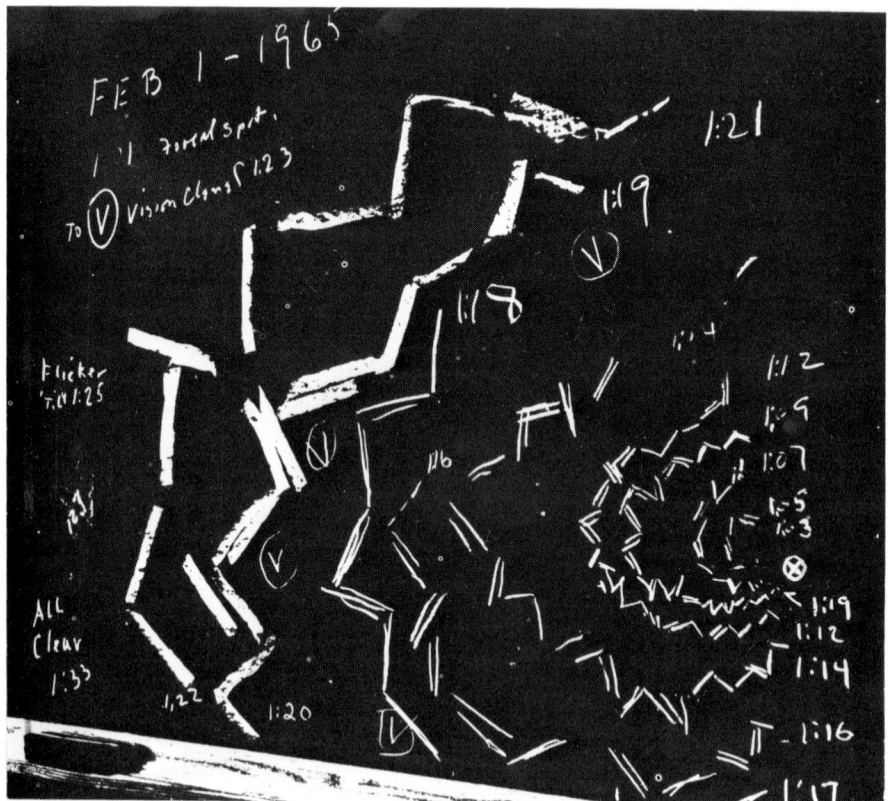

Fig. 8.1   Sketch of the spread of fortification spectra (⊗= point of fixation; numbers refer to time (1·03–1·33)).

followed by a scotoma, in which occasionally filling-in processes were described. In only 7 patients were fortification illusions with scotoma reported without preceding simple, uncharacteristic visual defects, scintillations or translucent spots. Different phases of this process could occur simultaneously in different regions of the visual field so that it is often very difficult to obtain an unambiguous description. Colour phenomena within the zig-zag lines of the fortification spectra, and motion illusions of the spots, were frequent but irregular and are not considered further.

(b) Sensory symptoms

Thirty six patients reported paraesthesiae (pin prick sensations) at the onset of migraine attacks. In 9 patients the paraesthesiae slowly spread and anaesthesia developed. 23 patients reported unilateral symptoms, mostly in the arm and the face, 10 patients described a slow sequence of the cortical type (thumb, hand, perioral) and 6 patients reported paraesthesiae circumorally or in both hands.

(c) Motor dysfunction

Eighteen patients complained of motor disturbances which often consisted of a feeling of tension in the face, tongue or limb and this could be followed by paresis. In 10 patients the dysfunction was localized in one arm, one leg or one half of the body. The descriptions of the further 8 patients were not clear enough to indicate a paresis. Paresis in different regions of the body, for example, in the facial and arm region, did not occur simultaneously, but successively within 1–2 minutes.

(d) Impairment of speech

Nineteen patients reported difficulties of speech and in 11 of these the disturbance followed paraesthesiae of the lips and tongue. In these patients, it was not clear whether the disturbance was dysarthric or aphasic. In 8 patients there was an expressive aphasia with paraphasia and dysfunction of writing and reading; in 4 of these, additional transient dyspractic symptoms were experienced. All patients confirmed that speech comprehension had remained intact.

(e) Sequence of visual and complex focal symptoms

It is unlikely that entoptic or other subjective phenomena are reported identically by different individuals. However, if one neglects qualitative differences and concentrates on the sequence and propagation of the

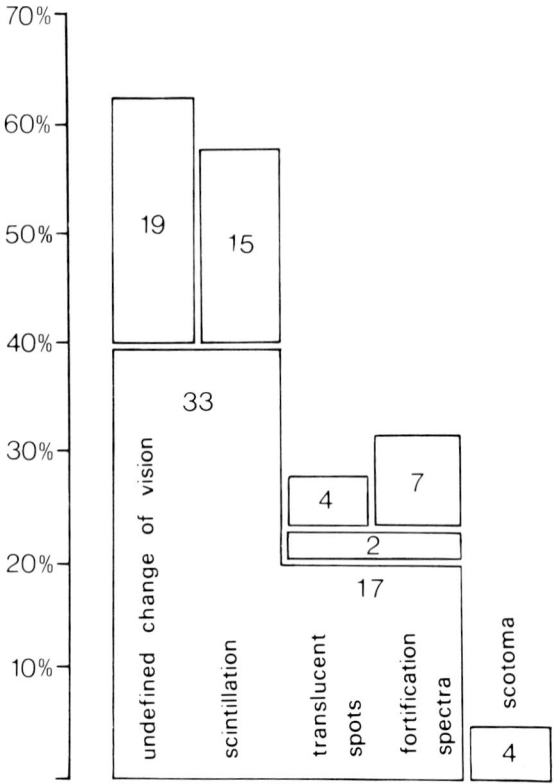

Fig. 8.2 Frequency and sequence of visual disturbances (84 = 100%; numbers within the graph correspond to patients). Patients with different components in succession are shown in the lower unseparated part; the rectangular columns correspond to patients with isolated symptoms.

symptoms, some order becomes obvious in the evolution of the visual disorder and of the complex neurological symptoms. The visual disturbances are characterized by a first phase of slight impairment of vision and scintillations in the entire visual field. In the second phase, grouped dysopsias (spots) and scintillating scotomas, predominantly in one half of the visual field, appear (Fig. 8.2).

The sensory symptoms begin with paraesthesiae and can be followed by a loss of surface sensibility. It could not be determined whether, in cases of paresis, the description of increased muscle tension shortly before the onset of weakness indicates a transient intensified innervation. In migraine accompagnée the symptoms never occurred synchronously, but showed predominantly first visual, then sensory, then motor, and finally aphasic

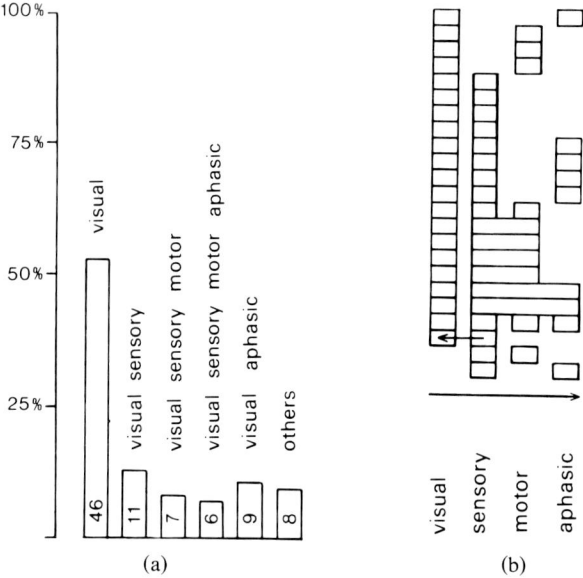

Fig. 8.3a Grouping of focal symptoms (n = 87, 87 = 100%).

Fig. 8.3b Read from left to right. Each rectangle on the same ordinate indicates one patient. Sequence of focal symptoms in 23 cases of classical migraine. In six patients, the sequence after the visual symptoms could not be recorded separately. In one patient, the sequence was sensory-visual (←).

symptoms. There is a clear dominance of visual events occurring as first symptoms with sensory disturbances second (Fig. 8.3a and b).

Neuronal mechanisms

In order to correlate pathological perceptions in migraine with neuronal mechanisms it is necessary to describe briefly the phenomenon of spreading depression, the behaviour of cortical neurones during hypoxia, and the functional organization of the cortex.

Spreading depression of Leào

Spreading depression of activity in the cerebral cortex was first described by Leào (1944, 1947). He found that after electrical, mechanical or chemical stimulation of a cortical area, a local reduction of the spontaneous electrical activity occurred and this slowly propagated in all directions. The spread of the depression within the cortex is about 2 to 6 mm per minute and following this, there is a slow recovery of local activity within 5 to 10 minutes.

Since Leào's description, spreading depression has been examined in many laboratories and is used as an experimental tool to study transient disconnection but the cause is still not clear. A loss of intra-cellular potassium, especially in the region of the dendrites, has been suggested and could explain the accompanying surface electro-negativity (van Harreveld & Ochs 1957, Ochs 1962). Grafstein (1956a,b) and Morlock *et al* (1964) have found that at the margin of the spreading depression, a brief phase of augmented neuronal activity precedes the depression. In the centre of the depression there is no neuronal activity, the neurones being depolarized.

Neuronal activity during hypoxia

Kolmodin and Skoglund (1959) have found that following asphyxia, motoneurones show a membrane depolarization of 5 to 10 mV after a latent period of about 30 seconds; in the succeeding 30 seconds, there is a more rapid depolarization with complete cessation of spike discharges. In cortical neurones we have found four different phases of neuronal activity in acute anoxia after N_2-respiration or local retinal ischaemia. After a latent period of 10 to 20 seconds, a second period of the same duration occurs, during which the neurones show anoxic activation, concomitant with an arousal reaction in the EEG. In the following third phase, the EEG pattern changes to delta-activity and the neurones are silent or have an irregular burst activity for 5 to 10 seconds. There is then complete silence of neurones with disappearance of EEG-waves (Baumgartner *et al* 1961). One has to conclude that the reduction of membrane potentials in the beginning of hypoxia facilitates the activity of the neurones. If hypoxia continues, the membranes become completely depolarized and accordingly there is complete cessation of electrical activity (Fig. 8.4).

Functional organization of the cortical visual receiving area

Our understanding of cortical circuits and of the data processing strategies in the second and higher visual areas (V2–V6) is still insufficient. On the other hand, there is some agreement on the functional organization of the first visual area and other primary receiving areas. Hubel and Wiesel (1962) have shown in cats and later also in monkeys (1968), that the cortex is organized in a mosaic with elements of 0·5–1 mm diameter. These elements correspond to columns of cells; each cell within a column responds only to specifically oriented stimuli. Cortical neurones do not respond to diffuse light but require stimulation by light or dark bars of specific orientation. This response characteristic is a consequence of the rearrangement of the visual input in the cortex.

It is thought that several concentric receptive fields of geniculate fibres

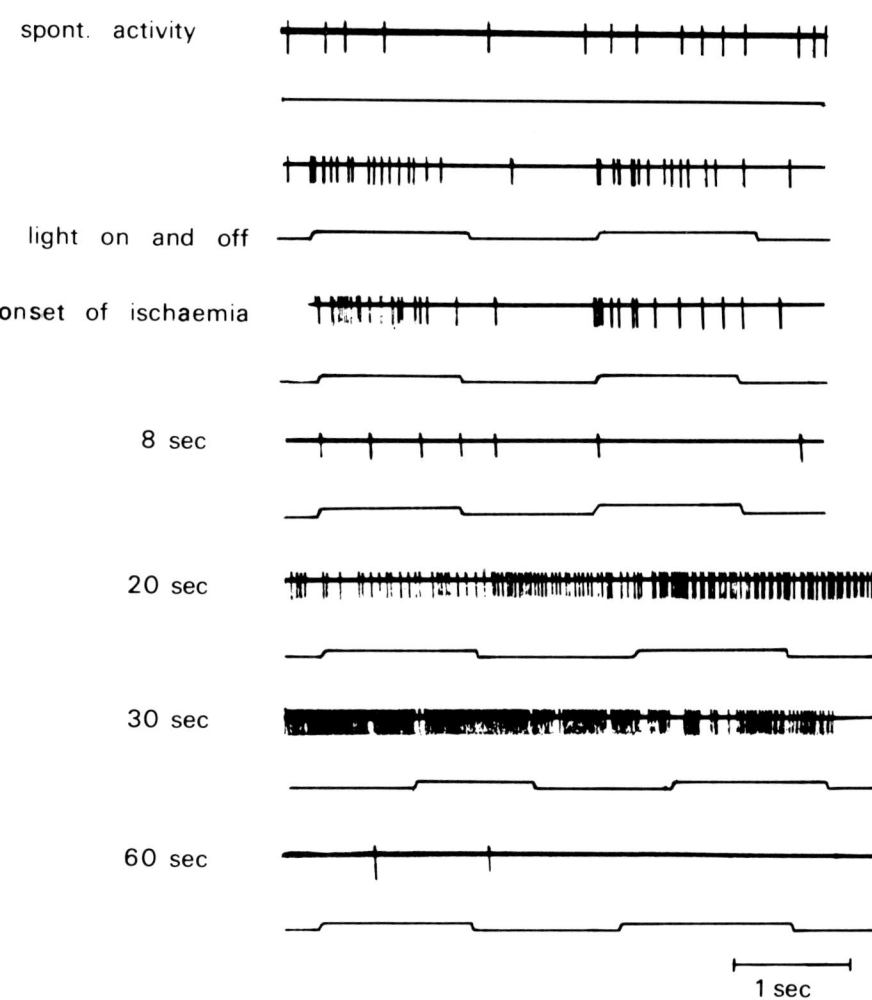

spont. activity

light on and off

onset of ischaemia

8 sec

20 sec

30 sec

60 sec

1 sec

Fig. 8.4 Single neurone response to light and retinal ischaemia recorded in Area 17 from a projecting fibre from the lateral geniculate body.

are arranged to converge on one cortical cell to reproduce the elongated receptive field typical of the simplest form of cortical neurone.

The discovery of cortical cells which respond only to stimulation with line elements and their columnar arrangement has been confirmed in many laboratories since the original description and there are many studies regarding the effects of line patterns in human perception (Campbell & Kulikowski 1966, Gilinsky 1968, 1969, Blakemore & Campbell 1969, and others). The results of these studies suggest a similar organization in the human cortex and support the hypothesis that a lateral inhibition exists between neighbouring cortical neurones with similar detector functions (Blakemore *et al* 1970).

Discussion

If one assumes that migraine attacks begin with a cortical hypoxia of still unknown origin, one has to expect a state of progressively disordered neuronal activity. One can easily understand that in such a condition neuronal responses triggered internally by hypoxia will interfere with neuronal responses triggered by external visual stimuli. This could explain the frequency of uncharacteristic defective vision in the beginning of an attack. Uncontrolled discharges in only a few neurones will probably not reach perceptual threshold, but nevertheless will influence perception. If hypoxia continues, the following hyperactivity of a larger amount of neurones could explain the scintillation phenomena. Since normal connectivity is preserved, one may expect that the increased activation of a functional column could inhibit its neighbouring columns via lateral inhibition and vice versa. The summated result would be a scintillating perception in the visual field. Since this scintillation is often reported as having a grain of small elongated structures, one is tempted to assume that cortical orientation detectors are free running in this condition.

The scintillation phenomena are usually observed covering the entire visual field. Since the neurones of the visual receiving area along the vertical meridian are connected via callosal fibres with the contralateral hemisphere and higher visual areas have massive callosal connections to homologue areas in the other hemisphere, the hyperactivity of visual neurones in one hemisphere will be transmitted to the contralateral side, and therefore produce scintillations in the entire visual field.

In more intensive migraines translucent spots and finally scintillating scotomas develop. Both of these phenomena are predominantly occurring in one half of the visual field, indicating that they are caused by dysfunction in the contralateral hemisphere. The scintillation scotomas again propagate slowly and if they spread from the centre to the visual periphery, a characteristic evolution (Fig. 8.1) is perceived. Lashley (1941) has mapped his own scintillating scotoma in brief intervals. By calculating the approximate cortical distance representing the corresponding points in the visual field, he concluded that the scotoma was spreading across the cortex with 3 mm per minute. Approximately the same value (3·3 mm per minute) was found in another person by Richards (1971). Hare (1966) published personal observations similar to Lashley. The sketch of the scintillating scotoma on Fig. 8.1 is from the late W. S. McCulloch and confirms the other observations and the impressive drawings of fortification spectras by Airy (1870).

Milner (1958) connected Lashley's observation to the spreading depression of Leào and the hyperactivity of cortical neurones at the advancing margin of the depression shown by Grafstein (1956a,b). The corresponding time course of both phenomena and the behaviour of neurones during spreading depression let him propose the possibility that scintillating scotomas in migraines could be the equivalent of a spreading depression triggered in the beginning of a migraine. Since then, spreading depression-like mechanisms as bases of scintillating scotomas were discussed several times (Baumgartner 1962, Basser 1969, Bücking & Baumgartner 1974, Jung 1973).

Until now, the evidence for such a mechanism is only based on the analogue time course and therefore very weak. It was not yet possible to induce spreading depression by hypoxia, and a common factor which would produce hypoxia in migraine and spreading depression as well has not been shown. However, a spread of excitation with following inactivity can be derived from entoptic phenomena.

Daniel and Whitteridge (1961) have presented a study of the representation of the visual field on the cerebral cortex in monkeys. They could demonstrate that the magnification factor, i.e. the linear extent of striate cortex devoted to each degree of visual field, falls off smoothly from the centre to the periphery parallel to the visual acuity. Cowey and Rolls (1974) have measured the magnification factor in patients with implanted stimulating electrodes on the striate cortex, who could map their phosphenes and came to the same conclusion. Daniel and Whitteridge indicated that the minimal angle of resolution is always represented by approximately 65 μm cortex. This would mean that the amount of cortical cells for one discrimination task is constant. The resolution therefore depends on the number of discriminating cells per unit-area of visual field. Correspondingly the size of the receptive fields of peripheral and cortical neurones is increasing towards the periphery. This again permits us to predict that the line elements of the scintillating scotomas have to become larger when they move towards the periphery. At the same time, although the velocity of cortical spread does not change, the perceived velocity of the spread has to accelerate. Richards (1971) has proposed that the zig-zag characteristics of the fortification illusions in scintillating scotomas could be a consequence of the cortical matrix of orientation detectors.

In the line of this reasoning, one could account for the additional symptoms in migraine accompagnée by further spread of the depression from visual to the sensory-motor areas.

Considering the gap between single neurone activity and perception, and especially entoptic phenomena with no possibility of psycho-physical control, such an interpretation may be judged as premature. But since the design of single neurone experiments on the base of psycho-physical data is very rewarding, the inverse way may be permitted, but with the risk of possible total failure.

Summary

The sequence of focal neurological symptoms preceding classic migraine are described. Possible connections between the neuronal activity during hypoxia and spreading depression and the preceding signs are discussed.

References

AIRY G.B. (1870) On a distinct form of transient hemiopsia. *Philos. Trans. roy. Soc.* **160**, 247–64.

BASSER L.S. (1969) The relation of migraine and epilepsy. *Brain* **92**, 285–300.

BAUMGARTNER G. (1962) Zur Klinik und Pathophysiologie der Migräne. *Mediz. Welt (Stuttgart)* **37**, 1915–18.

BAUMGARTNER G., CREUTZFELDT O. & JUNG R. (1961) Microphysiology of cortical neurones in acute anoxia and in retinal ischemia. In: Meyer J.S. & Gastaut H. (Eds) *Cerebral Anoxia and the Electroencephalogram*, pp. 5–34. Charles C. Thomas, Springfield, Illinois.

BLAKEMORE C. & CAMPBELL F.W. (1969) Adaptation to spatial stimuli. *J. Physiol.* **200**, 11–13.

BLAKEMORE C., CARPENTER R.H.S. & GEORGESON M.A. (1970) Lateral inhibition between orientation detectors in the human visual system. *Nature (London)* **228**, 37–9.

BÜCKING H. & BAUMGARTNER G. (1974) Klinik und Pathophysiologie der initialen neurologischen Symptome bei fokalen Migränen. *Arch. Psychiat. Nervenkr.* **219**, 37–52.

CAMPBELL F.W. & KULIKOWSKI J.J. (1966) Orientational selectivity of the human visual system. *J. Physiol.* **187**, 437–45.

COWEY A. & ROLLS E.T. (1974) Cortical magnification factor and its relation to visual acuity. *Exp. Brain Res.* **21**, 447–454.

DANIEL P.M. & WHITTERIDGE D. (1961) The representation of the visual field on the cerebral cortex in monkeys. *J. Physiol.* **159**, 203–21.

GILINSKY A.S. (1968) Orientation specific effects of pattern of adapting light on visual acuity. *J. Opt. Soc. Amer.* **58**, 13–18.

GILINSKY A.S. & DOHERTY R.S. (1969) Interocular transfer of orientational effects. *Science* **164**, 454–5.

GRAFSTEIN B. (1956a) Mechanism of spreading cortical depression. *J. Neurophysiol.* **19**, 154–71.

GRAFSTEIN B. (1956b) Locus of propagation of spreading cortical depression. *J. Neurophysiol.* **19**, 309–16.

HARE E.H. (1966) Personal observations on the spectral marche of migraine. *J. neurol. Sci.* **3**, 259–64.

VAN HARREVELD A. & OCHS S. (1957) Electrical and vascular concomitants of spreading depression. *Amer. J. Physiol.* **189**, 159–66.

HUBEL D. & WIESEL T. (1962) Receptive fields, binocular interaction and functional architecture in the cat's visual cortex. *J. Physiol.* **160**, 106–54.

HUBEL D. & WIESEL T. (1968) Receptive fields and functional architecture of monkey striate cortex. *J. Physiol.* **195**, 215–44.

JUNG R. (1973) Visual Perception and Neurophysiology. In: Jung R. (Ed.) *Handbook of Sensory Physiology*, Vol. VII/3A. Springer, Berlin, Heidelberg, New York.

KOLMODIN G.M. & SKOGLUND C.R. (1959) Influence of asphyxia on membrane potential level and action potentials of spinal moto- and interneurons. *Acta physiol. scand.* **45**, 1–18.

LASHLEY K.S. (1941) Pattern of cerebral integration indicated by scotomas of migraine. *Arch. Neurol. Psychiat.* (Chicago) **46**, 331–9.

LEÀO A.A.P. (1944) Spreading depression of activity in the cerebral cortex. *J. Neurophysiol.* **7**, 391–6.

LEÀO A.A.P. (1947) Further observations on the spreading depression of activity in the cerebral cortex. *J. Neurophysiol.* **10**, 409–14.

MILNER P.M. (1958) Note on a possible correspondence between the scotomas of migraine and spreading depression of Leào. *EEG & clin. Neurophysiol.* **10**, 705.

MORLOCK N.L., MORI K. & WARD A.A. Jr. (1964) A study of single cortical neurons during spreading depression. *J. Neurophysiol.* **27**, 1192–8.

MOUNTCASTLE V.B. (1957) Modality and topographic properties of single neurons of cat's somatic sensory cortex. *J. Neurophysiol.* **20**, 408–34.

OCHS S. (1962) The nature of spreading depression in neuronal networks. *International Review of Neurobiology* New York, London **4**, 2–65.

RICHARDS W. (1971) The fortification illusions of migraines. *Sci. Amer.* **224**, 89–96.

SHORT- AND LONG-TERM STABILITY OF CORTICAL ELECTRICAL PHOSPHENES

D. N. RUSHTON AND G. S. BRINDLEY

A useful visual prosthesis depending on electrical stimulation of the occipital cortex will be possible only if the positions of cortical electrical phosphenes in the visual field are to some extent stable; and the more stable they are, the better.

The blind patient who received the second visual prosthetic implant (Brindley *et al* 1972, Donaldson 1973, Brindley & Rushton 1974) has been intensively tested on nine 'visits' between November 1972 and November 1975. Each 'visit' lasted about a week, and testing occupied about 5 or 6 hours on each day of that week. The present paper will consider the degree of stability of mapping revealed by this testing.

Full maps

Part of each visit was used to make a full map of all the phosphenes then obtainable. The nine maps are shown in Figs. 9.1–9.9 and the layout of the cortical electrodes in Fig. 9.10. The number of phosphenes plotted decreases from map to map because of failures in the extracranial part of the implant.

To make a map, the position of each posphene was fixed by observing its relation to several of its neighbours, and the overall scale and shape of the map was established by making observations between phosphenes in different quadrants. The size and shape of each phosphene is given as described by the subject, and the maps take account of supplementary observations as to whether particular phosphenes touch or overlap each other. Full maps take a day or more to make, and even then it is not practicable to check the relation of every phosphene with every other that is near to it; the relations actually observed will vary from one map to another.

The possibility of making maps and the general agreement between the maps for different visits show that the positions of phosphenes in the visual field are to some extent stable. The differences of detail between maps suggest that the stability is not absolute; they do not prove instability, because they could perhaps be due to errors of mapping. To examine this question further,

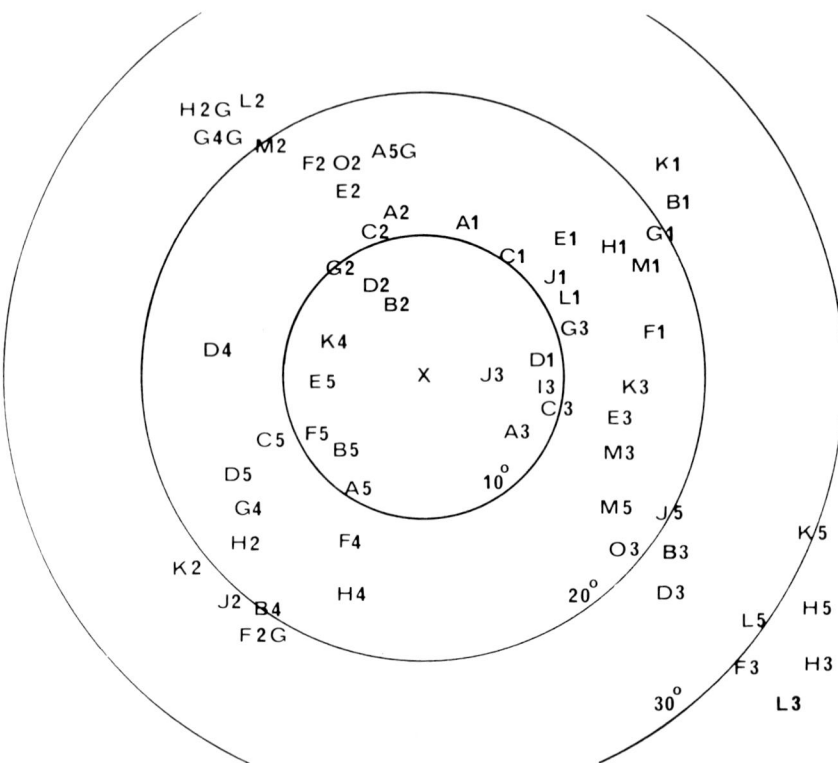

Fig. 9.1 Map of phosphenes made in November 1972. The shapes of the phosphenes on this visit were not carefully recorded, and are not shown. High threshold second phosphenes ('ghosts') are labelled with the suffix G. All maps are shown as seen by the subject, and not as would be plotted to confrontation.

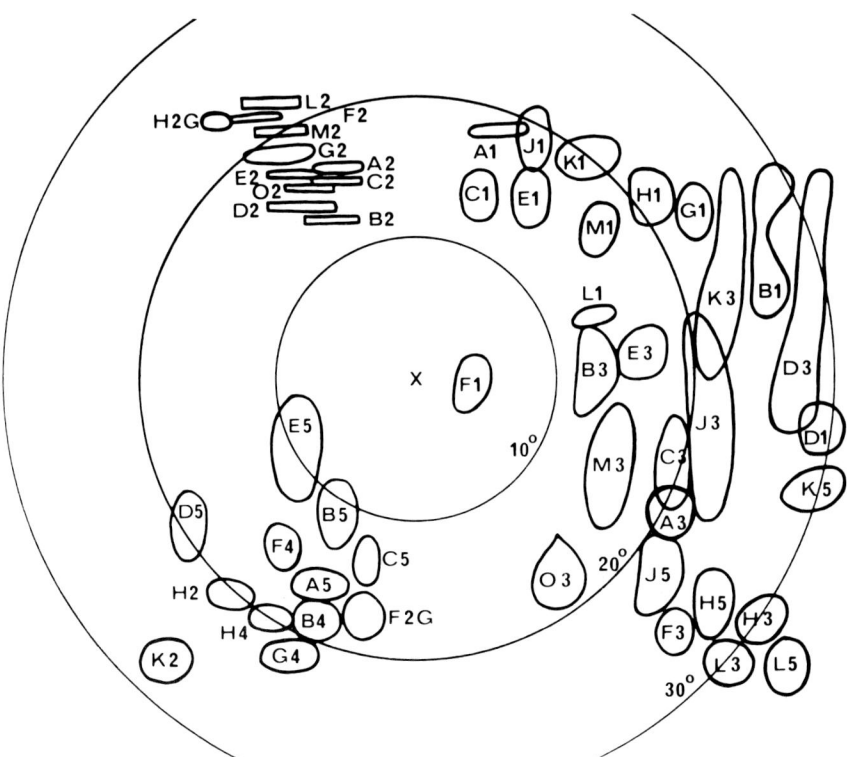

Fig. 9.2   Map of phosphenes made in February 1973. Outlines roughly indicate the size and shape of phosphenes, but many have indistinct edges, and all become larger with strong stimulation.

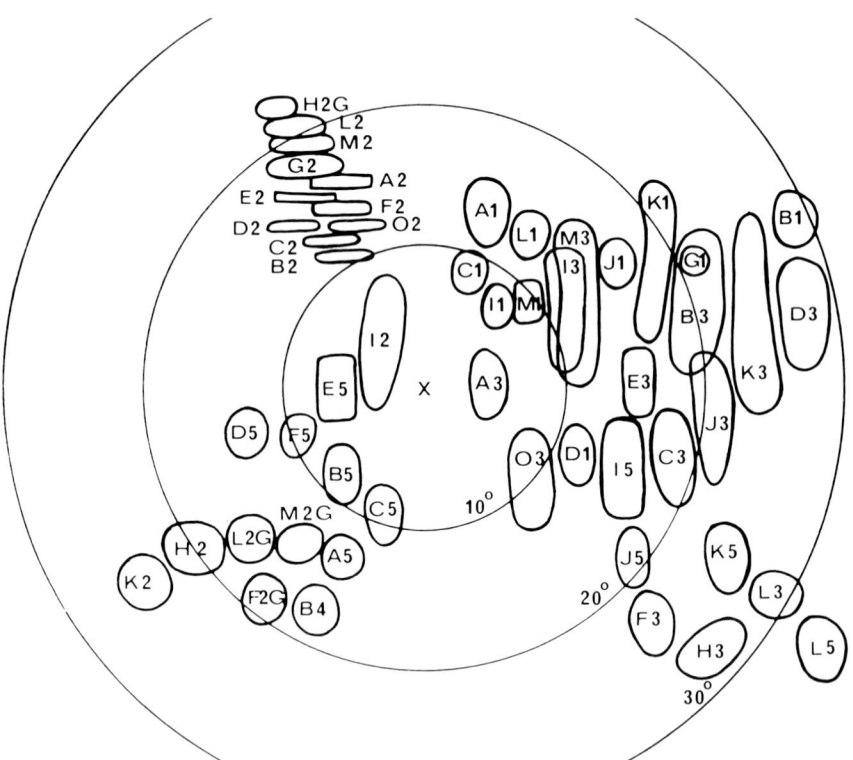

Fig. 9.3   Map of phosphenes made in May 1973.

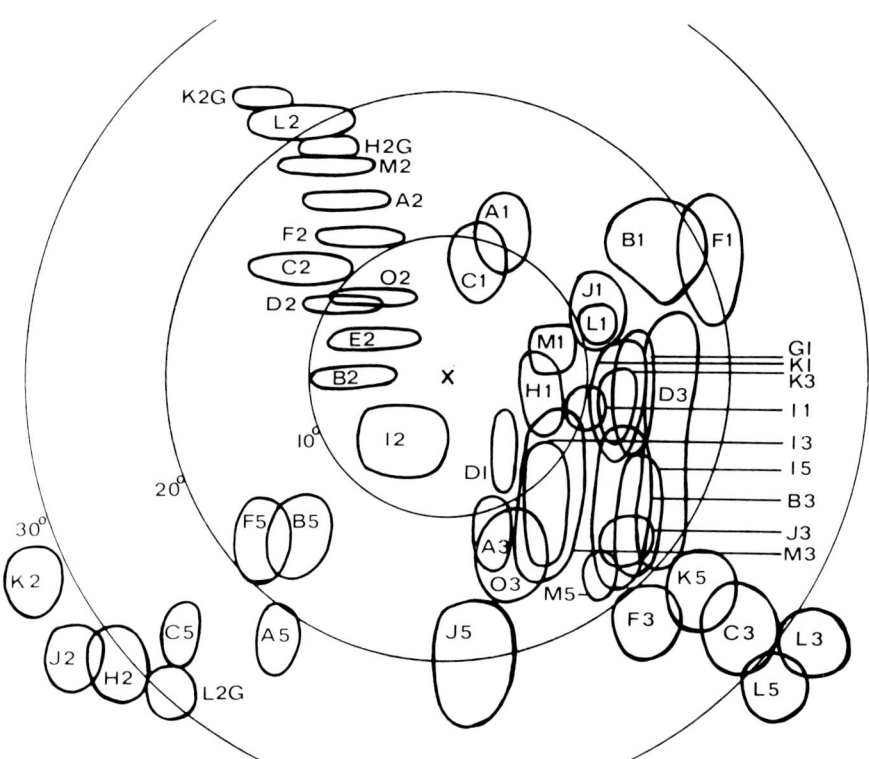

Fig. 9.4   Map of phosphenes made in September 1973.

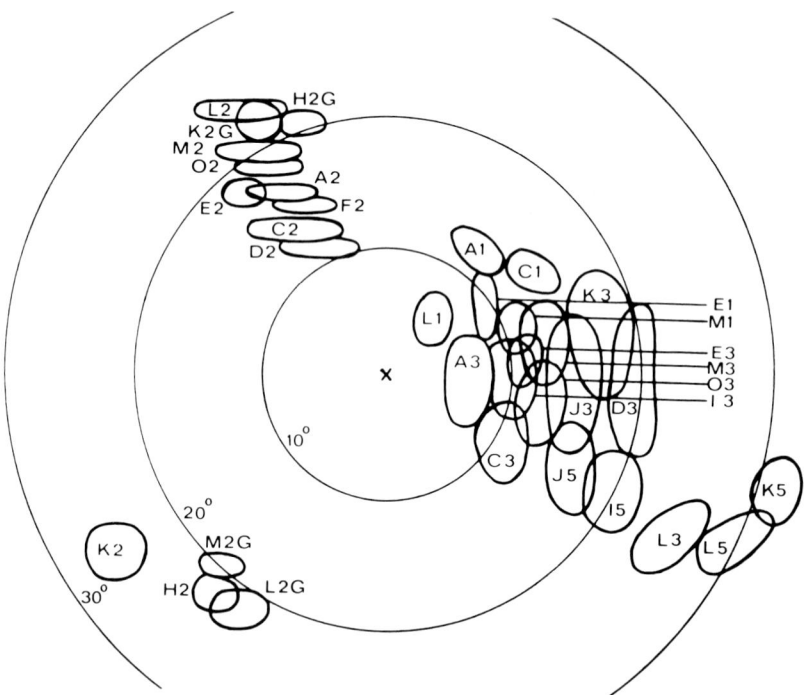

Fig. 9.5   Map of phosphenes made in January 1974.

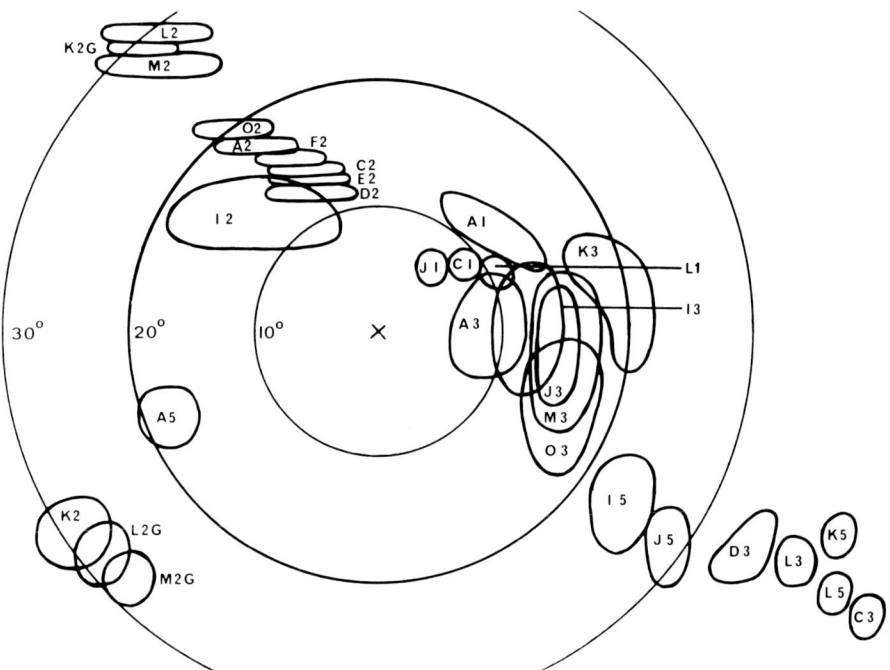

Fig. 9.6 Map of phosphenes made in June 1974.

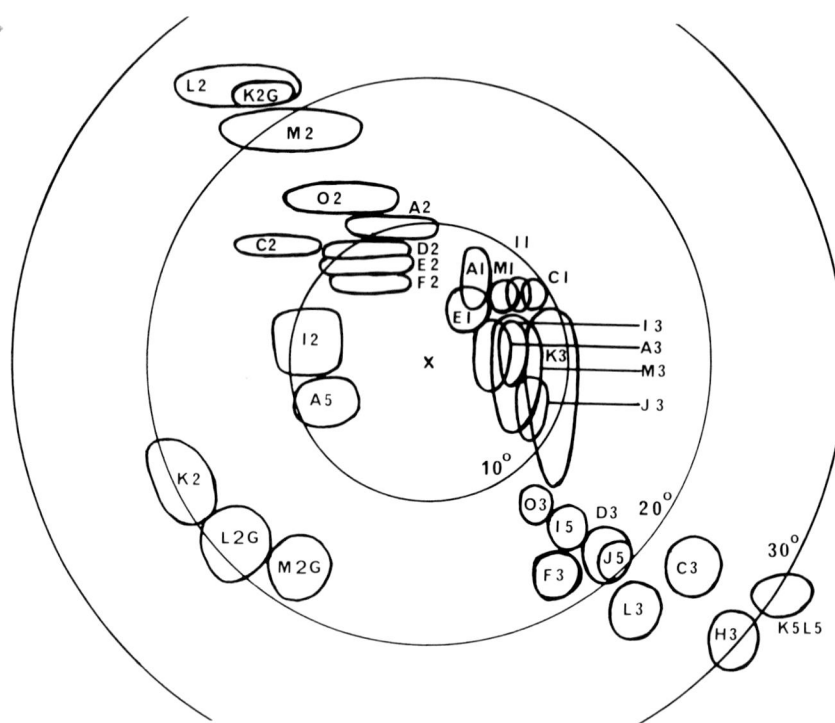

Fig. 9.7 Map of phosphenes made in November 1974.

During this visit, K5 and L5 did not give a phosphene singly, but did when stimulated together.

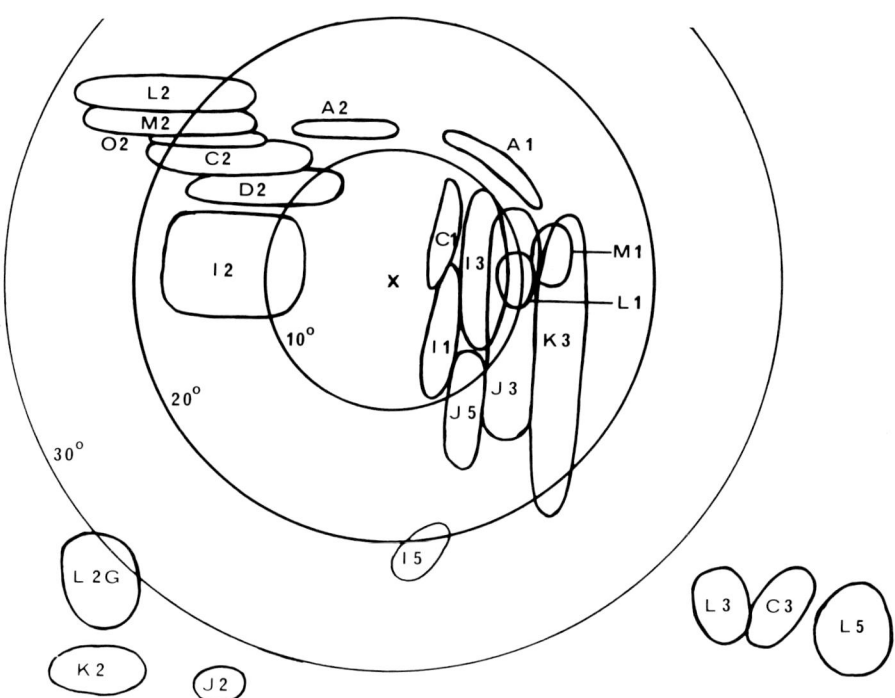

Fig. 9.8 Map of phosphenes made in May 1975.

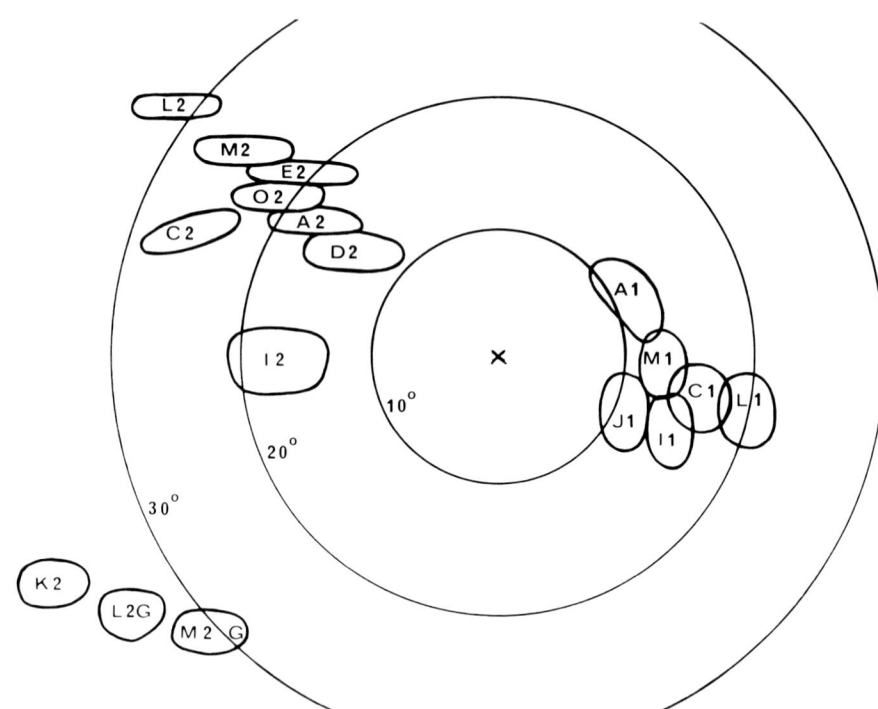

Fig. 9.9   Map of phosphenes made in November 1975.

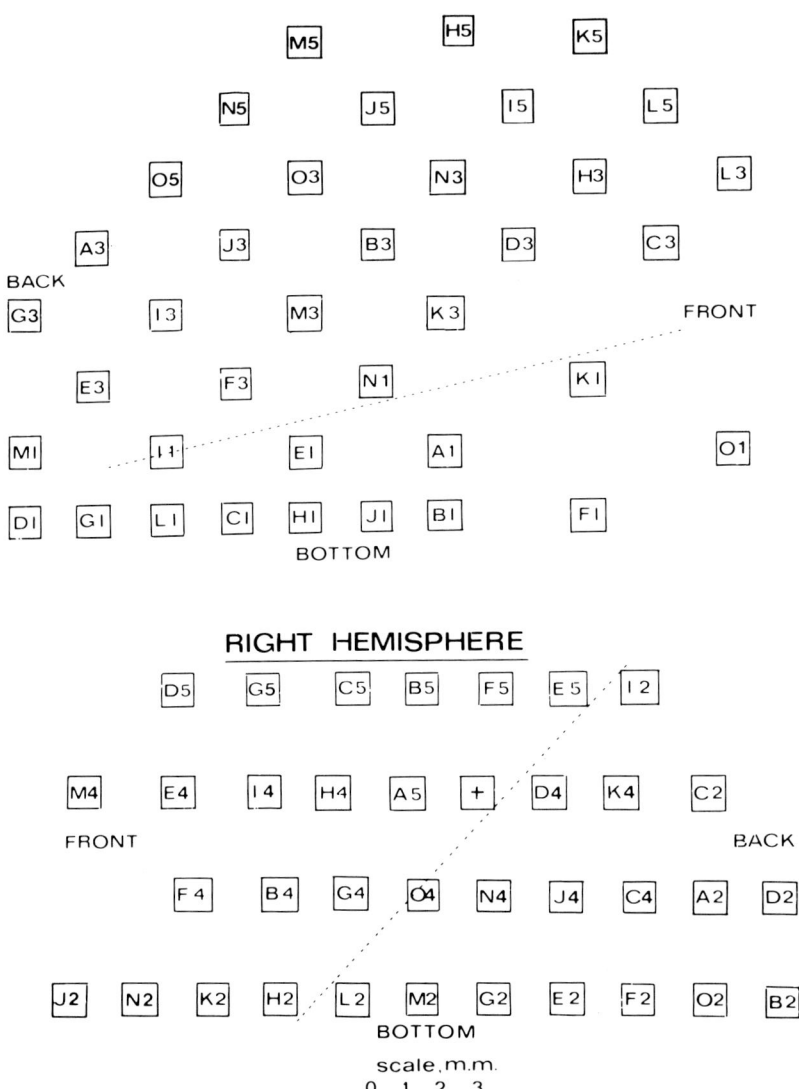

Fig. 9.10 Diagram of arrays of electrodes in contact with medial surfaces and occipital poles of the hemispheres.

we decided to make repeated observations of certain features of the map, and compare the changes over different time intervals. We took a limited set of phosphene pairs ('standard observations'), and repeated observations of their relative position at intervals of minutes, hours, days and months in order to discover the contributions made to changes in the map by real movement of phosphenes, and by the various kinds of error.

Standard observations

In making standard observations, as in making observations in the construction of a full map, the following technique is used. Phosphene A is presented, and is followed after an interval of less than a second by phosphene B. The subject gives the direction and distance of the centre of B from the centre of A. The direction is given as minutes past the hour, 0–59, treating phosphene A as if at the centre of a clock face. The distance is given in inches and fractions of an inch, as would be measured with a ruler at the distance at which the phosphenes are seen. This distance is not always constant, and the effects of changes in it are discussed later.

Standard observations are often made in groups of three, in the form:

> Phosphene A→Phosphene B
> Phosphene B→Phosphene C
> Phosphene C→Phosphene A.

Such a group of three forms a triangle, and a triangle of observations is self checking in that its failure to close gives an estimate of changes or errors operating in the few seconds required to make the observations.

Several such observations are made in a few minutes, and the whole set is then repeated. Pairs of sets of observations are made, up to three times in a day, at intervals of approximately two hours. These observations are repeated daily during a visit by the subject, which usually lasts for about a week, and is repeated every 3–6 months.

Standard observations have been made in nine visits, between November 1972 and November 1975, so that clusters of observations separated by minutes, hours, days and months are available. Short- and longer-term clusters can be compared to discover the time course of any changes in the observed relations of the selected phosphenes. The means and confidence of the means of the positions of phosphenes in clusters of observations can be calculated in order to determine which changes are significant.

Owing to the failure of certain radio receivers in the implant, few of the original standard pairs of phosphenes survived the nine visits. When one phosphene of a triangle failed, a neighbouring phosphene was, where possible, recruited to replace it.

Possible sources of error and variation in mapping and standard observations

Possible sources of difference between maps were listed by Brindley and Rushton (1974), but no attempt was there made to assess the contributions made by real changes in the map, and by errors of different kinds.

Table 9.1 (p. 149) lists some possible sources of internal inconsistency within the observations that comprise a standard triangle, and of differences between successive observations of the same phosphene pairs. The expected character of each kind of variation is given on the right in Table 9.1. The problem is to distinguish real changes in the phosphene map from the other causes of variation. Any real changes in the map are likely to be random, if the map is viewed for a sufficiently long time; phosphenes are unlikely to move in regular paths. Changes may seem, when the map is observed for a shorter time, to be sudden or progressive, or random, depending on the time scale over which they become random. Those changes that occur in a time less than that taken in observing a triangle will give rise to internal inconsistency within that triangle, which will fail to close.

Medium-term changes that are too slow to interfere with the making of a triangle of observations, but are rapid enough to appear random on successive visits (or some shorter interval), will be observed as sources of additional variance occurring over that time interval.

Changes that occur more slowly than the time between visits ('Long-term changes') will appear to be systematic with time, and will be observed as a significant difference between the mean observed relations for successive visits.

Range of data

Twenty-five phosphenes were used in those 42 pairs which survived for standard observations through more than one visit. Many of these pairs were assembled into the triangles discussed above.

Table 9.2 gives, as an example, the 82 observations of the pair C2-L2 made during visits 4 to 8 inclusive.

Table 9.3 shows, for the 7 longest-observed pairs, the overall frequency of observation of different angular relations. Several of the close pairs show a double maximum, either at 20 and 25, or at 50 and 55. The two maxima are scattered throughout all visits, and probably represent a tendency for our subject to give round numbers for the angular relation between phosphenes that are near to each other, rather than being caused by the movement of a phosphene between two alternative positions.

Observed errors and variations in standard observations

A. Internal inconsistency within a triangle of observations

Those sources of variation that act rapidly, during the course of an observation, will cause failure of closure of the triangle of observations in which it occurs. Causes of triangle closure failure can be subdivided into those in which the inconsistency is expected to be repeatable (3b, 4, 5 and 6 in Table 9.1), and those in which the inconsistency is expected to occur at random (1d, 3a and 7 in Table 9.1).

Some of these sources of variation are much more likely than others. Our subject is sure that phosphenes very seldom move during the time required to make an observation (1d) and that a phosphene does not affect the position of a phosphene subsequently given (6). On the other hand, he is aware that seeing a phosphene tends to provoke eye movements directed towards it, and hence to alter the position, on a fixed frame of reference, of a phosphene subsequently given (3). He is also aware that he tends to underestimate large separations in comparison with small ones (5), and that large differences between the apparent distances of two phosphenes from the eye makes estimation of their angular separation difficult (4).

The size and direction of the error by which a triangle of observations fails to close can be represented by a vector, as in Fig. 9.11a, and Fig. 9.11b gives the collection of error vectors obtained in the 82 observations of the longest-observed triangle (L2-D2-C2) through 5 (visits 4–8).

It can be seen that there is a strong tendency towards consistency in the

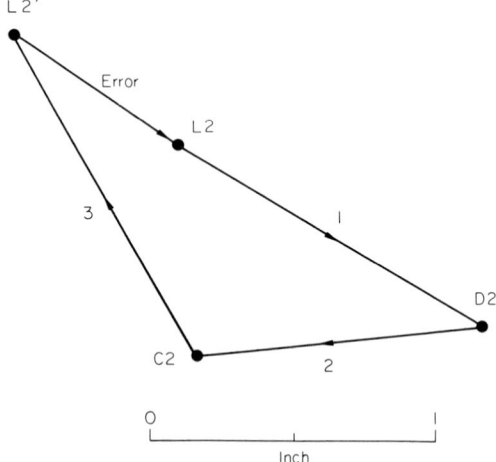

Fig. 9.11a   Closure error vector for one observation of the triangle L2–D2–C2. The observations were made in the order shown, from L2 to L2′.

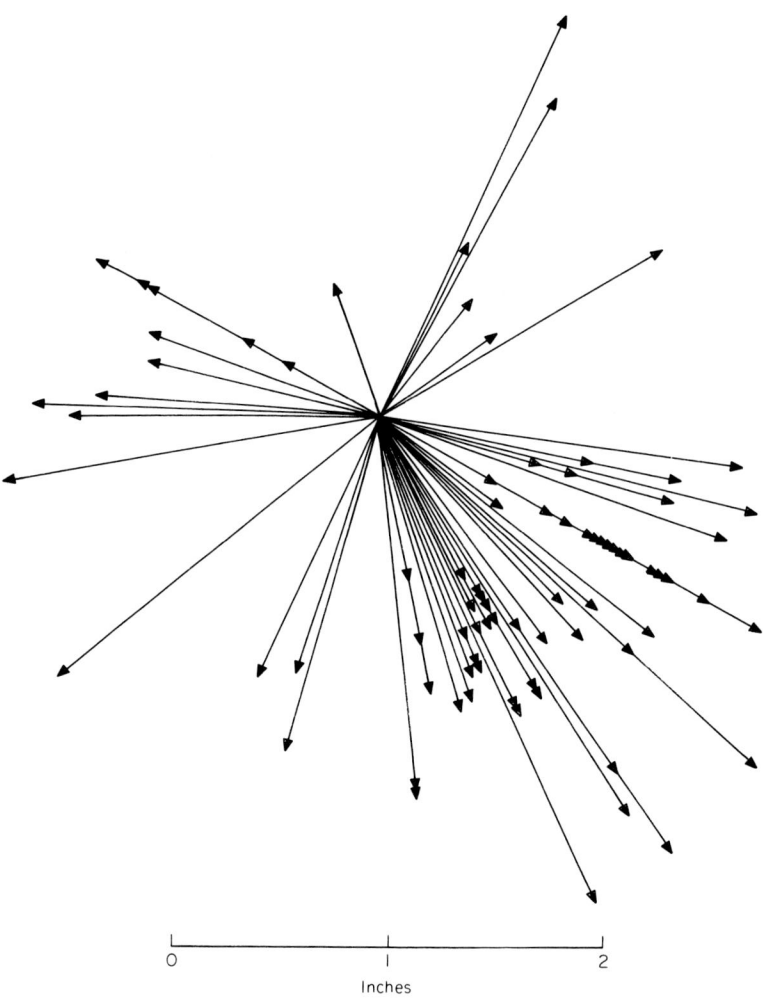

Fig. 9.11b Collection of triangle closure error vectors for the 82 observations of the triangle L2–D2–C2 during visits 4–8. Each arrow head represents the end of one vector.

direction of the error vectors. They tend to lie in the direction of the longest side of the triangle of observations, suggesting either that the underestimation of longer distances is an important source of error in this instance, or that the most peripheral phosphene (L2) has an increased tendency to provoke eye movements towards itself; or both of these.

B. Medium-term variation of standard observations

Phosphenes might move at random about a mean position, in a time much less than the time between visits. The mean position during a visit would then be unaffected by such movements. The movements could not be large, or they would be detectable as changes in the observed relation from hour to hour, or day to day; but if small they would remain undetected, because too few observations are made in a short time interval for an accurate mean.

Certain phosphenes are particularly likely to *appear* to move in this fashion. The large vertical phosphenes in the right-half field tend to vary from day to day in their shape, and in which part of their area is brightest and appears at lowest current threshold. We ask our subject to make his standard observations between the 'centres of gravity' of two phosphenes, and a change in the shape or distribution of brightness in a phosphene will change his estimate of its 'centre of gravity'.

This kind of random variation is potentially detectable by examining the data for sources of extra variance between observations separated by longer time intervals. However, even where such extra variance is found, it remains possible that the better agreement over short intervals is due to our subject's recollection of the figures he gave for his previous observation. The reason for this is that, although we do not tell our subject which of his standard observations is to be presented next, his phosphenes are so familiar to him that he can nevertheless often recognize them. This is likely to be the explanation for any extra variance added by an interval of hours.

Table 9.4 shows, for the seven longest-observed phosphene pairs, which time intervals were sources of significant extra variance. Extra variance introduced merely by changes in separation and not angle is marked by a letter D, and may represent changes in the scale of the map. Changes in the scale of the map are likely in themselves to cause changes in the direction of observations involving K2 and perhaps other low phosphenes, for reasons that are discussed later. After these exceptions are allowed for, the two long-observed pairs that show extra variance over days or months both include C2 (C2-L2 and D2-C2).

C. Long-term variation of standard observations

Long-term variation in a standard observation pair will be seen to have occurred when a consistently obtained relation gives place to a different relation that is also consistent, or when a significant progressive change occurs. In Table 9.1, hypotheses (1a), (1b), (2) and (8) are expected to give changes of this character. The effects of (8) are discussed later. In (1) the phosphenes may move singly, while in (2) all the phosphenes would be expected to move, although not equally, owing to variations in the cortical magnification factor (Daniel & Whitteridge, 1961).

We do not believe that such movement of the electrode array over the cortex ever actually occurred, after the first few days, because the electrode array would be expected to have become encapsulated by secondary dura (Brindley & Lewin 1968, Craggs & Rushton 1976). There has been no visible shift of the electrode arrays on X-rays taken during the 4 years since implantation.

Visit means

We looked for long-term changes by calculating the mean angle and separation between each standard pair for each visit. Table 9.5 gives the means for the seven longest-observed phosphene pairs, and the number of observations on which each mean is based. In order to determine whether the changes are significant, we calculated, for each visit mean, the size and shape of the ellipse of 95% confidence in the mean position of the second phosphene of each pair, arbitrarily taking the position of the first as being fixed. The ellipses were calculated on the assumption of bivariate normality of the observations. The overlap of the 95% confident ellipses around the visit means is given for the seven long-observed pairs in Fig. 9.12, a–g.

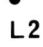

L2

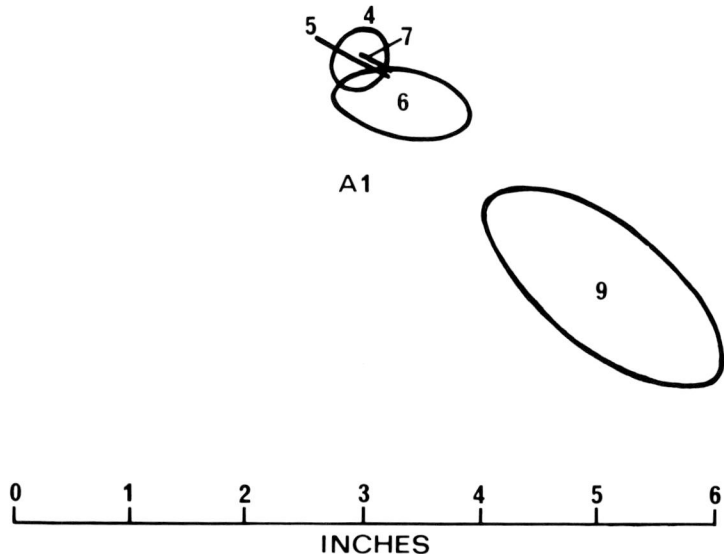

Fig. 9.12a Ellipses of 95% confidence in the mean relation L2–A1, for each of visits 4, 5, 6, 7 and 9. L2 is arbitrarily taken as fixed for this purpose, but turning the figure upside down shows the result where A1 is taken as fixed. For visits 5 and 7, the ellipse is of zero width, since the observed angle was unvaried throughout these visits.

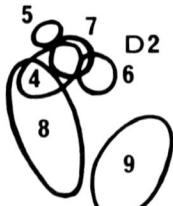

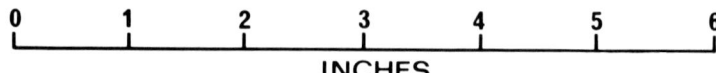

INCHES

Fig. 9.12b Ellipses of 95% confidence in the mean relation L2–D2, for each of visits 4, 5, 6, 7, 8 and 9.

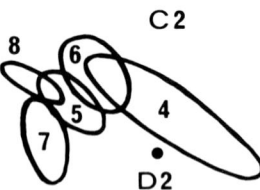

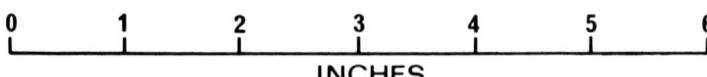

INCHES

Fig. 9.12c Ellipses of 95% confidence in the mean relation D2–C2, for each of visits 4, 5, 6, 7 and 8.

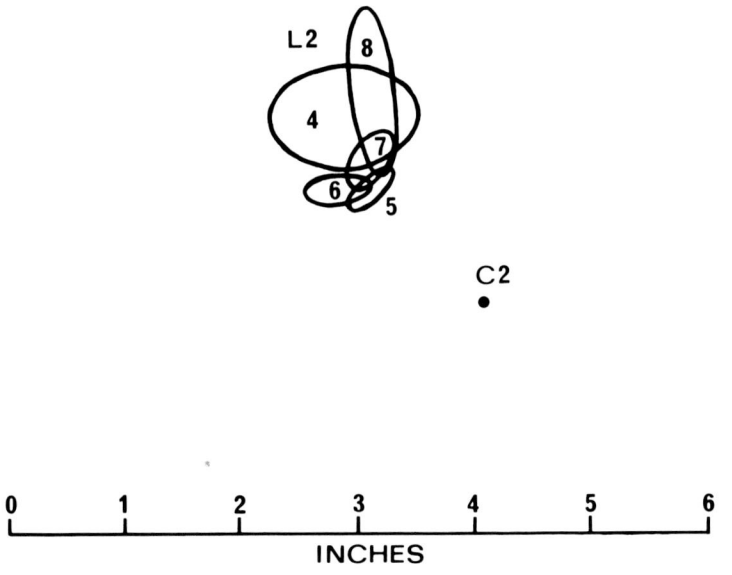

Fig. 9.12d Ellipses of 95% confidence in the mean relation C2–L2, for each of visits 4, 5, 6, 7 and 8.

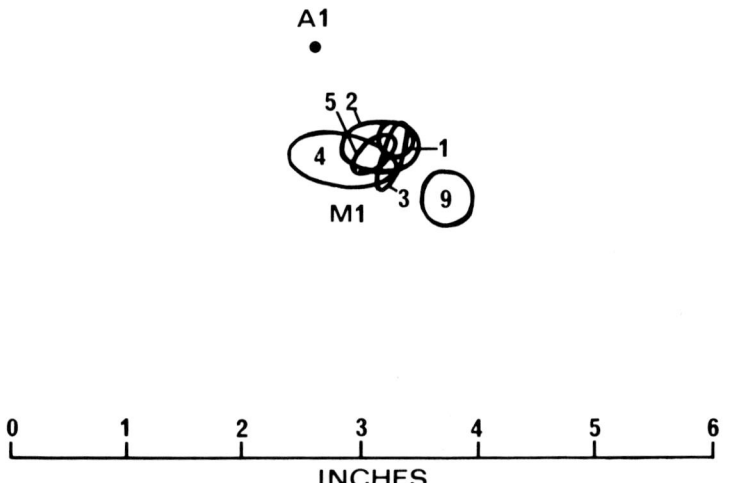

Fig. 9.12e Ellipses of 95% confidence in the mean relation A1–M2, for each of visits 1, 2, 3, 4, 5 and 9.

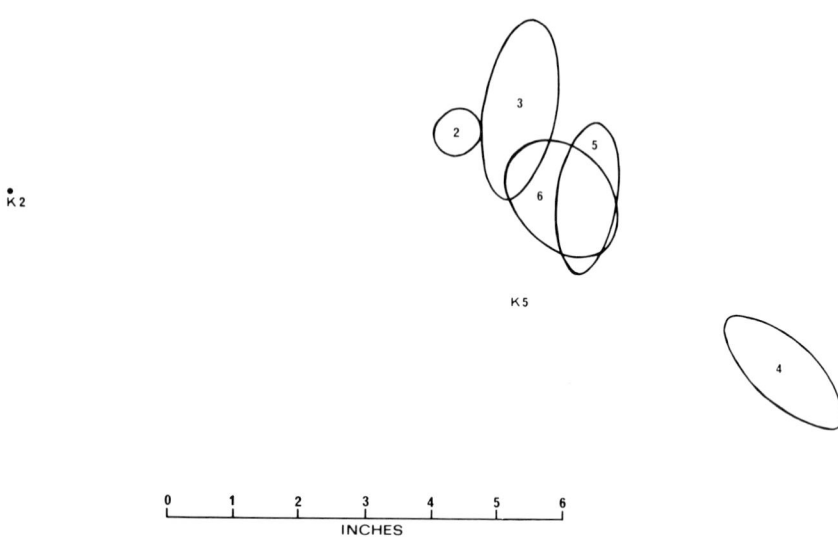

Fig. 9.12f Ellipses of 95% confidence in the mean relation K2–K5, for each of visits 2, 3, 4, 5 and 6. There were insufficient observations in visit 1 to calculate the confidence of the mean value.

We expected observations of angle to be more reliable than observations of separation, both within and between visits. We therefore expected that visit mean ellipses would in general have their long axes along a line joining the two phosphenes, and that the various visit mean ellipses would be spread out mainly along the same line. Both of these expectations were fulfilled in the case of L2-A1, and the latter for L2-D2 and A1-M1.

Visit means for C2-L2, A1-M1 and L2-D2 were very consistent. D2-C2 is the only short-distance pair that appears unstable, the mean for visit 4 being different from that for later visits. As may be judged from the size of the ellipse for visit 4, its observations were then highly variable (and rather few). A suspicion that D2-C2 may have changed is compatible with their rather variable relation on the full maps, and with the analysis shown in Table 9.4.

The three long-distance observations L2-A1, K2-K5, K2-L2, all varied significantly, the first in separation only, and the others in both angle and separation. The variation in direction of observations involving K2 is probably attributable to the great and variable difference between the distance of K2 from the eye and the distances of the other phosphenes.

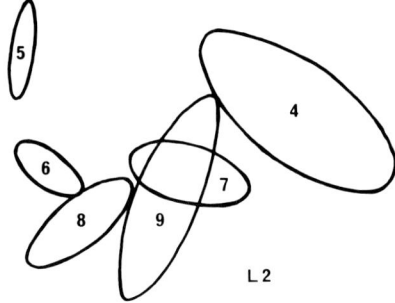

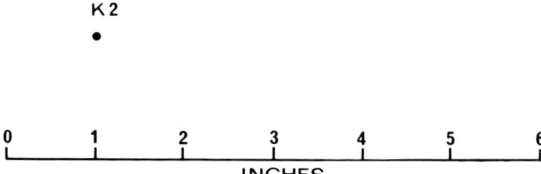

Fig. 9.12g Ellipses of 95% confidence in the mean relation K2–L2 for each of visits 4, 5, 6, 7, 8 and 9.

Variations in the scale of the map and the apparent distance of phosphenes

A tendency for visit means to vary more in separation than in angle has been noted above. If this variation is caused by changes in the overall scale of the map (which would be most plausibly explained by changes in the apparent distance of the phosphenes from the observer), then all phosphene separations should vary in proportion. This is not always the case, as is shown by Table 9.5, which gives the mean separation for each visit for each of the seven longest-observed phosphene pairs. Although there is a tendency for the separations to increase in later visits, this does not apply to all phosphene pairs.

The explanation for this may be that our subject does not see all phosphenes as being at the same distance, or as varying in distance in the same way. In particular, the lowest phosphenes are seen as being much closer than the higher phosphenes. This is shown in Fig. 9.13 for the most recent

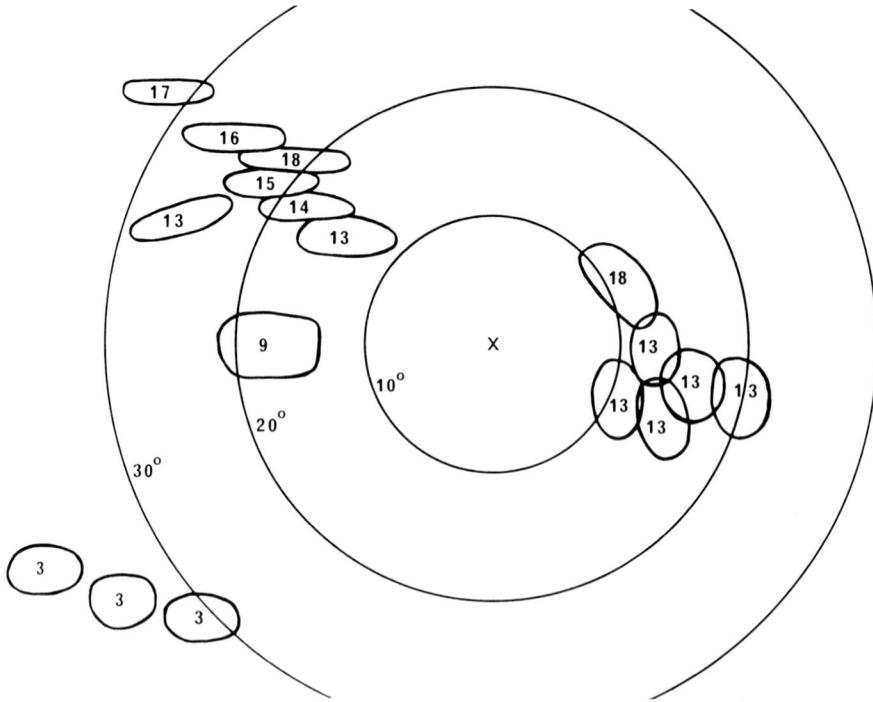

Fig. 9.13 Map of phosphenes made in November 1975. The identity of the phosphenes is as given in Fig. 9.9, but they are labelled with their stated apparent distance from the eye in inches, as observed by the subject.

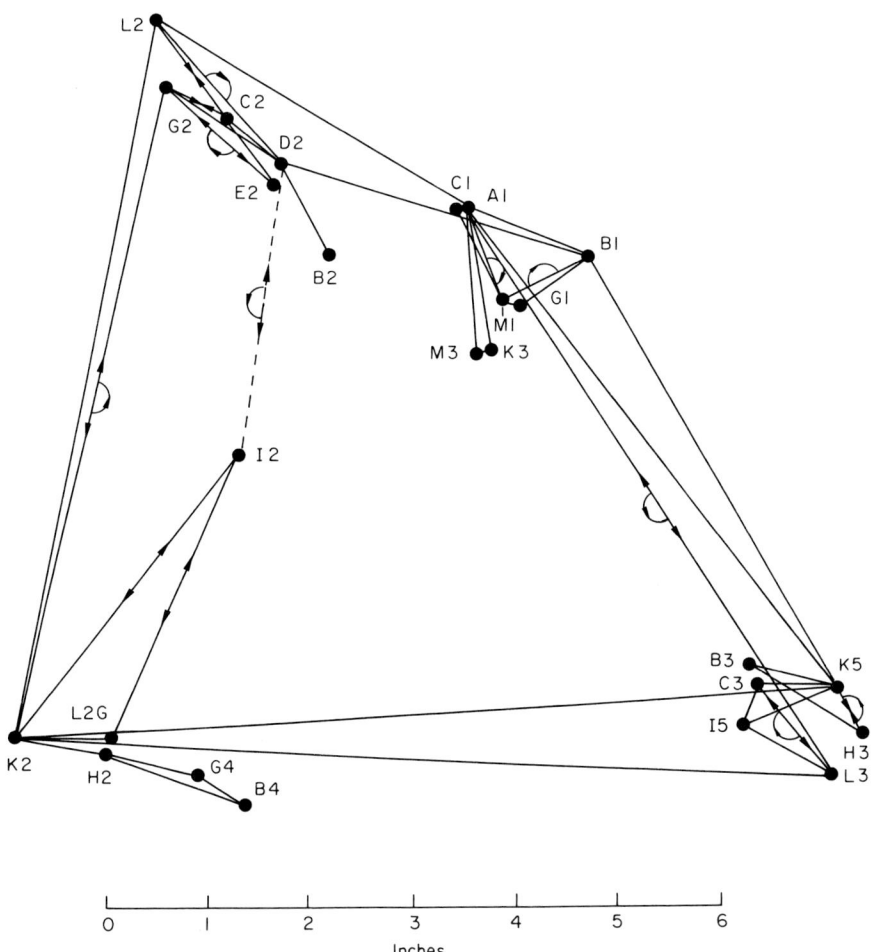

Fig. 9.14 Map obtained by triangulation of the mean relations of those 42 standard observation pairs (25 phosphenes) that were observed many times during more than one visit. Distortion introduced in the fitting, of more than 10° (in angle) or more than 10% (in separation), is shown for the relations in which it was necessary.

⟳ indicates that the angle had to be changed in a clockwise direction, in order to fit; and vice versa.

⋮ indicates that the separation had to be reduced, in order to fit; and vice versa.

The relation D2–I2, which was never a standard observation, but which has been observed on 11 occasions, is dotted in, since it fills an important gap in the skeleton map.

map (November 1975, visit 9), which is the only visit in which the distances of phosphenes from the eye were carefully recorded.

Compatibility between the means for the different standard observations

If the phosphene map is considered to be stable, subject to the exceptions discussed above, then it is permissible to calculate a grand mean for all observations of each standard pair. These pairs can then be fitted together into a many-times observed skeleton of a map. The random, but not the systematic, causes of error listed in Table 9.1 will be reduced in this way, and the goodness of fit of the parts of the skeleton will give an indication of the size of the systematic causes of error.

The result of this procedure applied to those 42 standard pairs (25 phosphenes) that were observed during more than one visit is shown in Fig. 9.14. Certain distortions of angle and separation had to be introduced, in order to make the skeleton fit together into a two dimensional map. Where the distortions were larger than a 10° angle or 10% of separation, the way in which they had to be distorted is shown.

Conclusion

Most of our subject's phosphenes have remained in the same part of the field throughout the time that we have studied them. The main exception to this general statement is K2, which moved from a very high to a very low position in the left field during the last week of February 1972, three weeks after implantation. A high threshold second phosphene remained in the original position, and it seems likely that the change was due to a slight early shift of the electrode array, which happened to move the electrode K2 from the lower to the upper lip of the calcarine fissure.

Certain phosphenes seem to be unstable, and to move about at random within a small area. Of the 42 phosphene pairs that were repeatedly observed over more than one visit, ten showed a signficant extra variation in direction that was added by an interval of days, while two of these, and nine others, showed a significant extra variation in direction that was added by an interval of months.

Although significant, none of these changes was very great, and the largest of them are included in the longest-observed pairs shown in Fig. 9.12, and Tables 9.4 and 9.5.

Twenty-three pairs gave no significant extra variation of direction with intervals of days or months, when compared with shorter intervals, and were, as far as we could tell, perfectly stable.

Acknowledgments

We are grateful to our subject, F.R.B., for his patient cooperation and careful observations throughout many hundreds of hours of testing; and to D. G. Clayton for statistical advice and for performing the bivariate analyses.

Table 9.1 Left column lists some possible causes of differences between successive observations of a triangle of cortical phosphenes, and of internal inconsistencies within such triangles of observations. On the right are shown the expected features of the change or inconsistency

Source of difference between maps	Expected result in Standard observations
1. Real changes in the map	
a. Slow, progressive (long term)	Systematic drifts in observed relation
b. Rare, sudden (long term)	Stepwise changes in observed relation
c. Random (medium term)	Random variation in observed relation
d. Random (short term)	Random failure of triangle closure
2. Movement of electrode array	Systematic change affecting all phosphenes
3. Eye movements	
a. Random	Random failure of triangle closure
b. Phosphene-provoked	Systematic failure of triangle closure
4. Phosphenes appearing to be at different distances from the eye	Systematic failure of triangle closure
5. Errors of judgement of small as against large separations	Systematic failure of triangle closure, where the sides of triangles are unequal
6. Phosphene A affecting the subsequent position of Phosphene B	Systematic failure of triangle closure
7. Random errors of judgement of angle or separation	Random variation of observed relations, and random failure of triangle closure
8. Changes in the apparent distance of phosphenes from the eye	Change in the observed separation of phosphene pairs, without necessarily any change in their angular relationship

Table 9.2 The table lists all 82 observations of the standard pair C2-L2, made during visits 4–8. Observations separated by minutes are placed together, and intervals of hours are represented by a space

	Visit				
Day	4	5	6	7	8
1	53′, 2″	55′, $1\frac{1}{4}$″	50′, $1\frac{1}{4}$	55′, 2″	55′, 1″
	55′, $1\frac{3}{4}$″	57′, $1\frac{1}{2}$″	50′, $1\frac{1}{2}$″	52′, 2″	55′, $1\frac{1}{2}$″
	50′, 1″	55′, $1\frac{1}{2}$″			50′, $1\frac{1}{2}$″
	59′, 2″	58′, $1\frac{1}{2}$″			53′, $1\frac{1}{2}$″
2	55′, $1\frac{1}{2}$″	50′, $1\frac{1}{2}$″	50′, $1\frac{1}{2}$″	50′, $2\frac{1}{4}$″	53′, $1\frac{3}{4}$″
	50′, 2″	50′, 2″	55′, $1\frac{1}{4}$″	55′, $1\frac{1}{4}$	55′, 2″
	50′, 3″	55′, $1\frac{1}{2}$″	50′, $1\frac{1}{2}$″	55′, 2″	
	55′, 3″	50′, $1\frac{1}{2}$″	50′, $1\frac{1}{2}$″	58′, $1\frac{1}{4}$″	
3		55′, $1\frac{1}{2}$″	53′, $1\frac{1}{2}$″	57′, 2″	55′, $2\frac{1}{2}$″
		50′, $1\frac{1}{2}$″	55′, $1\frac{1}{2}$″	55′, $1\frac{3}{4}$″	
		50′, $1\frac{1}{2}$″	50′, $1\frac{3}{4}$″		
		55′, $1\frac{1}{2}$″	55′, $1\frac{1}{4}$″		
		50′, $1\frac{1}{4}$″	50′, $1\frac{1}{2}$″		
			50′, 2″		
4		53′, $1\frac{1}{2}$″	55′, 2″	55′, $1\frac{3}{4}$″	55′, $1\frac{1}{4}$″
		50′, $1\frac{1}{2}$″	50′, 2″	55′, $1\frac{3}{4}$″	56′, 3″
		50″, $1\frac{1}{4}$″	50′ $2\frac{1}{2}$″	50′, $1\frac{1}{4}$	57′, $3\frac{1}{2}$″
		50′, $1\frac{1}{2}$″	55′, $1\frac{1}{2}$″	55′, $1\frac{3}{4}$″	57′, $3\frac{1}{2}$″
			59′, $1\frac{1}{4}$″	50′, $1\frac{1}{2}$″	
			53′, $1\frac{3}{4}$″	55′, $1\frac{3}{4}$	
5		53′, $1\frac{1}{2}$″	50′, $1\frac{1}{2}$″	50′, $1\frac{3}{4}$″	
		50′, $1\frac{1}{2}$″	50′, $1\frac{1}{2}$″	55′, $1\frac{3}{4}$″	
				50′, $1\frac{3}{4}$″	
				55′, $1\frac{3}{4}$″	
6			50′, $1\frac{1}{2}$″		
			50′, 2″		
			50′, 2″		
			50′, $2\frac{1}{2}$″		
			50′, $2\frac{1}{2}$″		
			50′, $2\frac{1}{4}$″		

Table 9.3 The table shows the overall frequency of observation of different angular relations, for the seven longest-observed standard phosphene pairs. The angle is shown in minutes past the hour, as observed by the subject, treating the first phosphene of each pair as if at the centre of a clock face, and the second as at the edge

Minutes	L2–A1	L2–D2	D2–C2	C2–L2	A1–M1	K2–K5	K2–L2
00							1
01							39
02							19
03			1				24
04							4
05							16
07							1
08							1
10						4	
12						7	
13						25	
14					3	16	
15						2	
16			1			9	
17			1			14	
18					1	4	
20	89	68	5		24		
21					1		
22					3		
23		14			11		
24					2		
25	6	17	1		29		
26		1			4		
27	1	3			5		
28					5		
29		1			5		
30					2		
31			1		1		
35			1				
39	1						
40			6		2		
43			1		1		
44			1		1		
47			1				
48			2				
50			38	37			
52				1			
53			3	7			
55			17	28			
56				1			
57				4			
58				2			
59			2	2			
Total	97	104	82	82	100	81	105

Table 9.4 The table gives the mean, for each visit, of the angle and separation of the seven longest-observed phosphene pairs. The angle from the first to the second is given as minutes past the hour, 0–59, to one decimal. The mean separation is given in inches and decimals, to three significant figures. The number of observations contributing to each mean is given. The right-hand column gives the overall bivariate means, for each of the seven pairs

Pair			Visit							Overall mean
	1	2	3	4	5	6	7	8	9	
L2-A1				20·0′	20·0′	20·6′	20·0′		21·1′	20·6′
				3·19″	3·00″	3·65″	3·25″		5·95″	4·06″
				N = 8	N = 19	N = 26	N = 18		N = 26	N = 97
L2-D2				21·6′	20·6′	20·8′	20·9′	24·1′	22·8′	21·8′
				1·49″	1·28″	1·82″	1·58″	1·88″	2·62″	1·82″
				N = 8	N = 19	N = 26	N = 18	N = 11	N = 22	N = 104

	1	2	3	4	5	6	7	8	9	10
D2-C2				03·4' 0.33" N=8	50·3' 0.89" N=19	53·6' 0.87" N=26	46·2' 0.97" N=18	49·8' 1·25" N=11		50·6' 0.83" N=82
C2-L2				53·7' 2·00" N=8	52·4' 1·42" N=19	51·3' 1·67" N=26	53·6' 1·65" N=18	55·1' 2·05" N=11		52·9' 1·67" N=82
A1-M1	23·0' 1·03" N=15	24·3' 1·02" N=28	23·3' 1·18" N=5	27·4' 0.97" N=8	25·2' 1·04" N=19				23·1' 1·71" N=25	24·3' 1·32" N=100
K2-K5	10·0' 13·5" N=2	13·4' 7·32" N=28	13·2' 8·34" N=8	17·2' 13·1" N=8	14·8' 9·39" N=19	14·9' 8·99" N=16				14·4' 8·85" N=81
K2-L2				04·2' 9·52" N=8	01·0' 9·36" N=19	01·5' 7·99" N=26	03·4' 8·33" N=18	02·1' 7·48" N=8	03·2' 7·96" N=26	02·4' 8·31" N=105

Table 9.5 The table shows, for the seven longest-observed phosphene pairs, which time intervals add significant extra variance to the observations, when compared with the next shorter time intervals. The observations were subjected to a hierarchical bivariate analysis of variance, assuming bivariate normality of the observations. The probability that any extra variance is attributable to chance was calculated.

P   0·05 represented as*
P   0·01 represented as***

Where the extra variance was attributable to changes in the apparent separation, and not the angle between phosphenes, it may be due merely to changes in the scale of the map. The suffix D (for distance) is added in these cases

Pair	Interval		
	Hours	Days	Months
L2-A1		***D	
L2-D2	***	*D	***D
D2-C2	***D		***
C2-L2		*	
A1-M1	***		
K2-K5	***		***
K2-L2	***D	***	***

References

BRINDLEY G.S., DONALDSON P.E.K., FALCONER M.A., & RUSHTON D.N. (1972) The extent of the region of occipital cortex that when stimulated gives phosphenes fixed in the visual field. *J. Physiol.* **225,** 57–58

BRINDLEY G.S. & LEWIN W.S. (1968) The sensations produced by electrical stimulation of the visual cortex. *J. Physiol.* **196,** 479–93.

BRINDLEY G.S. & RUSHTON D.N. (1974) Implanted stimulators of the visual cortex as visual prosthetic devices. *Trans. Amer. Acad. Ophthalmol. Otolaryngol.* **78,** OP 741–OP 745.

CRAGGS M.D. & RUSHTON D.N. (1976) The stability of the electrical stimulation map of the motor cortex of the anaesthetised baboon. *Brain* **99,** 575–600.

DANIEL P.M. & WHITTERIDGE D. (1961) The representation of the visual field on the cerebral cortex in monkeys. *J. Physiol.* **159,** 203–21.

DONALDSON P.E.K. (1973) Experimental visual prosthesis. *I.E.E. Proc.* **120,** 281–98.

PART II
THE MOTOR SYSTEM

CEREBELLAR FUNCTION IN THE CONTROL OF MOVEMENT

(WITH SPECIAL REFERENCE TO THE PIONEER WORK OF SIR GORDON HOLMES)

SIR JOHN ECCLES

Introduction

After a distinguished career in neurology from 1900 Sir Gordon Holmes had the good fortune to serve as a consulting neurologist with the British Army in France during the First World War. More than anybody else he realized the great significance of clinical studies on cases with local gunshot wounds of the brain. My lecture relates to the result of his investigations on cerebellar lesions. Extensive reports on 40 cases were published in *Brain* in 1917. In 21 cases there were repeated examinations over periods of many months. Later (1927) he reported that the total collection comprised 80 localized gunshot wounds of the cerebellum and in addition about 20 cases of localized cerebellar lesions that had been fully examined.

The opportunity to give a detailed evaluation of this most important material came in 1921 with his 4 Croonian Lectures to the Royal College of Physicians. Many years later (1939) in the Hughlings Jackson Lecture he reviewed again his classical findings and related them to the newer physiological discoveries. It is remarkable how his clinical investigations have stood the test of time. F. M. R. Walshe wrote in the Royal Society Obituary Notice on Holmes in 1966: 'His clinical studies still remain the most careful and detailed record of dysfunction of the human cerebellum'.

My initial idea in planning this chapter was to give an account of the principal clinical observations of Sir Gordon Holmes and then to show how our present understanding of cerebellar function allows us to continue on from the explanations that he developed. However, on further consideration it seemed best to give initially the present story of cerebellar function and on this basis to attempt an interpretation of Holmes' observations. Undoubtedly he would have done this if he had had the advantage of these new insights. I am not going to attempt a comprehensive survey, but will restrict my account to those aspects of the modern story that form an essential basis for the discussions of Holmes' remarkable investigations. That such an enterprise is worth undertaking is the best tribute I can offer in respect of the excellence of Holmes' studies, which stand out even to this day as the most comprehensive and best documented clinical observations on human cerebellar lesions. For example the great cerebellar authority, R. S. Dow, stated in 1970: 'As a matter of fact the kymograph tracings, which Gordon Holmes made in 1918, still remain about the only graphic records of cerebellar deficiency. I think it is a great misfortune that more has not been done'. To this I would add the unique photographic studies of movements by a technique still unrivalled today.

Principles of cerebellar functioning in the control of movement

Preliminary review of the neuronal machinery

It is not relevant to give an account of the way in which the cerebellar cortex processes the information coming to it by the two distinct inputs, the climbing fibres that come exclusively from the inferior olive and the mossy fibres coming via all the other inputs (cf. Eccles 1973). We still do not have a coherent and detailed understanding of the mode of operation of the neural machinery of the cerebellar cortex in this computation. For our present purposes it is sufficient to recognize that there is an incessant input by both mossy and climbing fibres to all regions of the cerebellar cortex, and from moment to moment the Purkinje cells signal the computed data by changes in the frequency of discharge of impulses, which in turn converge onto and inhibit the cells of the cerebellar nuclei. This inhibition is measured against a background excitation of the nuclear cells that is generated by the many input lines to the nuclei. It is important to realize that in the circuits to and from the cerebellum there are many lines in parallel, the only exception being the unitary climbing fibre input to each Purkinje cell. Otherwise there are convergence and divergence at each synaptic relay and always from moment to moment the clash of synaptic excitation and inhibition. This clash is the essential mechanism for computation in the central nervous system, and *par excellence* in the cerebellum. It is now necessary to describe the neuronal circuits, particularly the cerebro-cerebellar circuits which in man are pre-eminently concerned in cerebellar function.

As indicated diagrammatically in the transverse section of the cerebellum and brain stem (Fig. 10.1), three main subdivisions of the cerebellar cortex and its convectivities lie in a parasagittal array. Most medial is the vermis whose Purkinje cells project to the fastigial nucleus. The vermis is relatively very small in the human cerebellum, less than 5%. Next is the pars intermedia which is also small in the human cerebellum, and which projects

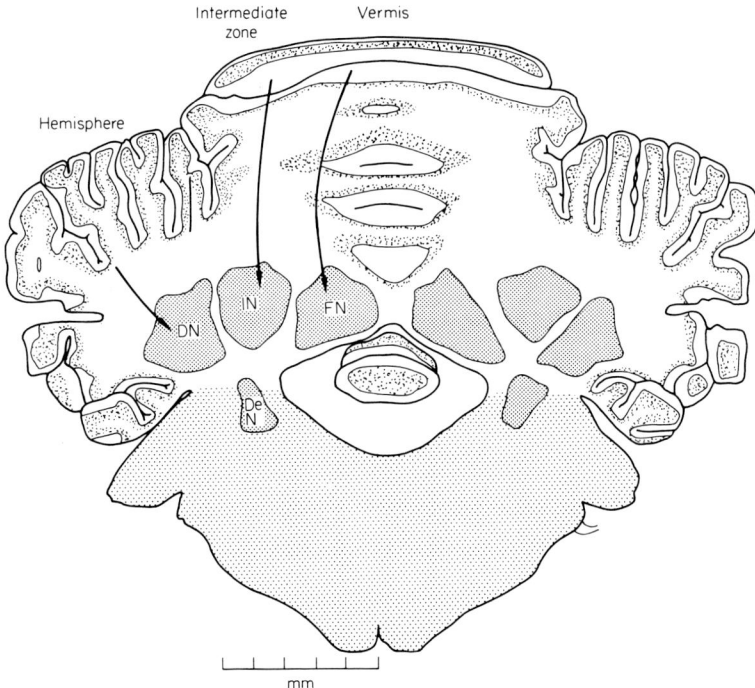

Fig. 10.1 Section of cerebellum and brain stem along the transverse plane. The large arrows indicate the lines of projection from the cerebellar cortex to the cerebellar nuclei. FN, fastigial nucleus; IN, interpositus nucleus; DN, dentatus nucleus; DeN, Deiters' nucleus.

to the nucleus interpositus (IP) or in man to the nuclei globosus and emboliformis. Finally there are the large cerebellar hemispheres that comprise about 88% of the human cerebellum and that project to the nucleus dentatus. Cerebellar circuitry has been most investigated in the cat, but there are now enough primate investigations to justify the attempt to use studies on the cat and primate in order to interpret the clinically observed results of lesions of the human cerebellum.

Cerebro-cerebellar pathways

The closed loop via the pars intermedia of the cerebellar cortex

Figure 10.2 is a very greatly simplified diagram to show how the motor cortex and the pars intermedia of the cerebellum are linked together. All the

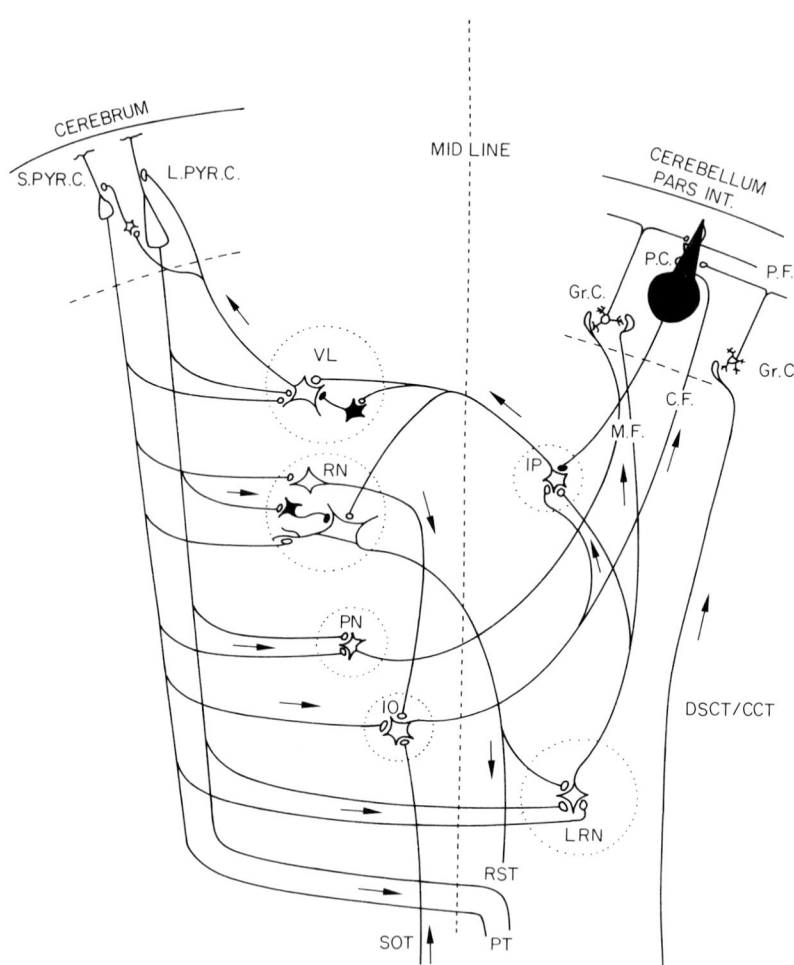

Fig. 10.2 Pathways linking the sensorimotor areas of the cerebrum with the pars intermedia of the cerebellum. Full description in the text. (Eccles 1977.)

neuronal pathways drawn in Fig. 10.2 are securely based on anatomical and physiological investigations. Simplification is achieved by having the individual species of cells reduced to just one example. However, each species shown has been recorded as individual cells, and the connectivities shown have all been checked by the timing of their discharges in each of the pathways. So this is a fairly complete diagram as far as it goes but, of course, it misses all the operational features deriving from the enormous numbers of cells in parallel with the wealth of convergence and divergence that has been already mentioned above. Thus Fig. 10.2 should be regarded merely as a skeleton drawing!

Let us start the operative sequence of Fig. 10.2 by the firing of a large pyramidal cell (L.Pyr.C.) of the motor cortex. These cells are the principal cells of origin of the pyramidal tract (PT). There is also shown one small pyramidal cell (S.Pyr.C.). Axons of these cells form small fibres of the pyramidal tract, but it is not known how effective these fibres are in the spinal cord. In Fig. 10.2 the large pyramidal tract fibre sends off branches that after synaptic relay in the nuclei pontis (NP) and the lateral reticular nucleus (LRN) give mossy fibre (MF) inputs to the cerebellar cortex (pars intermedia). Thus impulses fired down the pyramidal tract in order to begin a movement will at the same time go to the cerebellar cortex on the opposite side from the cerebral cortex, and on the same side as the movement. So there is an extremely fast and reliable input from the cerebrum to the cerebellum. The motor cortex cannot begin instituting any action without the cerebellum immediately 'knowing' about it. There is I think no doubt that the cerebrum is the command centre, but all instructions it fires to the motor machinery of the spinal cord are immediately fired into the computational machinery of the cerebellar cortex via the two mossy fibre pathways. In addition, impulses fired from the small pyramidal cells go to these two nuclei, presumably aiding in their responses. More importantly, small pyramidal cell discharges go to the inferior olive (IO), which is the exclusive source for the climbing fibre (CF) input to the cerebellar cortex.

After the stage of interaction in the cerebellar cortex there is the final stage of the return circuit to the motor cortex of the cerebrum. In Fig. 10.2 the Purkinje cell inhibits the nuclear cell in the interpositus nucleus (IP), which is also excited by collaterals from mossy and climbing fibres as shown for the LRN and IO pathways respectively. Here is a further site for computation in the clash of excitatory and inhibitory actions on the IP cells. Thence the pathway is very fast and direct, there being only one synaptic relay in the ventrolateral thalamus (VL Thal) on the way to the pyramidal cells of the motor cortex. Another pathway for action is also shown in Fig. 10.2, namely from IP to RN (the red nucleus) and so via the rubrospinal tract (RST) to the motoneurones of the spinal cord.

We can thus appreciate the authority of the cerebellar influence on the course of all movements that are initiated by the motor cortex. There is a very rapid and complete signalling to the pars intermedia of the whole array of impulse discharges down the pyramidal tract. We can assume that the input is computed in the cerebellar cortex with utilization of its memory stores, and after a further computation in the cerebellar nuclei (IP) it is returned to the same motor area of the cerebrum. In the cat the circuit time for this complete loop would be less than one hundredth of a second. With man it would be longer, about one fiftieth of a second. With respect to the motor cortex this system operates in a closed loop manner.

The open loop system of the cerebellar hemispheres

The cerebellar hemispheres comprise almost 90% of the human cerebellum, the principal cerebro-cerebellar circuits being shown in Fig. 10.3. In contrast to the pars intermedia, the cerebellar hemispheres receive most of their cerebral inputs from extensive areas of the cortex, such as the motor association cortex (Brodmann area 6) and less from the motor cortex via collaterals of pyramidal tract fibres (dotted lines in Fig. 10.3). This distinctive circuitry is well developed in primates, and is pre-eminent in man, where widespread zones of one cerebral hemisphere provide 20 million fibres passing to lower levels, as against only 500,000 pyramidal tract fibres. As shown in Fig. 10.3, impulses discharged from the pyramidal tract cells of the association cortex pass to the contralateral cerebellar hemisphere via relays in the pontine nuclei (PN) and the inferior olive (IO). After computation in the cerebellar hemisphere the return circuit is via the VL thalamus to the motor cortex and so down the pyramidal tract (PT) to effect the movement. Thus the cerebro-cerebellar circuit is essentially an open-loop system.

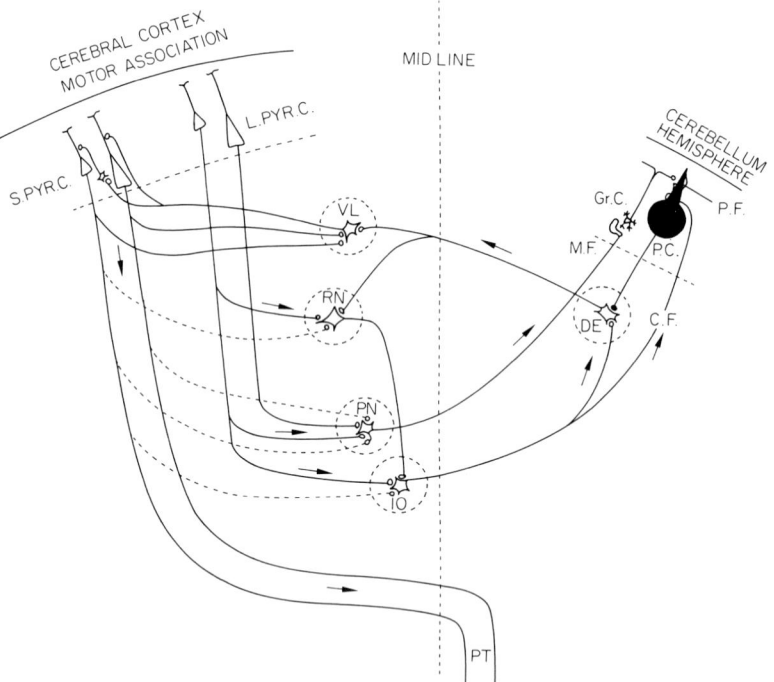

Fig. 10.3 Cerebro-cerebellar pathways linking association and motor cortices with the cerebellar hemisphere. DE is nucleus dentatus. Other symbols are as in Fig. 10.2. In the red nucleus only a small cell is shown. (Allen & Tsukahara 1974.)

Moreover there is evidence that some of the return from the dentatus nucleus goes to the VA thalamus and thence to association cortex, which again can project down the pathways to the cerebellar hemisphere. Hence there is the possibility of reverberatory operation of the cerebro-cerebellar circuits.

Dynamic operation of the cerebro-cerebellar circuits

The circuit operations are best appreciated by the very simplified diagrams of Fig. 10.4, in which lines of communication are shown by arrows that substitute for all the synaptic connectivities of Figs. 10.2 and 10.3. Fig. 10.4a illustrates the mode of operation of the pars intermedia that has already been considered in relation to Fig. 10.2, but it adds the input–output components of spinal centres and the evolving movement.

Let us recapitulate and simplify: when pyramidal cells of the motor cortex (area 4) are firing impulses down the pyramidal tract (PT) in order to bring about a voluntary movement (a motor command), the patterns of this discharge (the evolving movement) in all details are transmitted to the cerebellum (pars intermedia) by virtue of the collateral branches of the

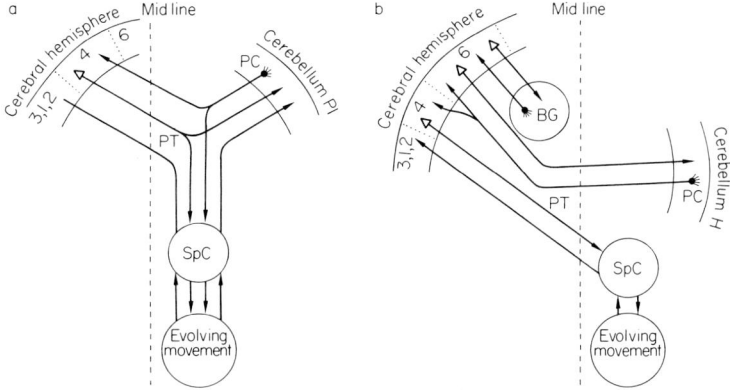

Fig. 10.4 Cerebro-cerebellar circuits in motor control are shown simplified by omission of the synaptic connectivities. a Shows the circuits from pyramidal cell in motor cortex (4) via pyramidal tract (PT) to spinal cord, and so to the evolving movement, and with collateral to the pars intermedia (PI) of the cerebellum. The Purkinje cell (PC) in PI communicates (via synaptic relays) back to the motor cortex and also down the spinal cord to the spinal centres (SpC). Also shown is the projection from spinal centres to PI and to the somaesthetic area (3, 1, 2). In b the circuits are shown from the cerebrum (principally area 6) to the hemisphere (H) of the cerebellum. The return circuit from the Purkinje cell, PC, is back to areas 4 and 6. From area 4 there is the projection down the spinal cord by the pyramidal tract, PT, as in a, and the return circuit from the evolving movement via the spinal centres to areas 3, 1, 2. Additionally there is shown the circuit from area 6 to the basal ganglia (BG) and the return to the cerebrum. (Eccles 1976.)

pyramidal tract fibres. Computation occurs in the cerebellar cortex (PI) and the resulting output is returned to the motor cortex so that there is an on-going 'comment' from the cerebellum within 10 to 20 msec of every motor command. We may regard this 'comment' as being in the nature of an on-going correction continuously provided by the cerebellum and being immediately incorporated in the modified motor commands issued by the motor cortex. Figures 10.2 and 10.4 also illustrate a longer feedback loop that operates through the same region of the cerebellum. When the motor command brings about a movement, this evolving movement excites a wide variety of peripheral receptors, in muscles, skin, joints, etc., and these signal back to the same regions of the cerebellar cortex (up-going arrow) that were concerned in the more direct loop. A computation of the two sets of input forms the basis of the cerebellar response. Thus this cerebellar discharge provides to the motor command centres an on-going cerebellar comment synthesized from these two loops. In addition the pars intermedia has a more direct path for influencing the spinal centres via the red nucleus (RN) and the rubrospinal tract (RST), as indicated in Fig. 10.2 and by the downward arrow in Fig. 10.4a.

In summary we can regard the pars intermedia of the cerebellum as acting like the controlling system on a target-finding missile. It acts similarly in that it does not give a single message for correction of a movement that is off-target. Instead it delivers sequences of correcting messages, so providing a continuously updating control by closed dynamic loops.

In the primate there is no peripheral input to the cerebellar hemispheres such as that for the pars intermedia (cf. Fig. 10.4a with b). Hence the only feedback information into this open-loop system is via the sensory pathways to the cerebral cortex from peripheral receptors in muscle, skin, joints, etc., that project to the somaesthetic areas, Brodmann, 3, 1, 2. Because of these special features of connectivity Allen and Tsukahara (1974) have proposed that the cerebellar hemisphere is concerned in the planning of a movement rather than in its actual execution and correction by follow-up control. Its function is largely anticipatory based upon learning and previous experience, and also upon preliminary, highly digested sensory information transmitted from areas of the association cortex.

In Fig. 10.4b there is indicated another dynamic loop system that operates via the basal ganglia (BG). The principal cortico-nuclear pathways are from other cortical areas, 6 and 3, 1, 2. The further projection is to the globus pallidus and thence to the VA and VL thalamus. There are subsidiary looping circuits to the substantia nigra and to the nucleus subthalamicus. However, the main circuit is another open-loop system from the association cortex to the basal ganglia and so to the motor cortex via the thalamic nuclei. It will be suggested that this open loop system is in parallel with the open loop through the cerebellar hemisphere. The close analogy between these two open loop systems is of particular interest because the control of movement is disordered when either one is defective. Degenerations of the basal ganglia result in Parkinsonism or in Huntington's chorea, while cerebellar lesions give cerebellar ataxia and tremor. However, the mode of operation of the neural machinery of the basal ganglia is still poorly understood.

Synthesis of the various neuronal mechanisms concerned in the control of voluntary movement

Figure 10.5 gives an imaginative illustration of the interacting loop controls that have been illustrated in Figs. 10.2, 10.3 and 10.4 (Allen & Tsukahara

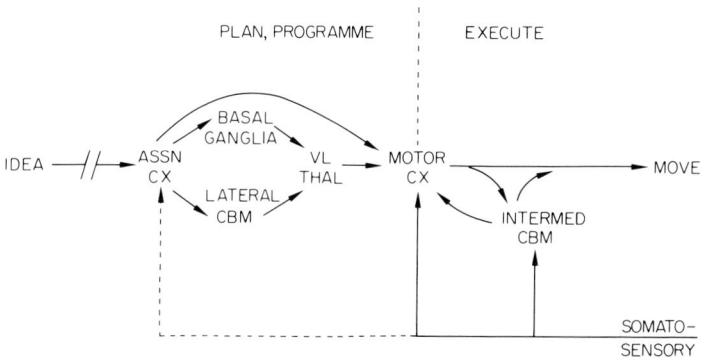

Fig. 10.5 Diagram showing pathways concerned in the planning, execution and control of voluntary movement. ASSN CX, association cortex; lateral CBM, cerebellar hemisphere; intermediate CBM, pars intermedia of cerebellum. Full description in text. (Modified from Allen & Tsukahara 1974.)

1974). As discussed in relation to Kornhuber's (1974) experiments, the idea of a movement achieves expression in patterns of excitation in the association cortex, which are recognized as the 'readiness potential' in diffuse scalp recordings. At the same time there are the two systems of dynamic loops illustrated in Fig. 4B with projection back to the motor cortex via the VL thalamus. In addition these loop systems project back to association cortex (area 6 in Fig. 10.4b) with the opportunity of further dynamic loop circuitry. The synthesis of all these loop inputs with the on-going activities of the association cortex provides what we may call pre-programmed information for the motor cortex that as a consequence generates the appropriate discharges down the pyramidal tract (the motor command) for bringing about the desired movement.

At the stage of motor discharge, by the two closed loops illustrated in Figs. 10.4 and 10.5, the pars intermedia makes an important contribution by updating the movement that is based upon the sensory description of the limb position and its velocity, and upon this description the intended movement is superimposed. This closed loop operation is a kind of short-range planning as opposed to the long-range planning of the association cortex and the cerebellar hemispheres. Certainly both of these cerebellar zones must cooperate in the performance of every skilled movement (Allen & Tsukahara 1974).

In learning the movement we first execute the movement very slowly because it cannot yet be adequately pre-programmed. Instead it is performed largely by intense cerebral concentration as well as with the constant updating via the pars intermedia of the cerebellum. With practice and the consequent motor learning a greater amount of the movement can be pre-programmed and the movement can be executed more rapidly. With very rapid movements, e.g. piano playing or typing, we rely entirely on pre-programming by the circuits to the left of Fig. 10.5 because there is no time for on-target correction by the pars intermedia once a fast movement has begun.

We may thus conjecture that trained movements are largely pre-programmed, whereas exploratory movements, which constitute an important fraction of our movement repertoire, are imperfectly pre-programmed, being provisional and subject to continuous revision. The role of the cerebellum, presumably the pars intermedia, in untrained exploratory movements is attested to by the clumsiness and slowness with which they are performed when, after cerebellectomy, the cerebrum has to function in the absence of cerebellar cooperation both in pre-programming and updating.

Let us now try to visualize what would be happening in the cerebro-cerebellar circuits during some skilled action, for example a golf stroke, or a stroke in billiards. There will be initially a voluntary motor command with a pre-programming of the movement by circuits shown to the left of Fig. 10.5. This pre-programming mobilizes all the learnt skills and leads on to the pyramidal tract discharges with the consequent report of this discharge in detail to the pars intermedia. At the next stage there will be a report back to the motor cortex of corrective information in accord with its learned skills. There will be a consequent modification of the pyramidal discharge which also reaches the pars intermedia for further revision. But meanwhile the pre-programming circuits will also be in continual action, for the movement is not just some staccato action, but a smooth highly integrated performance with a duration of hundreds of milliseconds. Thus we have to envisage that, in the carrying out of a skilled movement, there is an immense integration of neuronal activities in interacting dynamic loops.

Experimental evidence relating to the operative features of the circuits of Figs. 10.2, 10.3, 10.4 and 10.5 is illustrated in the experiments of Evarts (1967) and Thach (1968). In an initial operation the monkey in Fig. 10.6a had an electrode implanted in his motor cortex in the right place for

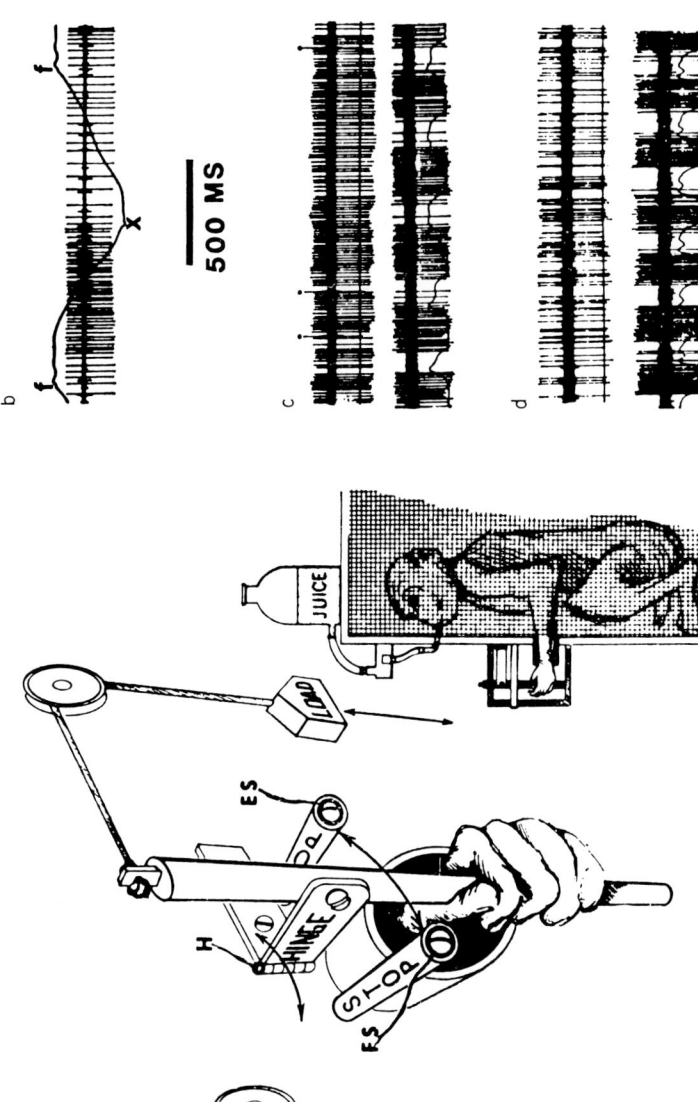

Fig. 10.6 a. Illustration of experiment on monkey hand movement. b, Motor pyramidal cell discharges (Evarts 1967). c, Purkinje cell discharges. d, nuclear cell discharges (Thach 1968). Note that in c and d the sweep speed is much slower.

recording pyramidal cells concerned in an action he has been trained to do. During an experimental run, he is seated comfortably in a cage (a) and has to move the control bar from one stop to the other, shown in detail in a, backwards and forwards in a time that must be between 0·4 sec and 0·6 sec, else he is not rewarded by grape juice. In Fig. 10.6b you can see the traces of the movement and the firing of the pyramidal cell which clearly is related to the downward movement that he is doing. There is no doubt that this particular pyramidal cell is concerned with a particular movement, with flexion and not extension. Doubtless, there are many more pyramidal cells in that location of the motor cortex also firing in effective relation to the movement. In Fig. 10.6c the upper trace shows the rapid background firing of a Purkinje cell in another experiment (Thach 1968) and in the lower trace it exhibits a modulated increase and decrease of firing rate in phase with the movement, just as with the pyramidal cell in B. Figure 10.6d shows similar responses of a cerebellar nuclear cell. The phased relationship of these firing patterns for the three species of neurones is exactly in accord with the diagrams of Figs. 10.2 and 10.4a.

Cerebello-spinal connectivities

These connections have been far more intensively studied than the cerebro-cerebellar connections so far considered. They are specially concerned in walking, standing, reacting, balancing and in all the postural adjustments that follow active movements—stabilizing the positions attained thereby. Essentially it can be seen from Fig. 10.7 that the same general circuits from the spinal cord act on the cerebellar cortex as those diagrammed in Figs. 10.2 and 10.4a. There are first the two main tracts up the spinal cord that end as mossy fibres (MF), the fast dorsal spinocerebellar tract (DSCT) and the slower tract (bVFRT) up to the lateral reticular nucleus (LRN). Second, there are the slow tracts to the inferior olive (IO) and so to the cerebellum as climbing fibres (CF). The inhibitory outputs by the Purkinje cells go initially to the fastigial (FN) or Deiters' (DN) nucleus and secondarily via FN either to DN or to the reticular nucleus (ReN) and so down the spinal cord to motoneurones via the vestibulospinal (VST) or reticulospinal (ReST) tracts, respectively.

   The important feature of these connections of the cerebellar vermis is that there is only one loop in the dynamic control system. The evolving movement results in the discharge of various kinds of receptors that project via the several ascending pathways to the cerebellar cortex thus modifying the Purkinje cell output to the cerebellar nuclei and so via the ReST and VST to the motoneurones. In this way the cerebellum is able to control posture and movements by the simplified version of dynamic loop operation. We have studied intensively most of the stages in the neuronal system illustrated in

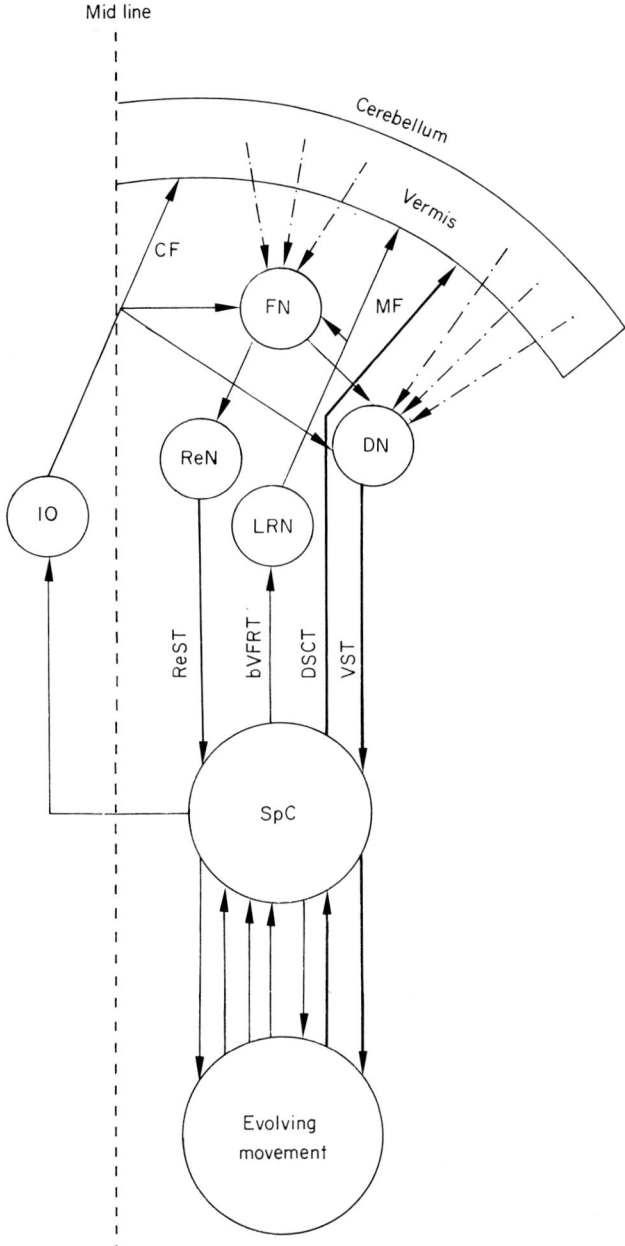

Fig. 10.7 Pathways linking the cerebellar vermis with the spinal centres and so to the evolving movement. Further description in text. (Eccles 1977.)

Fig. 10.7 and find that the various species of neurones show the responses that would be expected for inputs from receptor organs of skin and muscle via the DSCT and bVFRT. It should be mentioned that Fig. 10.7 is a diagram for the hindlimb. For the forelimb the cuneocerebellar tract (CCT) substitutes for the DSCT.

The clinical findings reported by Holmes (Holmes 1917, 1922a, b, c, d, 1927, 1939)

The most striking investigations of Holmes were on subjects that had a sharply defined lesion of the cerebellum on one side only. The best patients were those with a small bone depression giving a well localized injury. Such lesions gave the opportunity that he fully utilized to compare the movements on the normal side with the movements on the affected side. Another advantage of Holmes' work was that he developed remarkable clinical recording techniques. Holmes classified the disorders arising from cerebellar lesions under 4 main headings.

1. Hypotonia and diminished postural tone of muscle. As a consequence there are flail-like movements of limbs, pendular knee jerks, etc. Holmes (1939) summarized this by stating that cerebellar lesions give diminution of 'postural tone which alone or by reinforcing voluntary effort, tends to fix each part of the body in the attitude which it occupies, and they show that volitional contraction of the muscles alone is not adequate to maintain posture'. The postural tone is equally important in movement which, as Hughlings Jackson states, can be regarded as a succession of postures. An excellent demonstration of hypotonia is illustrated by Holmes (1939, Figs. 1, 2), where he recorded the movements of the two arms supported by a bar that was suddenly removed. The affected arm fell at once through a larger angle and developed an irregular tremor.

2. Asthenia and muscle fatigue were found by Holmes (1939) to be a major symptom of cerebellar lesions. He used special dynamometers to measure strengths of a wide range of limb movements for both arm and leg. The power on the affected side may be reduced to as low as half the control. The feebleness was often recognized by the patients, who also noted the tendency of the affected limb to tire more readily in some repetitive task.

3. Abnormalities in the rate, regularity and force of voluntary movements. The accounts Holmes (1922b, c, 1939) gave of his investigations lead to most fruitful considerations in the light of our present knowledge and also provide guidance for further laboratory investigations. It is important to reproduce some of Holmes' excellent illustrations. Holmes developed a very simple but effective technique in studying the disorders of movement and obtaining simple photographic pictures where it was possible to compare the normal with the disordered movement.

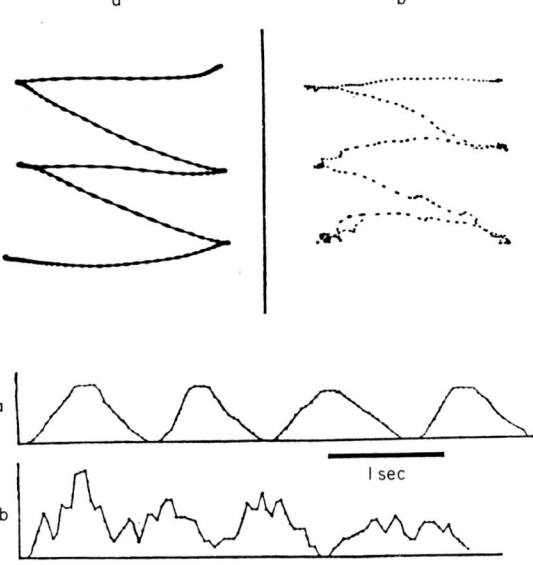

Fig. 10.8 a and b are records obtained as described in text. The range of movement was about 75 cm. The plotted curves below are calculated from the traces above to show movements on normal and abnormal sides in a and b, respectively. The range of movement is plotted vertically and there is 0·04 sec in the horizontal scale between the dots. In contrast to the normal side a, there is in b gross irregularity and failure to reach target dots in the later three movements. (Holmes 1939.)

In Fig. 10.8 the subject was asked to move his arm so that a finger pointed accurately and in smooth sequence to a series of red spots arranged in two vertical rows of 3 each. On the tip of his finger there was a small bulb giving flashes of light at 25 per sec. This flashing technique ensured a photographic record of both the course and the speed of movement. On the normal side in a the subject moved his finger from point to point fairly directly and slowed up smoothly in approaching the target then accelerated to the next target and so on. A quite different record is shown in b on the side of the cerebellar lesion, where the movements were irregular in direction and showed evidence at each of the turning points of inaccuracy and indecision and tremor. This is well illustrated by the plotted measurements below. I do not know of a more effective display of the essential disorders of movements in a cerebellar lesion.

Holmes gave many other impressive illustrations. I select two examples. For example (Fig. 10.9) the subject had to move his finger from spot A above his head to his nose at B. Here we have an example of the decomposition of movement described by Holmes. The subject did not move his finger directly from A to B, but first lowered it to about the level of his nose and then moved

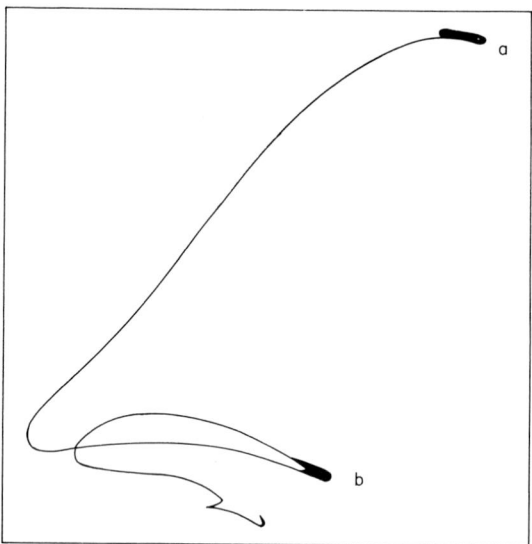

Fig. 10.9 Movement of finger from a above head to nose at b in subject with cerebellar lesion as described in text. (Holmes 1939.)

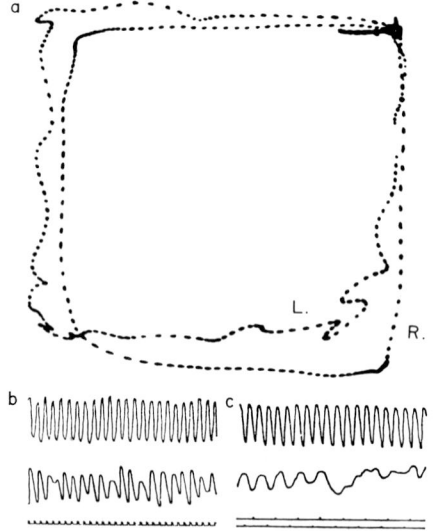

Fig. 10.10 In a the subject with a left cerebellar lesion attempts to outline by finger of outstretched arm a square on the wall of the room, there being as in Fig. 8 a flashing light at 25 per sec on his finger tip. In b and c there are tracings of the alternating pronation and supination of the arm on the normal (upper) and on side of cerebellar lesion (lower). In c there is a faster rate of alternation with a corresponding further disorder of movement on the affected side. Time in seconds for b and c. (Holmes 1939.)

it towards the nose in an uncontrolled manner hitting it sharply, as may be seen by the rapid rebound and the uncertain attempt to go back more gently but with disorder. Another striking example of Holmes' illustrations is shown in Fig. 10.10a where the light flash technique is also used with the subject outlining with his finger a square which is projected on the wall of the room. On the normal right side there is a reasonably good trace of a square with again the slowing up at the corners and then acceleration. With the left side the disordered movement is apparent in the irregularity and uncertainty of direction, particularly in approaching and departing from a corner of the square. Fig. 10.10b and c illustrates the disorder on the affected side of movement in alternate pronation and supination (adiadokokinesis). Holmes (1939, Figs. 4, 5, 6, 9) also illustrated graphically the delays in onset and in cessation of movement on the affected side, which also displayed a slowing in execution. The type of cerebellar disability illustrated in Figs. 10.9 and 10.10 is often called hypermetria because of the overshooting of the movement with respect to the target. Alternatively it is called cerebellar ataxia. The essential feature is the failure of smooth control.

Holmes rightly concluded that the irregularities in movement were due to a disorder in the innervation of the prime movers and could not be attributed merely to hypotonia. The decomposition of movement (Fig. 10.9) indicates the same kind of disorder of smooth control. The patient evidently cannot carry out a movement of complex integration, but has to decompose the movement into action at one joint after another in order to bring about the desired position of the limb. As Holmes states: 'It is an invariable rule that the more component movements there are in any action, the more irregular that action is'. Simple actions are the movements at a single joint, e.g. bending finger or elbow. Compound movements in one direction only, e.g. Fig. 10.9, are next in order of complexity. The most complex movements he analysed were compound movements in which there were changes in direction, as for example in Figs 10.8 and 10.10. It is of great interest that delicate finger movements were most affected. Holmes (1922c) also attributed the defects of speech to failure of the fine control of movement, but, because of the bilateral innervation of the speech mechanisms, recovery is good when the cerebellar lesion is restricted to one side.

4. Disorders associated and automatic movements. This fourth category is I think linked with disorders of posture and gait and involves loss of the coordinating influence of the cerebellar vermis as diagrammed in Fig. 10.7. Of course when walking is not an automatic action, but it is a deliberate and carefully controlled action, as when walking on ice or over a rough terrain, its control is from the motor cortex and the cerebellar control is via the cerebro-cerebellar circuits depicted in Figs 10.2, 10.3 10.4 and 10.5.

The disorders in eye movements and nystagmus involve special structures of the paleocerebellum, the floccular-nodular lobe with control by visual and vestibular inputs. It is a distinct highly specialized field taking us beyond the main contributions of Holmes to cerebellar performance.

Holmes clarified a much debated subject when he so clearly disproved all suggestions that the cerebellum is concerned in sensation. He reported that his patients never suffered from loss of cutaneous sensation, both superficial and deep and also had no defects in recognition of movements at joints or in weight discrimination. The tendency to feel a weight to be heavier on the affected side he plausibly attributed to the hypotomia and asthenia, which resulted in a greater sense of effort in hefting weights.

More debatable is his fairly complete rejection of all functional localization in the cerebellum except for three fairly general statements (Holmes 1927). '1. Each lateral lobe influences the motor functions of the same side of the body only. 2. When the vermis is injured or both lateral lobes are involved, articulation and the postures and movements of the head and trunk are more affected than when one lateral lobe only is damaged. 3. No local lesion affects only or exclusively one limb or a portion of a limb.' At the most he would agree to a 'prevalence of representation, in Rossi's sense (1913), the arm being represented in the hemispheres more anteriorly and the leg more posteriorly' (Holmes 1922d).

The interpretations of symptoms of human cerebellar deficiency

I will first attempt to give an imaginative account of the cerebro-cerebellar activities during some relatively simple planned movement, such as placing finger on nose from a position above the head (Fig. 10.9). The initial posture as maintained by the continuous operation of the cerebro-cerebellar circuits is illustrated in Figs. 10.2, 10.3, 10.4 and 10.5. The steadiness is not static, but is the result of a balanced operation of muscle contractions that are the final result of the thousands of lines in parallel, particularly those of Figs. 10.2 and 10.4a with their closed loop operation. The voluntary initiation of the movement occurs by the mysterious operation of the self-conscious mind on special areas (the liaison areas) of the cerebral cortex as indicated to the left of Fig. 10.5. The immense build up of neuronal activity in the cerebral hemispheres can be recognized by the readiness potential (Kornhuber 1974), which for this movement would have a duration of more than 1 second before there is any discharge from the motor cortex. In this latent period we can envisage the immense dynamic operation of loops within the cerebral cortex with superimposed thereon the loops to the cerebellar hemispheres and basal ganglia as indicated in Figs. 10.3, 10.4b and 10.5. This is the operation of pre-programming whereby there is a spatio-temporal ordering in the neuronal machinery of the sequence of motor actions required for the smooth movement. Kornhuber goes so far as to suggest that, if the cerebral cortex were deprived of the dynamic loops through both the basal ganglia and the cerebellar hemispheres, no voluntary movements could be carried out. Once the movement is under way the loops of Figs. 10.2 and 10.4a come into action in a corrective capacity to keep the movement smoothly on target. So throughout the movement there are the superimposed operations of the 2 systems diagrammed in Fig. 10.4a and b, and the combined neuronal performances being beyond imagination. The slowing of the movement when the target (nose) is being approached and the eventual finish on the target require detailed control by the two cerebellar systems. It has to be recognized that, as indicated in Figs. 10.4a and b, essential sensory information from muscle, joints, skin, etc., is being provided to the cerebrum and the pars intermedia of the cerebellum during all stages of the movement.

The defects of voluntary movement in human cerebellar deficiency (cf. Figs 10.8, 10.9 and 10.10) are so overwhelming that both Holmes (1922b, c, d) and Walshe (1927) came to focus on these defects as the primary disability, other associated phenomena such as disorders in tone, posture and gait being secondary. Thus the symptoms were disorders of movement resulting from the reactions of the intact parts of the brain after the cerebellar ablation. Of particular interest were Holmes' observations (1922b) on the conscious corrective efforts of patients. For example, the movements of the affected limb become more irregular if the patient's attention is diverted, as by making him perform actions by the two limbs at the same time, or when he suffered from fatigue. Furthermore we have the most pertinent comment of a patient as quoted by Holmes (1940). 'The movements of my left arm are done subconsciously, but I have to think out each movement of the right (affected) arm. I come to a dead stop in turning and have to think before I start again.' I suggest that this is one of the most penetrating statements that can be made with respect to the disability produced by a cerebellar lesion.

I now quote an excellent hypothesis that Holmes (1922b) developed for cerebellar function as disclosed by his immense analytical experience of the deficiencies. 'The accurate combination and correlation of the phasic and tonic elements of every movement demand the active intervention of the cerebellum, and that the tonic supplement to tetanic contractions as well as the modifications of tone in the antagonistic, synergic, and fixating muscles are excited or controlled through it in every stage of every movement.' Essentially this is the hypothesis that I was expressing above in relation to our modern understanding of cerebellar function.

I now attempt explanations of the three main symptoms of cerebellar deficiency as defined by Holmes.

1. *Hypotonia.* Rossi's (1913) observation that stimulation of the cerebellum causes a lowered threshold of the motor cortex to stimulation has been repeatedly confirmed. The cerebellar inputs to the motor cortex are thus preponderantly excitatory; hence loss of the cerebro-cerebellar circuits (cf.

Figs 10.2, 10.3, 10.4 and 10.5) would result in diminished activity of the motor cortex, and a diminished tonic discharge down the pyramidal tracts with a consequent hypotonia.

2. *Asthenia and muscle fatigue* can be similarly explained. Because of a reduction of motor cortical activity due to loss of cerebellar reinforcement the subject will have to exert stronger voluntary commands in order to evoke a given muscular contraction. With continued activity fatigue will be experienced at an earlier stage because of the increasing and eventually prohibitive voluntary efforts required. Thus it can be envisaged that by the cerebro-cerebellar circuits of Figs 10.2, and 10.3 and 10.4 there is a continuous reinforcement of motor cortical activity.

3. *Abnormalities in rate, regularity and force of voluntary movements* (cf. Figs 10.8, 10.9 and 10.10). It is proposed that errors arise in the first place from a failure in pre-programming so that the motor cortex does not receive from moment to moment the fully tailored inputs from the association cortex and the cerebellar inputs (cf. Figs 10.3, 10.4b and 10.5) that give patterns of pyramidal discharge more or less adequate to carry out the desired movements. Superimposed on this continuous pre-programmed input there are, once the motor cortex begins discharging, the on-going comments via the pars intermedia that give finer corrective information. The patient can of course learn to become more efficient in substituting for the loss of cerebellar controls, but this requires continuous conscious effort as stated above and only a partial recovery is possible. The loss of fine skills is permanent, as is well illustrated by two case reports by Holmes (1922b): 'A professional musician with a tumour of the left side of the cerebellum complained that with his left hand he "could not strike the four notes of a chord in proper sequence or time" on the piano, and one of my patients with a long-standing gunshot wound was no longer able to play the flute, although the movements of his arm were apparently normal to other tests.'

The failure to discover any precise localization of function in the cerebellar hemispheres (Holmes 1922d) is I think to be attributed to the unlikelihood that gunshot wounds would give sharply defined lesions. There is evidence by Allen and associates (Allen & Tsukahara 1974) that there is a fairly well-defined topographic relationship between the cerebrum and the cerebellum. Certainly highly specific connectivities have to be postulated if one is to account for the immense number of fine skills that are dependent on cerebro-cerebellar circuitry. There is an appalling hiatus in our knowledge with regard to the topographic relations of cerebrum to cerebellum, particularly in the primate.

The other great deficiency lies in the rudimentary state of the attempts to give an account of learning processes in the cerebellum. The vague hypothesis of Marr (1969) that the climbing fibres act as teaching instructors for the mossy fibre inputs is most attractive, and at last Ito (1975) is providing effective experimental testing. We can hope for a full elaborated hypothesis in the near future.

In appraisal of the attempt to account for the symptoms of cerebellar lesions in the light of our modern knowledge, I am cognizant of the great deficiencies in this knowledge. There has been a successful analysis of the neuronal interactions in the cerebellar cortex (Eccles 1973), but this does not help to any appreciable extent in the attempt to develop an understanding of the mode of operation of the cerebellum in the control of movement. At the best it can form the basis for building models. Explanations based on the skeletal circuits of Figs 10.2, 10.3, 10.4, 10.5 and 10.7 give no more than vague statements of generalities. The immensity of the neuronal machinery and the amazing finesse and reliability of its performance completely escapes our comprehension. I am sure that Holmes would have felt that we have not advanced very far beyond the explanations he was able to develop before the analytical successes of recent times. The understanding of cerebellar function can be attempted only when there have been synthetic studies to match the analytical. But this is an age where analysis attracts the attention and the rewards! The much more demanding and visionary task of synthesis is being attempted in far too few laboratories. Holmes would have been very unhappy at this grave unbalance, as also would have been Sherrington.

References

ALLEN G.I. & TSUKAHARA N. (1974) Cerebrocerebellar communication systems. *Physiol. Rev.* **54**, 957–1006.

DOW R.S. (1970) Discussion on p. 470. In: Fields W.S. & Willis W.D. (Eds) *The Cerebellum in Health and Disease.* W. H. Green, St. Louis, Mo.

ECCLES J.C. (1973) The cerebellum as a computer: Patterns in space and time. *J. Physiol.* **229**, 1–32.

ECCLES J.C. (1977) *The Understanding of the Brain*, 2nd edn McGraw-Hill Book Company, New York.

EVARTS E.V. (1967) Representation of movements and muscles by pyramidal tract neurons of the precentral motor cortex. In: Yahr M.D. & Purpura D.P. (Eds) *Neurophysiological Basis of Normal and Abnormal Motor Activity*, pp. 215–53. Hewlett; Raven Press, New York.

HOLMES G. (1917) The symptoms of acute cerebellar injuries due to gunshot injuries. *Brain* **40**, 461–535.

HOLMES G. (1922a) The Croonian Lectures on the clinical symptoms of cerebellar diseases and their interpretation. *Lancet* **100**(1), 1177–82.

HOLMES G. (1922b) The Croonian Lectures on the clinical symptoms of cerebellar diseases and their interpretation. *Lancet* **100**(1), 1231–7.

HOLMES G. (1922c) The Croonian Lectures on the clinical symptoms of cerebellar diseases and their interpretation. *Lancet* **100**(2), 59–65.

HOLMES G. (1922d) The Croonian Lectures on the clinical symptoms of cerebellar diseases and their interpretation. *Lancet* **100**(2), 111–15.

HOLMES G. (1927) Discussion in Symposium on the cerebellum. *Brain* **50**, 385–8.

HOLMES G. (1939) The cerebellum of man. *Brain* **62**, 1–30.

ITO M. (1975) Cerebellar learning control of the vestibulo-ocular mechanisms. In: *Mechanisms in Transmission of Signals*

For Conscious Behavior. 26th International Physiological Congress, New Delhi.

KORNHUBER H.H. (1974) Cerebral cortex, cerebellum, and basal ganglia: An introduction to their motor functions. In: Schmitt F.O. & Worden F.G. (Eds) *The Neurosciences: Third Study Program.* Cambridge MIT Press, 267–80.

MARR D. (1969) A theory of cerebellar cortex. *J. Physiol.* **202,** 437–40.

ROSSI G. (1913) Sui rapporti funzionali del cerveletto con la zona motrice della corteccia cerebrale. *Arch. Fisiol.* **11,** 258–64.

THACH W.T. (1968) Discharge of Purkinje and cerebellar nuclear neurons during rapidly alternating arm movements in the monkey. *J. Neurophysiol.* **31,** 785–97.

WALSHE F.M.R. (1927) The significance of the voluntary element in the genesis of cerebellar ataxy. *Brain* **50,** 377–85.

DISORDERS OF MOVEMENT IN CEREBELLAR DISEASE IN MAN

C. D. MARSDEN, P. A MERTON, H. B. MORTON, MARK HALLETT, JANE ADAM AND D. N. RUSHTON

Introduction

Figure 11.1 from Holmes' classical paper (1922) summarizes many of the errors in movement that characterize cerebellar deficit. The patient, who had a wound in the left side of the cerebellum, was asked to extend springs of equal strength by flexing his two arms at the elbow on a signal and to maintain the stretch at a level indicated by the line A–B.

The affected arm starts the movement late (delay in contraction). The velocity of movement is less and the movement itself consists of a series of irregular jerks and pauses (astasia). The arm overshoots the point of aim (dysmetria). What cannot be shown in the figure is the subject's statement 'I cannot put force into it' or 'I have to put more effort into it to move it' (asthenia).

The simple movement illustrated in Holmes' experiment is a continuous event from start to finish, but it is useful to consider three stages in its execution; initiation, transit, and termination. The initiation of the movement may or may not be under control from peripheral receptors in the limb, while transit and termination almost certainly are. The distinction is emphasized by comparison of fast, or ballistic, limb movements and slow, or ramp, movements. Although most normal limb movements comprise a mixture of these two elements, ballistic movements are generated by bursts of firing of both agonist and antagonist muscles which, to some extent, occurs independently of feedback control; ramp movements are produced by continuous firing of the agonist muscle which is exquisitely sensitive to peripheral influence.

Normal ballistic movements

Figure 11.2 illustrates typical ballistic movements. In Fig. 11.2a the subject was asked to flex the elbow as rapidly as possible through 10°. In Fig. 11.2b

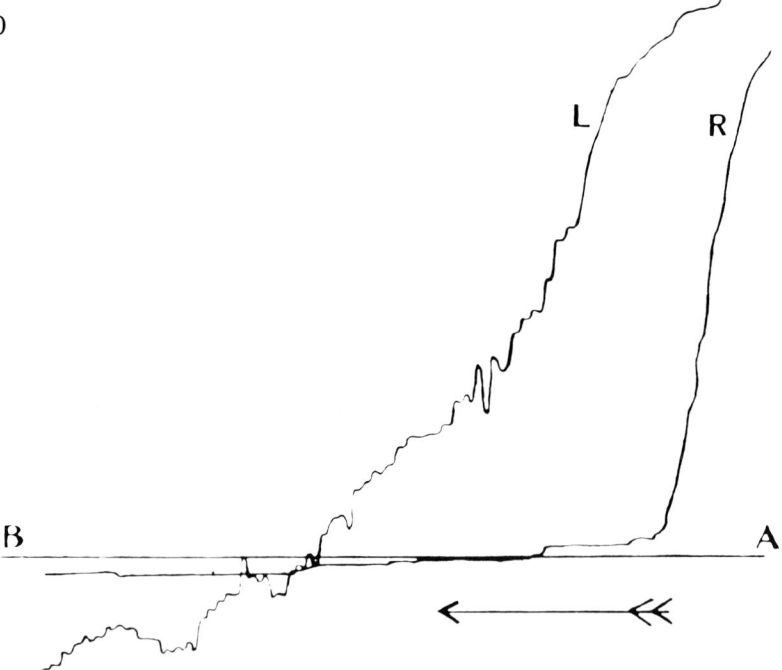

Fig. 11.1 Holmes' observation on errors in movement in a patient with left-sided cerebellar ataxy. The subject extended springs of equal strength with his two arms at a signal and tried to maintain the stretch at a level indicated by the line A–B. The records read from right to left. Holmes noted 'the slowness of the left arm in exerting power, the irregular tremulous character of the movement and the failure to maintain the final posture'. (From Holmes 1922, with permission.)

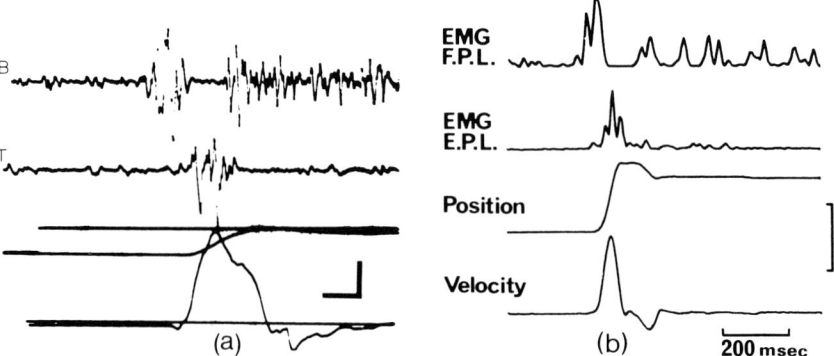

Fig. 11.2 Fast ballistic movements in man. In (a) the subject flexed the elbow through 10°. In (b) a different subject flexed the top joint of the thumb through 20°. In (a) and (b) the records are from above down, E.M.G. activity in the agonist (raw E.M.G. in biceps—B, rectified E.M.G. in flexor pollicis longus—F.P.L.), E.M.G. activity in the antagonist (raw E.M.G. in triceps—T, rectified E.M.G. in extensor pollicis longus—E.P.L.), position and velocity. The calibration in (a) is 50 msec and 500 μV; that in (b) is 200 msec and 200 μV, 27° or 336° per sec. (Figure 11.2a is from Hallett, Shahani & Young 1975a, with permission.)

the subject flexed the top joint of the thumb as fast as possible through 20°. In each case the position and velocity of the limb is shown, and the electromyographic activity of the agonist and antagonist muscles is displayed. (In the case of elbow flexion, E.M.G. activity was recorded through surface electrodes 3 cm apart over biceps and triceps. In the case of thumb flexion, E.M.G. activity was recorded from bipolar fine wire electrodes inserted via needles into flexor pollicis longus and extensor pollicis longus.)

The ballistic movement is generated in both proximal and distal arm muscles by a characteristic triphasic burst of activity in flexors and extensors (Wachholder & Altenburger 1926, Hallett, Shahani & Young 1975a). In the agonist there is an initial burst of activity, followed by a silent period, which terminates in a second burst of activity. In the antagonist there is a single burst which occurs at about the time of the agonist silent period.

In Fig. 11.2, the antagonist muscle (triceps or extensor pollicis longus) is relatively quiet prior to the movement. However, if the antagonist is tonically active, as shown for the thumb in Fig. 11.3, the first event in any movement is seen to be inhibition of the ongoing antagonist activity which occurs usually before the initial burst in the agonist. The same is seen in triceps before making the ballistic movement if the subject is asked to hold the elbow steady against a weight tending to flex it.

How is this triphasic pattern of activation of agonist and antagonist adapted to generate ballistic movements of different distances and against

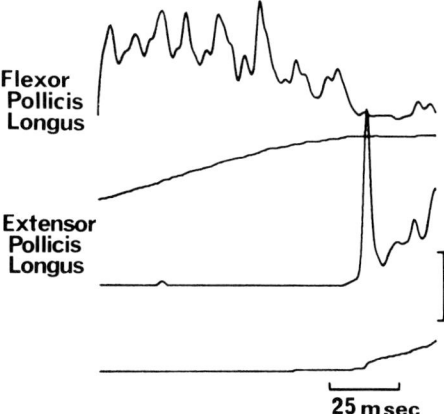

Fig. 11.3 Antagonist inhibition prior to a ballistic movement in man. The subject flexed the top joint of the thumb against a resistance (0·16 Nm). On a signal he extended the thumb as quickly as possible. The records are from above down, rectified E.M.G., then rectified and integrated E.M.G. from flexor pollicis longus; rectified E.M.G., then rectified and integrated E.M.G. from extensor pollicis longus. The average of 16 trials is shown. The calibration is 25 msec, and 300 μV. Note that ongoing E.M.G. activity in flexor pollicis longus begins to silence about 25 msec prior to the burst in extensor pollicis longus.

varying loads? Detailed experiments have been done on the human thumb. The subject rested his thumb on a bar connected to the spindle of a low inertia motor (Printed Motors Ltd). The force required to maintain the bar in a constant position could be varied by altering the current drive to the motor. The position of the thumb was recorded by a sensitive potentiometer attached to the other end of the spindle of the motor. Details of these experimental arrangements have been described elsewhere (Marsden, Merton & Morton 1976a).

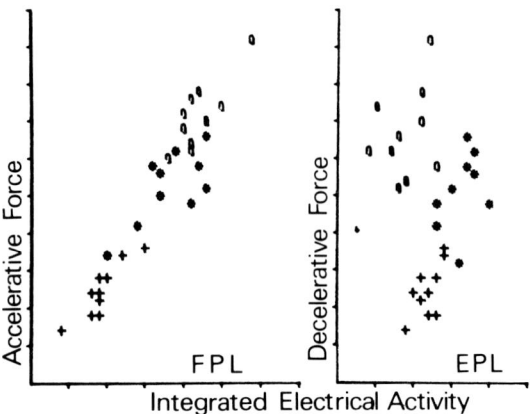

Fig. 11.4   Relation of E.M.G. activity in initial burst in the agonist (flexor pollicis longus—F.P.L.) and antagonist (extensor pollicis longus—E.P.L.) in ballistic thumb flexion movement to the accelerative and decelerative forces generated. Data for one subject are shown. A series of fast thumb flexions (as shown in Fig. 11.2) were made through 5° (+), 10° (*) or 20° (0). The forces produced were calculated from records of acceleration and are shown in arbitrary units. The integrated E.M.G. activity from the two muscles was measured directly and is also shown in the same arbitrary units.

The amount of electrical activity in the initial agonist burst (found by rectification and integration of the raw E.M.G.) is linearly related to the accelerating force exerted and, hence, to the distance moved (Fig. 11.4), but the duration of the agonist burst (some 50–100 msec) is independent of the distance moved, the initial angle of the joint and the background force against which the thumb works. Adjustments to compensate for these various conditions are made by altering the amount of activity within the predetermined time intervals.

The size of the antagonist burst of activity is not as closely related to the amplitude of the movement or the decelerative force and is probably of insufficient magnitude by itself to arrest the movement. The additional effect of an agonist burst of limited duration generating a pulse of force acting against the passive mechanical elements of the thumb working to arrest the movement also restricts the distance travelled. However, the antagonist burst of activity must assist in halting movements, particularly small brief movements, and like the initial agonist burst, it is of fixed duration (some 40–100 msec).

The duration of the silent period that follows the initial agonist burst is also fairly constant (some 50–110 msec), but the size and duration of the second burst of activity in the agonist are very variable. The latter appears to depend on the accuracy of the initial ballistic movement, and thus represents corrective action.

To what extent this pattern of activation of agonists and antagonists is pre-programmed and independent of peripheral feed-back can be examined by study of the effect of altering peripheral circumstances at the instant of movement. In the case of the elbow (Hallett, Shahani & Young 1975a), the initial bursts of activity in biceps and triceps were unaltered by passive extension of the elbow (which unloaded triceps and stretched biceps) just prior to the voluntary ballistic movement, and were unaffected in a patient with a sensory neuropathy of such severity as to render him functionally deafferented. Thus these initial components in a ballistic movement of the elbow would seem to be pre-programmed and relatively immune to peripheral influence (see also Garland & Angel (1971) and Hopf, Lowitzsch & Schlegel (1973) who arrive at the same conclusion from other experiments). However, extension of the elbow does cause an increase in the size of the second agonist burst in healthy subjects.

In the case of the thumb the situation is somewhat different, for a stretch of the long flexor suitably timed to preceed a voluntary ballistic thumb flexion can augment the initial agonist burst, while a similarly timed release can reduce it. The burst of antagonist activity is similarly modifiable. Thus the pattern of muscle activation in a ballistic thumb movement is subject to peripheral influence. This does not mean that it is not pre-programmed, but it is certainly modifiable.

The general conclusion is that the initial events in the generation of a ballistic movement (which are, in sequence, antagonist inhibition, agonist burst, and antagonist burst) are centrally pre-programmed. They are generated by signals from the brain direct to alpha motoneurones, and the timing and pattern of agonist and antagonist firing is determined by the brain. However, the force to be exerted, and hence the speed and distance moved, can only be computed by the brain on the basis of information on existing joint angle and muscle length. Patients with deafferented limbs, due to either peripheral nerve lesions or posterior column damage, cannot make accurate ballistic movements, nor can deafferented monkeys (Gilman & Denny-Brown 1969, Gilman 1975). Adjustments in the force exerted to achieve a given amplitude of ballistic movement are made by varying the size, but not the duration, of the initial bursts of activity in agonist and antagonist. The size of these bursts would appear to be computed by the brain on the basis of information received from the periphery and a knowledge of the desired goal. There is, too, the problem of adjusting burst size to existing resistance to movement. The size of the agonist burst required to move a given distance will depend on whether the limb is working free or lifting a weight. Two components in this judgement can be recognized. The brain clearly makes a guess at the resistance likely to be encountered, as is illustrated by the familiar suitcase illusion. The surprise at jerking an empty suitcase that one expects to be full is a commonplace. In addition, the brain is provided with some information on existing conditions by monitoring the force exerted prior to the movement. Thus, when holding a heavy weight, the brain must obtain information as to the mass to be moved from knowledge of the force required to support the weight. This might be achieved either by monitoring cortico-motoneurone discharge, or spindle feed-back (assuming $\alpha-\gamma$ co-activation), or by the central gain mechanism under μ input control proposed by Marsden, Merton and Morton (1976a).

Ballistic movements in cerebellar disease

Examination of the pattern of muscle activation during ballistic movements in patients with cerebellar disease reveals distinct abnormalities.

The normal reaction time of about 200 msec is considerably prolonged. In a study of fast elbow flexion in 18 patients with cerebellar ataxy due to various pathologies (Hallett, Shahani & Young 1975b), average reaction time was some 270 msec. These patients also exhibited a delay in onset of antagonist inhibition when asked to carry out a fast elbow flexion against a background of tonic triceps contraction. In particular, the activity in triceps commonly did not cease until biceps activity had begun.

The pattern of activation of biceps and triceps was similar to that in normal subjects, consisting of an initial agonist burst, followed by a period of silence which corresponds to a burst in the antagonist, followed by a second burst of activity in the agonist (Fig. 11.5a). However, the duration of the initial bursts in agonist and antagonist were distinctly abnormal. Both were prolonged in some patients, while in others, either the agonist burst or the antagonist burst was abnormally long.

Similar observations have been made on the thumb in cerebellar patients (Fig. 11.5b). The opportunity has also been taken to study the effects of acutely poisoning the cerebellum with alcohol in a normal subject. The ingestion of 200 ml of 50% ethanol in water resulted in marked slurring dysarthria, an ataxic gait, and obvious ataxia of arm movement with dysmetria, astasia and inability to carry out rapid tapping or alternating movements. Handwriting deteriorated to a scrawl. The effects on rapid

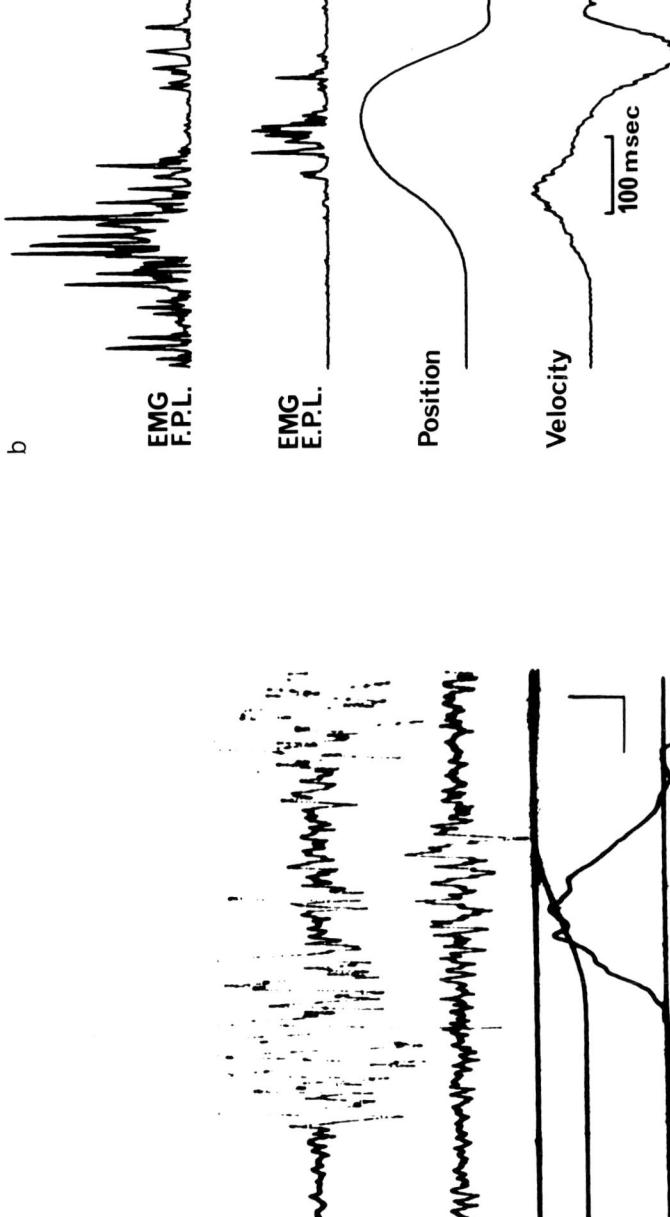

Fig. 11.5 Fast ballistic movements in patients with cerebellar ataxy. In (a), a fast elbow flexion from a 52-year-old man with a spino-cerebellar degeneration. The records shown are the same as those in Fig. 11.2a. Note, by comparison with the normal subject in Fig. 11.2a, the prolongation of the initial agonist and antagonist bursts of E.M.G. activity. The calibration is 50 msec and 200 μV. In (b), a fast thumb flexion is shown from a 62-year-old man with unilateral cerebellar ataxy due to a stroke. By comparison to the normal in Fig. 11.2b, note the slower movement, the inability to hold the final position, and the very prolonged bursts of activity in the agonist and antagonist muscles. The calibration is 100 msec and 100 μV, 25° or 313° per sec. (Figure 11.5a is from Hallett, Shahani & Young 1975b, with permission.)

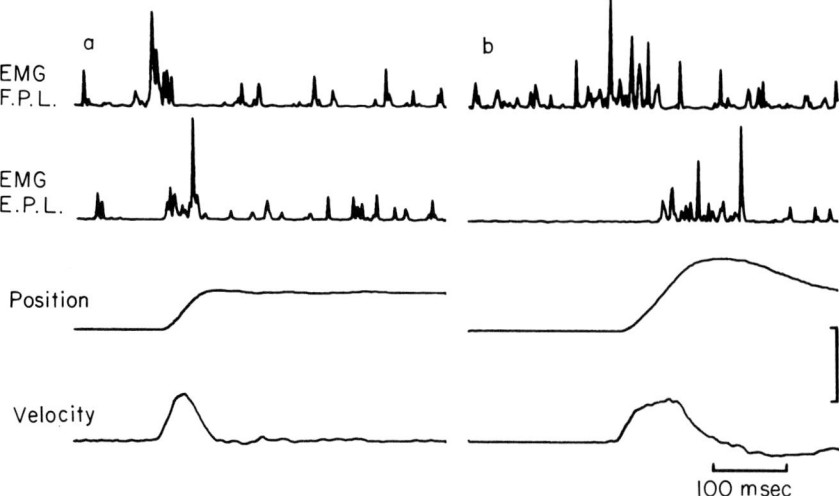

Fig. 11.6 Effect of ingestion of alcohol sufficient to cause cerebellar ataxy on fast ballistic thumb flexion. The records in (a) were taken in the morning prior to alcohol. Those in (b) were obtained 1½ hours after 200 ml of 50% ethanol by mouth. The signal to move occurred 50 msec in (a) and 100 msec in (b) prior to the start of the sweep. Note the delay in onset of movement, the slower movement, the overshoot of the target and inability to hold the final position, and the prolongation of the bursts of rectified E.M.G. activity in the agonist (F.P.L.) and antagonist (E.P.L.). The calibration is 100 msec and 100 μV, 20° or 250° per sec.

ballistic movements of the thumb are illustrated in Fig. 11.6. Reaction time was prolonged from mean control values of 146 msec to 218 msec. The duration of the initial agonist and antagonist bursts was also prolonged, and overshoot of the aiming mark was common (Fig. 11.6).

Thus, in summary, a number of abnormalities of agonist and antagonist activity in ballistic movements have been identified in cerebellar ataxy.

1. A delay in onset of contraction, as originally observed by Holmes (1917, 1922).

2. Delay in antagonist inhibition, which would contribute to dysdiado-chokinesia, and might be responsible for the pathological 'rebound' phenomena observed by Holmes (1917, 1922) in cerebellar patients when asked to flex a limb against a resistance which is suddenly released.

3. Abnormal durations of initial activity in agonist and antagonist. As argued by Hallett *et al* (1975b) this must result in the generation of inappropriate accelerative and decelerative forces and may be responsible for dysmetria (either hypometria or hypermetria). Furthermore, these inaccuracies in agonist–antagonist timing would grossly disrupt rapid alternating movements.

The feature common to all these abnormalities in cerebellar ataxy is an error in *timing* of the muscle activity generating ballistic movements. The pattern of agonist and antagonist firing is preserved, but the onset of antagonist inhibition is delayed and the duration of the initial bursts in agonist and antagonist muscles is prolonged. This suggests that the cerebellum times the bursts of muscle activity responsible for ballistic movements, as proposed by Braitenberg (1961, 1967, see also Kornhuber 1971). Braitenberg, on the basis of the lattice geometry of the cerebellar cortex proposed that the anatomical arrangement of climbing fibre input and mossy fibre input via granule cells and parallel fibres was such as to allow precise timing of Purkinje cell output appropriate to initial joint position and the desired distance of the movement. While the original theory does not fit all the facts of cerebellar physiology now known, Braitenburg's concept of the cerebellum and timing certainly is supported by the observed errors in ballistic movements in cerebellar patients.

The question arises as to whether these timing errors in ballistic muscle activity are related to the abnormalities in fusimotor discharge caused by cerebellar damage. Certainly, unilateral experimental cerebellar ablation in primates causes the hypotonia and slow pendular deep tendon reflexes observed in man by Holmes (1922). Gilman (see review, 1975) has demonstrated that such lesions increase the threshold to stretch required to evoke electromyographic activity in the affected limbs, and depresses the responses of primary spindle afferents (but not the secondaries) to both static and dynamic extension. Subsequent work showed that cerebellar ablation decreased activity in fusimotor efferents innervating muscle spindles. However, while such an effect of cerebellar damage on fusimotor discharge and primary spindle activity would explain the hypotonia and alteration in deep tendon reflexes in cerebellar disease, it would not account for the abnormalities in timing of muscle activation in ballistic movements. As indicated above, the initial components of a ballistic movement appear independent of peripheral influence. Liu and Chambers (1971) and Gilman (1970, 1975) have shown that while deafferented monkeys exhibit astasia and dysmetria, subsequently cerebellectomy considerably increases these errors in movement. Thus there appear to be mechanisms of cerebellar ataxy which are independent of the peripheral stretch reflex. The peripheral stretch reflex mechanism is, however, of critical importance in the control of slower ramp movements.

Normal ramp movements

For limb movements it is difficult to clearly separate fast ballistic movements from slow ramp movements. The fast ballistic thumb flexion shown in Fig.

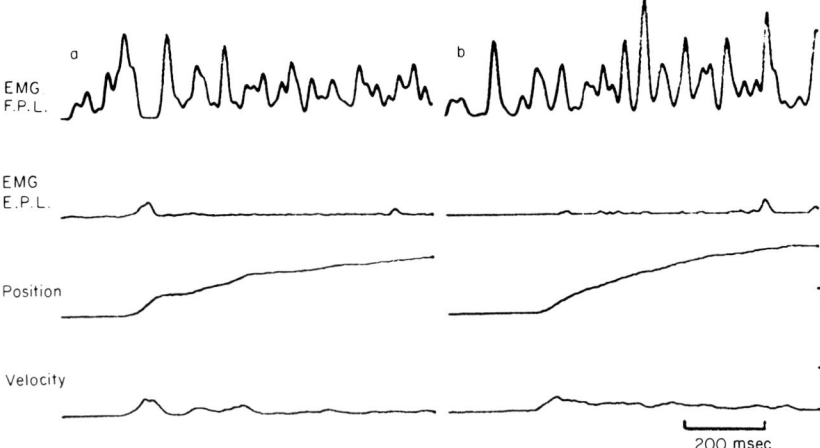

EMG
F.P.L.

EMG
E.P.L.

Position

Velocity

200 msec

Fig. 11.7 Attempts to generate slow ramp movements of thumb flexion for comparison with the fast ballistic movement in the same subject shown in Fig. 11.2b. As shown in a, such movements may begin with initial ballistic bursts in the agonist (F.P.L.) and antagonist (E.P.L.), but, with practice it was possible to obtain a relatively smooth onset of contraction with asynchronous activity in the agonist (F.P.L.) and little activity in the antagonist (E.P.L.). The calibration is 200 msec and 100 μV, 29° or 336° per sec.

11.2 can be compared with attempts to generate slow ramp thumb flexion through the same distance in Fig. 11.7. Often the movement was started by a ballistic pattern of muscle activation, with successive agonist–antagonist bursts (Fig. 11.7a). However, with practice and care it was possible to generate a smooth ramp movement (Fig. 11.7b) consisting of continuous agonist activity from the onset. This is the pattern of muscle activation that obtains throughout a slow tracking movement once it has started. These are the movements employed by Marsden, Merton and Morton (1972, 1973, 1976a, b, c) to investigate servo action in movement in man. Full details of the experiments and results are given in these papers.

The muscle most commonly employed was the long thumb flexor, and the experimental arrangements have been described briefly above. The subject was asked to make smooth flexion movements of the top joint of the thumb against a constant torque load offered by a low inertia motor. The rate of movement was standardized by giving the subject a tracking task. In some movements the load remained constant, but in others random perturbations were introduced in mid-course. By altering the current to the motor, the movement was halted, stretched or released. Muscle activity was recorded from surface electrodes or fine bipolar wire electrodes inserted into the active muscle, flexor pollicis longus, and in some experiments from its antagonist extensor pollicis longus. The muscle's response to halting, stretching or release during such ramp movements were obtained by averaging a number of trials, and are most clearly illustrated by rectification and integration of the raw electromyogram.

Figure 11.8a illustrates the effect of halt, stretch and release on the long thumb flexor. About 40 msec after a perturbation the muscle's activity alters so as to compensate, i.e. it increases to stretch and halt and decreases to release. The response to stretch is, by definition, a stretch reflex, but that to halt which occurs at the same time can be regarded as a stretch reflex without muscle stretch, and, hence, indicates servo action in response to the halt, probably due to fusimotor discharge. The response to release, in the form of the familiar silent period, also indicates servo support of the ongoing

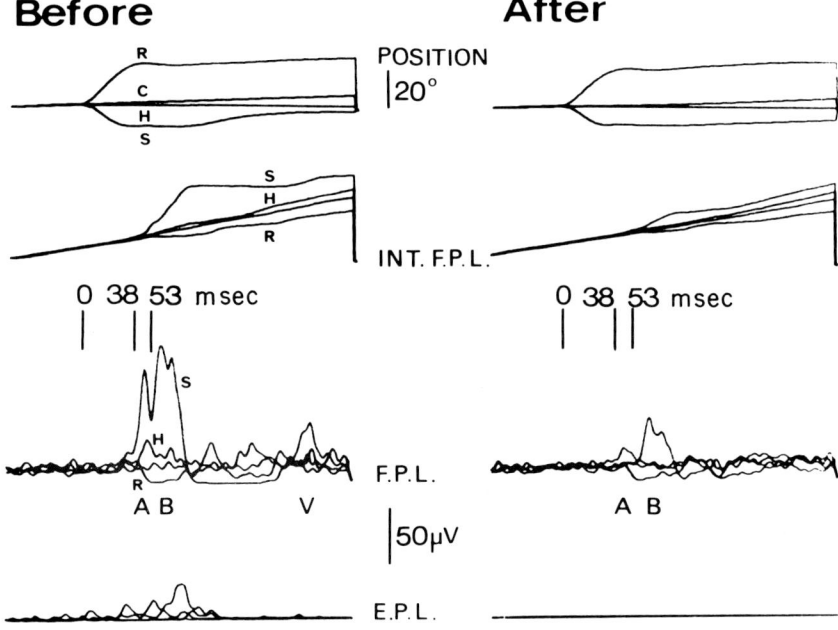

Fig. 11.8 Effect of stretch (S), halt (H) and release (r) on E.M.G. activity in the long thumb flexor (F.P.L.) and extensor (E.P.L.) during smooth thumb flexion tracking movements. Details of the experimental arrangements are given in the text. (a) Control records in a normal subject (C.D.M.), (b) two hours after ingestion of 200 ml of 50% ethanol which rendered C.D.M. very ataxic. The records are from above down, position of the thumb (with flexion upward), rectified and integrated E.M.G. activity of flexor pollicis longus (F.P.L.), rectified E.M.G. from F.P.L., rectified E.M.G. from extensor pollicis longus (E.P.L.). E.M.G. was recorded with fine-wire bipolar electrodes inserted into the muscles. The average of 24 individual responses to each perturbation is shown. The sweep duration is 250 msec, and perturbations were introduced at the time marker indicated as 0 (which is 50 msec after the start of the sweep). For further details see text.

movement. All these responses are interpreted as manifestations of automatic servo action based on the stretch reflex, for they occur too early to be voluntary and are independent of visual feedback.

A number of novel features of this servo action in human muscles have been discovered. An increase in the initial load against which the thumb works increases the size of the servo responses. Thus the gain of the servo is, to a first approximation, proportional to initial load and tends to zero in a relaxed muscle (Marsden, Merton & Morton 1976a). Gain appears to be determined by the level of muscle activation, rather than by the pressure exerted by the thumb. Such gain control also appears to compensate for fatigue in muscle, for it is boosted as the muscle has to be activated more strongly to keep up the same output. These servo responses, although based on the stretch reflex, are in the case of the thumb (but not the big toe) heavily dependent on sensation. They are abolished by anaesthesia of the naïve thumb, which leaves the active muscle in the forearm unaffected (Marsden, Merton & Morton 1976c)

The latency of these servo responses for the human long thumb flexor is about twice that of tendon jerks or F waves recorded from similarly placed muscles. This observation led us to consider whether they employed a cerebral cortical rather than a spinal arc (Marsden, Merton & Morton 1973), on the lines suggested by Hammond (1960) and Phillips (1969). If transcortical, such stretch reflexes would be expected to show an excess latency over that of a tendon jerk in proportion to the distance of the muscle from the brain not from the spinal cord. Thus the excess would be larger for the long flexor of the big toe and smaller for the jaw-closing muscles than for the long thumb flexor. This turns out to be the case, and the alternative hypothesis that these long latency stretch reflexes are mediated by slow-conducting afferents is unlikely since equally long latencies are found in the homologous component of the stretch reflex in proximal arm muscles. All this evidence is compatible with the notion that the functionally active long-latency stretch reflex is transcortical (Marsden, Merton & Morton 1976b). The notion receives further support from the available data on conduction time to and from the cerebral cortex in man, and from observation in human patients with a variety of neurological lesions affecting different portions of the nervous system. Thus such long latency servo responses are depressed by dorsal column lesions (Marsden, Merton & Morton 1973, Lee & Tatton 1975), and by damage to the sensori-motor cortex and capsular pyramidal pathways (Adam *et al* 1975, and unpublished data).

This data on human servo action suggesting the existence of powerful transcortical stretch reflex pathways, particularly for the hand, is supported and extended by similar studies undertaken in conscious primates. Single unit recordings from motor cortex neurones in monkeys trained to carry out arm movements have revealed distinct short-latency responses to changes in load

(Evarts 1973, Conrad *et al*, 1975). Units firing in relation to the movement were commonly excited by stretch and depressed by unloading of the active muscle after a short latency of some 20–40 msec. About 20 msec later an appropriate change in electromyographic activity occurred in the active muscle. Both Evarts and Conrad *et al* interpret these observations as indicating the operation of a transcortical load compensating servo pathway.

Further investigation has established that the long-latency stretch reflex in human muscle is composed of a number of identifiable events (Adam, Marsden, Merton & Morton unpublished observations). The initial burst following stretch of the human long thumb flexor at about 40 msec (A) is followed by a second burst (B) at about 55 msec, which terminates in a period of relative silence from about 80–150 msec, which is followed by a burst of activity (V) which is clearly voluntary. The voluntary burst (V) can begin around 80 msec and is equivalent to the M3 response to sudden wrist flexion described by Lee and Tatton (1975) and the V3 response produced by median or ulnar nerve stimulation on top of a voluntary contraction or combined with post-central cortical stimulation in man described by Milner-Brown, Girvin and Brown (1975).

The initial activity in A and B between 40 and 80 msec is a reflex involuntary stretch reflex. It corresponds in time to the M2 response of Lee and Tatton (1975) and the V2 response of Milner-Brown *et al* (1975) and Upton, McComas and Sica (1971). The two components A and B in this long-latency stretch reflex behave differently. This is illustrated in Fig. 11.9a, where small and large fast brief stretches of similar initial velocity are compared with a slower sustained stretch of similar amplitude to the large fast stretch. The A component is approximately similar in size with all the stretches; the B component is larger with the larger stretches, and biggest with the sustained stretch. Other evidence distinguishes A from B. Thus A cannot be altered in any way by the subjects 'set' or response to the stretch, while B can; a second stretch imposed soon after the first will only produce an A response; stretch of the long thumb flexor acting as the agonist causes both A and B responses, but a similar stretch of the same muscle acting as an antagonist causes only a B response; and while a severe sensori-motor cortex lesion in man abolishes both A and B, a lesion restricted to the cortical sensory areas may diminish only the A response. (In primates, Tatton *et al* (1975) have observed that ablation of the post-central cortex abolishes their M2 response.) The conclusion is that the long-latency stretch reflex is composed of two events (Adam *et al* 1975).

The question arises as to the basis of these two components. The loss of the initial A component with sensory cortical lesions may be correlated with the powerful projection of primary spindle afferents to area 3a of the primate cortex (Phillips, Powell & Wiesendanger 1971), but, as yet, no conclusive evidence exists to indicate that this projection area for low-threshold muscle

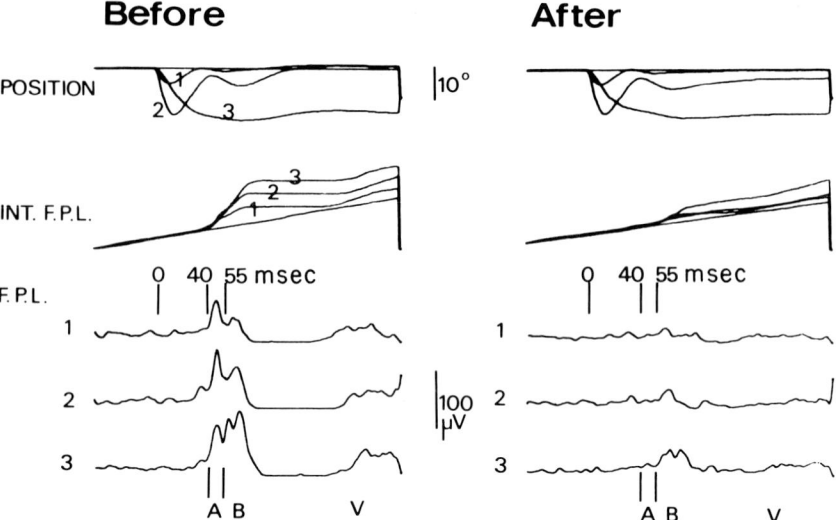

Fig. 11.9   The effect of a short fast stretch (1), a large fast stretch of similar initial velocity (2), and a slower sustained stretch (3) on E.M.G. activity in the long thumb flexor holding a steady position. (a) Control records in a normal subject (C.D.M.), (b) 2 hours after ingestion of 200 ml of 50% ethanol which rendered C.D.M. very ataxic. The records are from above down, position of the thumb (with flexion upwards), rectified and integrated E.M.G. activity from flexor pollicis longus (F.P.L.) recorded by fine-wire bipolar electrodes in the muscle, and rectified E.M.G. from F.P.L. with the responses to the three forms of stretch separated for clarity. The average of 24 responses to each form of stretch are shown. The sweep duration is 250 msec, and stretch was introduced at the time marker indicated as 0 (which is 50 msec after the start of the sweep). For further details see text.

afferents has output to cortical motoneurones or spinal cord. However, Wiesendanger (1973) was able subsequently to demonstrate electrophysiologically that electrical stimulation of muscle nerves at intensities above threshold for group II afferents did excite both pyramidal and non-pyramidal neurones in motor cortex. (That such neurones could also be excited by cutaneous stimulation may be relevant to the human observation that the long-latency stretch reflex in the thumb can be depressed by anaesthesia.) More recently, Lucier, Rüegg and Wiesendanger (1975) by the use of high frequency vibration obtained data in anaesthetized monkeys to suggest that signals from both primary and secondary muscle spindle endings from the forelimb reached the motor cortex. Lemon and Porter (1976) have been able to demonstrate in conscious monkeys trained to pull a lever, that joint movements, muscle movements and cutaneous stimulation all were capable of influencing motor cortex neurones, whose discharges were related to voluntary movement.

Thus it seems likely that both primary and secondary spindle afferents (as well as cutaneous and joint afferents) may excite cortical motoneurones. Either the primary or the secondary input to motor cortex, or both, could be responsible for the observed long-latency stretch reflexes in man. It is even possible that the early A response is generated by primary spindle afferents, while the later B response is due to slower group II afferent input. However, alternative pathways, perhaps via the cerebellum as suggested by Murphy, Kwan, MacKay and Wong (1975) on the basis of observations in the cat, must be considered (see Milner-Brown, Girvin & Brown 1975).

Ramp movements in cerebellar disease

Patients with cerebellar ataxy generally carried out smooth tracking movements of thumb flexion surprisingly accurately. So too did subjects who ingested sufficient alcohol to render them ataxic. Hallett, Shahani and Young (1975b) also noted that most cerebellar patients carried out a smooth elbow flexion normally. Both tasks involved a simple movement at a hinge joint, so that errors in direction could not occur, and visual feed-back was available to control the rate of movement.

Patients with cerebellar disease responded abnormally to a stretch introduced in the course of such smooth tracking movements. Figure 11.10

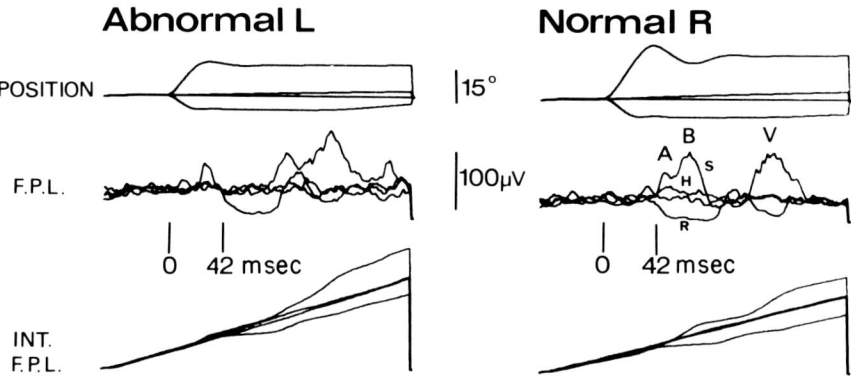

Ms PK 27.11.74 Age 43

Fig. 11.10 Effect of unilateral cerebellar ataxia of the left arm, due to an acoustic neuroma, on the E.M.G. responses of the long thumb flexor to stretch, halt and release during smooth tracking movement of thumb flexion. The records are from above down, position of the thumb (with flexion upwards), rectified E.M.G. from surface electrodes over flexor pollicis longus (F.P.L.) and rectified and integrated E.M.G. from F.P.L. The average of 24 individual responses to each perturbation are shown. See legend to Fig. 11.8 for further details.

illustrates a typical example of the effects of stretch, halt and release on smooth thumb flexion in a lady with unilateral cerebellar ataxy of the left arm due to an acoustic neuroma.

In the normal arm, stretch evoked a small spinal latency response at about 25 msec, followed by the typical, larger, long-latency response with onset of the first component at about 42 msec (A), and a later even larger burst of activity at some 55 msec (B). In the ataxic arm the stretch caused an obvious spinal response, but neither component of the long-latency reflex is apparent. A late response at 80 msec is evident, at a time when in the normal arm the silent period is beginning. Whether this is a delayed response, or an early voluntary component cannot be determined in this case, but in other cerebellar patients a clear response at B latency has been observed in the absence of an A response. This is also evident in the records shown in Figs 11.8b and 11.9b, which illustrate the effect of alcohol on a normal subject. At a time when cerebellar ataxy was evident, the normal A response recorded in control runs prior to alcohol has almost disappeared, but the B response is preserved although it is smaller than normal. Thus the most striking effect of cerebellar dysfunction seems to be a loss or diminution of the initial component of the long-latency stretch reflex, with relative preservation or delay of the later component.

With regard to the early response to halt, this also is reduced or lost in cerebellar patients, but the response to release is strikingly preserved. As is illustrated in Figs. 11.8b and 11.9b, the silent period following a release is at the usual latency around 45 msec, and is similar in degree and duration to normal. This preservation of the silent period in cerebellar patients contrasts with the effects of sensori-motor cortex lesions which usually cause loss of the long-latency response both to stretch and halt, and also that to release.

An explanation of these abnormalities in the response to stretch of the contracting thumb flexor in cerebellar ataxy invokes the known effects of cerebellar damage on muscle spindle function. Earlier it has been suggested that these responses to stretch are mediated by spindle input to cerebral cortex. The experimental evidence in animals indicates that both primary and secondary spindle afferent discharge may reach cerebral cortex and may evoke such transcortical stretch reflexes. The faster conduction velocity in primary spindle afferents would suggest that the earliest response seen, the A component, might be mediated via these fibres. The origin of the later B component is not clear; that this response is mediated via secondary spindle afferents is one possibility. On this interpretation, the loss of the initial A component of the long-latency stretch reflex could be explained by a reduction in primary spindle afferent sensitivity while the relative preservation of the later B component might indicate preservation of secondary spindle afferent action. This is, in fact, what has been demonstrated in experimental animals subjected to cerebellectomy. Gilman

(1969, 1975) has shown that acute cerebellectomy in primates depresses the response of muscle spindle primary afferents to both static and dynamic muscle stretch, but has no effect on the responses of spindle secondary afferents. However, the observation in cerebellar patients that the silent period to a release is preserved suggests that the muscle contraction is supported by spindle input. At present the roles of different spindle endings in the generation of the long-latency stretch reflex is a matter for speculation. At this stage in our understanding, such an explanation for the abnormalities in the response to perturbations during slow ramp movement in cerebellar disease must be tentative. An alternative explanation might involve an alteration in cerebellar action on the cortical neurones activated by muscle stretch (see, for example, Brooks 1975). Whatever the reason, the consequences of the observed abnormality in response to stretch would be to impair the servo regulation of muscle contraction, and to compromise such compensation for alteration in load during slow ramp movements. Such a failure of servo action may explain the irregularity of slow movements of the unsupported arm in cerebellar ataxy.

Discussion

We have described two basic abnormalities of muscle contraction in patients with cerebellar ataxy: (a) a breakdown in the normal timing of activation of agonist and antagonist muscles at the onset of fast ballistic movements, and (b) a failure of the normal long-latency load compensating reflexes, that may involve a transcortical stretch reflex pathway, during slow ramp movements. Since many normal human limb movements comprise a mixture of a ballistic initiation and a ramp execution, these abnormalities must cause the cerebellar patient to start moving with the wrong muscles and be subsequently inaccurate in correcting for the initial errors. The result is the disorder of movement illustrated by Fig. 11.11, taken from Homes (1922), in which slow movements are 'jerky, intermittent, or clonic' (Fig. 11.11a), and rapid repetitive movements are 'slower and of smaller amplitude than normal' and 'are irregular in rate and range' (Fig. 11.11b).

On this evidence the human cerebellum appears to be required for the initiation of movement and its subsequent control. Another question is whether with practice the cerebellum gets better at executing such functions. As expressed by Eccles (1974) are 'we learning throughout our lifetime, getting a wiser and wiser cerebellum to enable us to make more graceful and efficient movements'? Eccles (1973) has championed the view that the cerebellum may contain a repository of learnt motor patterns, at the command of the cerebral cortex (see also Allan & Tsukahara 1974). Marr (1969), on the detailed findings of Eccles and his co-workers (1967), has

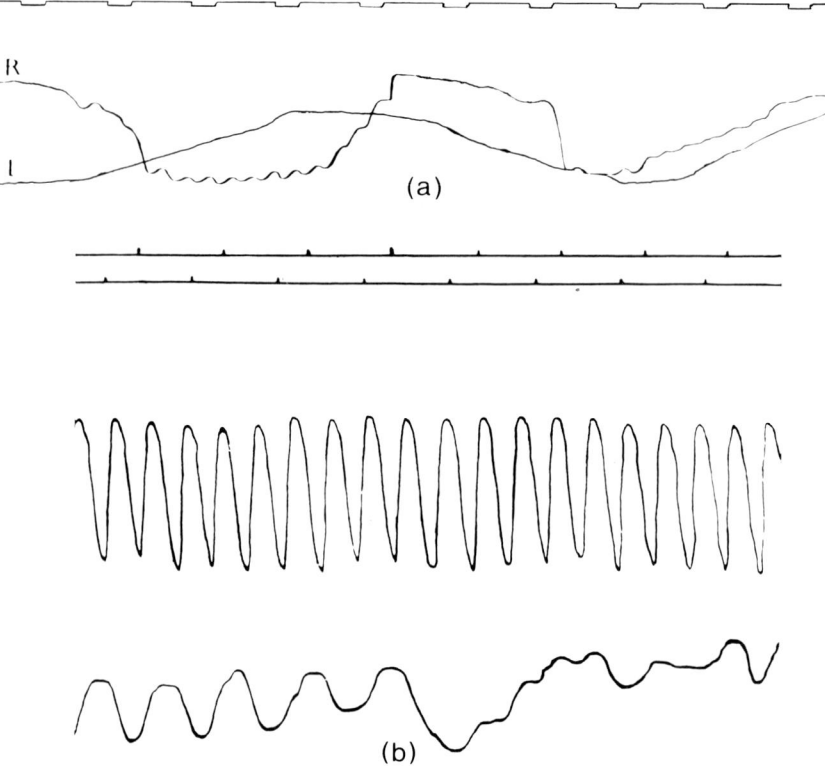

Fig. 11.11 Errors in movement in unilateral cerebellar ataxy as recorded by Holmes. (a) A patient with a right-sided cerebellar lesion flexing and extending each index finger at a slow and uniform rate. Holmes noted that 'the jerking and tremulous character of the movements of the right finger contrasts with the regular and uniform rate of those of the left'. (b) Tracings of rapid pronation and supination of each forearm. Holmes noted that 'the movements of the affected arm (below) were for a time regular though slower and of smaller amplitude that the normal, but grew irregular and the arm became more or less fixed in supination'. (From Holmes 1922, with permission.)

created a theoretical model of the cerebellum as a learning machine. While Marr's original theory is open to serious criticism, the notion that the cerebellum may learn to execute skilled movement is intriguing. In the course of our experiments, we have a singular experimental observation relevant to such a suggestion. In our early studies on servo responses of the long flexor of the human thumb, anaesthesia of the thumb regularly abolished or attenuated the long-latency reflexes to stretch, halt, or release during movement. Two of us (C.D.M. and P.A.M.) have now used our thumbs repeatedly for such experiments for close to six years. We now find that anaesthesia of the thumb no longer strikingly depresses such servo responses (Marsden, Merton & Morton 1976c).

The techniques available for study of human cerebellar function necessarily are indirect. However, very recently, the development of cerebellar stimulation as a treatment for intractible epilepsy has provided a new tool, giving the opportunity of direct access in conscious man. After implantation, the electrodes on the dorsal cerebellar surface are available to recording for a few days. Averaged evoked responses have been obtained to a biceps tendon tap, to median nerve stimulation at the wrist at group I strength, and to mechanical skin stimulation at the wrist, at latencies to the onset of the evoked wave of 13–15 msec, 25–30 msec, and 30–35 msec respectively. As yet, in the two patients studied, we have been unable to record cerebellar responses prior to voluntary movements, but responses some 100 msec after the onset of E.M.G. activity in the active muscle have been detected in one of the patients. It has not proved possible, yet, to identify cortical (scalp) evoked responses of short latency to cerebellar surface stimulation (stimulus artefact has proved a major problem). Such evoked responses have been identified from the contralateral hemisphere, but the latency to the earliest event is over 20 msec, and such waves appeared only at stimulus strengths sufficient to cause facial paraesthesia indicating excitation of the trigeminal nerve.

Electrical stimulation of the cerebellar surface may or may not alleviate epilepsy, but certainly would be expected to disrupt the normal activity of the cerebellar cortex. It is therefore very surprising that we have been unable to detect any effect of cerebellar cortical stimulation on the performance of tests that are regarded by neurologists as being tests of the integrity of the cerebellum and its connections. For example, unilateral cerebellar surface stimulation at 10 per sec or 70 per sec with pulses of 0·2 msec duration and at strengths up to those sufficient to cause dural pain and stimulation of cranial nerves as evidenced by facial paraesthesia and twitching, had no discernible effect on motor function. Muscle tone, deep tendon reflexes, accuracy and speed of rapid alternating limb movements, handwriting, reaction time, saccadic eye movements, physiological tremor and judgement of weights were unaltered during stimulation. Medial or bilateral cerebellar surface stimulation caused no detectable gait ataxia, nystagmus or disorder of speech. Pulses of this strength can hardly fail to stimulate the excitable elements of the cerebellar cortex near to the electrode. Current neurophysiology would suggest that effective surface stimulation at pulse rates of 10 per sec or above should block the greater part of spontaneous local Purkinje cell output. Some interference with cerebellar function would be expected, but none has been found. This disconcerting observation may be due to pre-existing cerebellar damage in the epileptic patients, but neither exhibited evidence of cerebellar deficit. Whatever the explanation, this clinical opportunity may allow novel means of studying cerebellar function in man.

References

ADAM J., MARSDEN C.D., MERTON P.A. & MORTON, H.B. (1976) The effect of lesions in the internal capsule and the sensorimotor cortex on servo action in the human thumb. *J. Physiol.* **274**, 27–28.

ALLEN G.I. & TSUKAHARA N. (1974) Cerebro-cerebellar communication systems. *Physiol. Rev.* **54**, 957–1006.

BRAITENBERG V. (1961) Functional interpretation of cerebellar histology. *Nature* **190**, 539–40.

BRAITENBERG V. (1967) Is the cerebellar cortex a biological clock in the millisecond range? *Prog. Brain. Res.* **25**, 334–46.

BROOKS V.B. (1975) Roles of cerebellum and basal ganglia in initiation and control of movements. *Canad. J. neurol. Sci.* **2**, 265–77.

CONRAD B., MEYER-LOHMANN J., MATSUNAMI K. & BROOKS V.B. (1975) Precentral unit activity following torque pulse injections into elbow movements. *Brain Res.* **94**, 219–36.

ECCLES J.C. (1973) The cerebellum as a computer; patterns in space and time. *J. Physiol.* **229**, 1–32.

ECCLES J.C. (1974) Conceptual models of neural organization. In: Szentágothai J. & Arbib M.A. (Eds) *Neurosci. Res. Prog. Bull.* **12**, 454.

ECCLES J.C., ITO M. & SZENTÁGOTHAI J. (1967). *The Cerebellum as a Neuronal Machine.* Springer-Verlag, New York.

EVARTS E.V. (1973) Motor cortex reflexes associated with learned movement. *Science* **179**, 501–3.

GARLAND H. & ANGEL R.W. (1971) Spinal and supraspinal factors in voluntary movement. *Exp. Neurol.* **33**, 343–50.

GILMAN S. (1969) The mechanism of cerebellar hypotonia: An experimental study in the monkey. *Brain* **92**, 621–38.

GILMAN S. (1970) The nature of cerebellar dyssynergia. In: Williams D. (Ed.) *Modern Trends in Neurology,* Vol. 5, pp. 60–79. Butterworths, London.

GILMAN S. (1975) Primate models of postural disorders. In: Meldrum B.S. & Marsden C.D. (Eds) *Primate Models of Neurological Disorders. Advances in Neurology* **10**, 55–76.

GILMAN S. & DENNY-BROWN D. (1966) Disorders of movement and behaviour following dorsal column lesions. *Brain* **89**, 397–418.

HALLETT M., SHAHANI B.T. & YOUNG R.R. (1975a) EMG analysis of stereotyped voluntary movements in man. *J. Neurol. Neurosurg. Psychiat.* **38**, 1154–62.

HALLETT M., SHAHANI B.T. & YOUNG R.R. (1975b) EMG analysis of patients with cerebellar deficits. *J. Neurol. Neurosurg. Psychiat.* **38**, 1163–9.

HAMMOND P.H. (1960) An experimental study of servo action in human muscular control. *Proc. 3rd Int. Conf. Med. Electron.* pp. 190–9. Institute of Electrical Engineers, London.

HOLMES G. (1917) The symptoms of acute cerebellar injuries due to gunshot injuries. *Brain* **40**, 461–535.

HOLMES G. (1922) Clinical symptoms of cerebellar diseases (The Croonian Lectures). *Lancet* **i**, 1177–82, 1231–7, and **ii**, 59–65, 111–5.

HOPF H., LOWITZSCH K. & SCHLEGEL H.J. (1973) Central versus proprioceptive influences in brisk voluntary movements. In: Desmedt J.E. (Ed.) *New Developments in Electromyography and Clinical Neurophysiology,* Vol. 3, pp. 273–6. Karger, Basel.

KORNHUBER H.H. (1971) Motor functions of cerebellum and basal ganglia: The cerebello-cortical saccadic (ballistic) clock, the cerebellonuclear hold regulator, and the basal ganglia ramp (voluntary speed smooth movement) generator. *Kybernetik* **8**, 157–62.

LEE R.G. & TATTON W.G. (1975) Motor responses to sudden limb displacements in primates with specific CNS lesions and in human patients with motor system disorders. *Canad. J. neurol. Sci.* **2**, 285–93.

LEMON R.N. & PORTER R. (1976) Natural afferent input to movement-related neurones in monkey pre-central cortex. *J. Physiol.* **258**, 18.

LIU C.N. & CHAMBERS W.W. (1971) A study of cerebellar dyskinesia in the bilaterally deafferented forelimbs of the monkey. *Acta Neurol. Exptl.* **31**, 263–89.

LUCIER G.E., RÜEGG D.G. & WIESENDANGER M. (1975) Responses of neurones in motor cortex and in area 3a to controlled stretches of forelimb muscles in Cebus monkeys. *J. Physiol* **251**, 833–53.

MARR D. (1969) A theory of cerebellar cortex. *J. Physiol* **202**, 437–70.

MARSDEN C.D., MERTON P.A. & MORTON H.B. (1972) Servo action in human voluntary movement. *Nature* **238**, 140–3.

MARSDEN C.D., MERTON P.A. & MORTON H.B. (1973) Is the human stretch reflex cortical rather than spinal? *Lancet* **i**, 759–61.

MARSDEN C.D., MERTON P.A. & MORTON H.B. (1976a) Servo action in the human thumb. *J. Physiol.* **257**, 1–44.

MARSDEN C.D., MERTON P.A. & MORTON H.B. (1976b) Stretch reflex and servo action in a variety of human muscles. *J. Physiol.* **259**, 531–560.

MARSDEN C.D., MERTON P.A. & MORTON H.B. (1976c) Anaesthesia and servo action in the human thumb. *J. Physiol.* (in press).

MILNER-BROWN S.H., GIRVIN J.P. & BROWN W.F. (1975) The effects of motor cortical stimulation on the excitability of spinal motoneurons in man. *Canad. J. neurol. Sci.* **2**, 245–53.

MURPHY J.T., KWAN H.C., MACKAY W.A. & WONG Y.C. (1975) Physiological basis of cerebellar dysmeria. *Canad. J. neurol. Sci.* **2**, 279–84.

PHILLIPS C.G. (1969) Motor apparatus of the baboon's hand. *Proc. R. Soc. B.* **173**, 141–74.

PHILLIPS C.G., POWELL T.P.S. & WIESENDANGER M. (1971) Projection of low-threshold muscle afferents of hand and forearm to area 3a of baboon's cortex. *J. Physiol.* **217**, 419–46.

TATTON W.G., FORNER S.D., GERSTEIN G.L., CHAMBERS W.W. & LIU C.N. (1975) The effect of postcentral cortical lesions on motor responses to sudden upper limb displacement in monkeys. *Brain Res.* **96**, 108–13.

UPTON A.R.M., McCOMAS A.J. & SICA R.E.P. (1971) Potentiation of 'late' responses evoked in muscles during effort. *J. Neurol. Neurosurg. Psychiat.* **34**, 699–711.

WACHOLDER K. & ALTENBURGER H. (1926) Beiträge zur Physiologie der willkürlichen Bewegung. 10. Einzelbewegungen. *Pflügers Archiv für Physiol des Menschen und Tiere* **214**, 642–61.

WIESENDANGER M. (1973) Input from muscle and cutaneous nerves of the hand and forearm to neurons of the precentral gyrus of baboons and monkeys. *J. Physiol.* **228**, 203–19.

RECONSIDERING THE 'ALPHA-GAMMA SWITCH' IN CEREBELLAR ACTION

RAGNAR GRANIT

Sir Gordon Holmes' summaries of 1922 in *The Lancet* and of 1939 in *Brain* discuss all of the cerebellar deficiencies seen in the clinic but I shall deal mainly with his fundamental ideas on hypotonia and its relevance for the rest of the symptomatology. I regard my particular task to be an attempt to try out present-day notions on motor control, as derived from physiological experimentation, on this aspect of his keen analytical thinking. Holmes himself did what was possible to do with the physiological knowledge of his own time but some advance has taken place since then justifying a renewed effort in the same direction.

One of Holmes' leading ideas was that full recognition of the part that tone plays in both active and passive attitudes and in movement has cut down enormously the number of special explanations needed for the medley of symptoms observed and described. This general conclusion can hardly be doubted. All movements are accompanied by tonic adjustments whose absence must be reflected in different clinical tests and in the patient's behaviour.

Unilateral hypotonia

Of singular importance were the observations on small, circumscribed lesions, as from gunshot wounds, because they showed so clearly that hypotonia ensued in all the muscles of the side on which the injury was inflicted. The contralateral side provided a valuable control for this conclusion. A total ipsilateral hypotonia after a very small wound would hardly seem possible unless the cerebellar signals converge towards a common site representing an integrated programme for the control and maintenance of basic tone. As such it seems reasonable to postulate a need for a mechanism correlating tonic adjustments of arm, trunk and leg in response to a shift of the centre of gravity. The common governor would be expected to exhibit a neatly balanced state of left–right equilibrium, controlled by proprioceptive and skin impulses, and hence to be highly sensitive to any asymmetry in this input.

The results of local lesions of the fastigial nucleus in the decerebrate cat suggest a paradigm that has been independently established in three laboratories (Chambers & Sprague 1955, Moruzzi & Pompeiano 1956, 1957, Stella *et al* 1955). A unilateral lesion in the rostral part of the *n. fastigii* produced an ipsilateral hypotonia, seen also in the chronic state (Batini & Pompeiano 1957). If the lesion was made in the caudal pole of the nucleus, crossed atonia was obtained; these results have been well reviewed by Dow and Moruzzi (1958). They imply that a balanced equilibrium between the rostral and caudal poles of this nucleus regulates tone in compensation for gravitational asymmetries.

The commonly seen statement that hypotonia is found only in primates and man, because it requires the large neocerebellar hemispheres of higher species, is thus shown to be without foundation. What matters is to select the right kind of lesion but it is, of course, not possible to compare cat and man, site for site. The upright posture has required readjustments of control so that, for instance, the vestibular influence on tone is likely to be relatively more important in the cat. The gist of my argument is that it may well prove profitable to think of extensive hypotonias from small lesions in the terms suggested by the results quoted, even though the corresponding symptoms in man are due to interference with the lateral lobes (Holmes). It presupposes that the dentate nucleus in man is designed on the same principles as the *n. fastigii* of the cat (for anatomical details, see Jansen & Brodal 1954, Evarts & Thach 1969).

Tonic and phasic motoneurons

A brief summary (taken from Granit 1970, 1972) of results covered by this subtitle should in the first instance draw attention to the fact that tonic or maintained motor activity must be restricted to muscle units actually capable of sustaining it. These units are mostly the first to be recruited into action; they produce modest amounts of force and this only at slow speed of contraction; they are provided with a dense capillary network and are richly supplied with oxidative enzymes. When greater force at higher velocity is required, the pale muscle units take over. Their tension drops quickly suggesting phasic types of employment. The metabolism of these fibres is based on anaerobic glycolysis. In man as in the cat there are likely to be muscle fibres intermediate in properties between the two main types, nowadays spoken of as Type I and Type II, roughly corresponding to tonic and phasic respectively. (For distribution of these types in human muscles, see Johnson *et al* 1973.)

The animal work has shown that motoneurons and muscle fibres are matched for cooperation. Large motoneurons, whose firing rates vary a great deal with input strength, send their axons to phasic muscle units; small motoneurons, chiefly governed by their recruitment threshold, innervate the slow muscle units and are relatively independent of input strength for their firing rates (cf. Gydikow & Kosarov 1973, on man). Partly their stable firing frequencies are membrane characteristics, as proved by intracellular transmembrane stimulation (Kernell 1966), partly it is upheld by the spinal mechanism of recurrent inhibition which acts more strongly in the direction phasic–tonic than the other way round (cf. Granit 1975). Clearly, since the tonic muscles contract slowly, it makes sense to find them run by their motoneurons at slow stimulus rates.

As to the other species of motoneurons, the fusimotor gamma cells, there is no reason to suspect that man differs from other mammals in which the gamma loop plays a prominent role in postural adjustments. It then acts in conjunction with the alpha output by a mechanism of alpha-gamma linkage. For the spinal cord of the cat we now possess wiring diagrams illustrating such linkages by relevant experiments. In man voluntary activity has been studied a great deal since the first reports by Hagbarth and Vallbo in 1967 and 1968 on microneuronographic recording from human nerves. Both single-fibre and multi-fibre records are available. Agreement prevails on the fact that in all voluntary contractions studies the muscle spindles are co-activated across the loop by alpha-gamma linkage. The effects are recorded from spindle fibres and so it is unknown to what an extent there is subthreshold gamma activity keeping the spindles under slight stretch prepared for action.

Hagbarth and his colleagues at Uppsala disagree with Struppler in Munich and Szumski in Richmond (Virg.) on the question of independent spindle activation in muscles distant from the ones voluntarily activated as, for instance, in the Jendrassik manoeuvre (Burg *et al* 1974, Hagbarth *et al* 1975*a*). When spindle activation is seen in this case, Hagbarth and his colleagues maintain that it, too, is due to co-activation by alpha-gamma linkage and not to selective mobilization of spindles alone. This is because they always find minute muscular contractions in the distant muscle from which the spindle impulses are recorded.

The diagnosis of hypotonia

'It is obvious', says Holmes (1939), 'that the hypotonic muscles do not respond by contractions to stretch suddenly imposed upon them as readily as the normal'. This statement is in perfect agreement with the notion of a suppression of co-activated tonic alpha and gamma motoneurons. If the suppression of the tonic motoneurons were a pure alpha symptom, there is no reason why a remaining normal gamma activity could not depolarize the motoneurons to a maintained firing level by sensitizing the spindles to stretching. When spindles are activated, the tendon jerk is modified by the so-called 'shortening reaction' which is absent in the hypotonic limb whose knee jerk is of the pendular type. The shortening reaction is a kind of spindle 'rebound' caused by a re-excitation of these receptors when the muscle is pulled out in the relaxation phase (Granit *et al* 1966). If the spindles are slack they are incapable of overcoming the combined effects of after-hyperpolarization and the recurrent inhibition following the jerk. The shortening reaction therefore disappears.

The hypotonia would necessarily have to be first visible in the low-threshold tonic motoneurons which activated by alpha-gamma linkage produce little but well-maintained tension. Purely passive spindles would not be able to support a sustained state of activity of these motoneurons, unless the muscle in question were much extended so as to produce by external stretch what is meant to be produced internally by the gamma motor fibres. The symptom that in the tonic motoneurons emerges as hypotonia would in their phasic partners betray itself as a deficiency of muscular force and some slowing of the force that is left. Luciani's symptom of asthenia from his well-known 'triad' would seem to correspond to this physiological postulate. Holmes found it in some patients and not in others and remarks that it may not be a primary effect.

The phasic motoneurons are perhaps not regularly subjected to testing at the necessary level of force required for their mobilization. In this matter I can have no opinion of my own. It seems to me that there are two alternatives. Either the hypotonic symptom—or rather, the deficiency behind it—is selectively restricted to the alpha-gamma linkage of the tonic motoneurons or else it includes that of all motoneurons. If the latter is believed to be the case, then why should the symptom in phasic motoneurons turn up as a hypotonia when these motoneurons do not participate significantly in postural tonic adjustments? Good voluntary contractions would have to be used to activate them. *A priori* one would like to think of the deficiency as a loss of facilitation for *both* phasic and tonic alpha-gamma linked motoneurons and to attribute the manifestations of hypotonia and asthenia to post-cerebellar differences between the properties of the two executives, as described above.

A patient, says Holmes, tries to compensate for the hypotonia by voluntary muscular contractions, but 'cannot supplement efficiently the loss of postural tone (which) is a necessary adjunct to those muscular contractions'. This is seen clearly when a patient with a unilateral lesion is requested to extend both arms horizontally. The affected arm drops more rapidly and evenly than its partner. This test makes use of the very kind of voluntary contraction that now has been proved to be executed in alpha-gamma linkage. The weight of the arm is perhaps not greater than that which tonic musculature alone could cope with for a while, provided that the spindles were activated to a normal degree through the gamma loop. The experimental evidence (to be discussed below) points to reduced spindle activity in cerebellar disease. Hence it appears that the average depolarizing pressure on the motoneurons is too low to support the 'maintenance' function to which the spindles by their maintained discharge add so much. Once alpha-gamma linkage is present, the most probable interpretation of Holmes' test is that the two excitatory routes, the indirect and direct one, have shared the same fate, common also for the two kinds of alpha motoneurons.

Normal cerebellar contribution to tone

The cat, used so much in this field of study, has a strong component of vestibular tone. As to cerebellar tone, the old view based on work with the decerebrate preparation (Dow & Moruzzi 1958) implied that its anterior lobe inhibits a postural tone facilitated by the efferents from the nuclei (*n. fastigii* and *n. interpositus*). This general explanation has not been superceded by anything better but we are somewhat better informed about the mechanisms engaged in preserving nuclear activity.

Circuit analysis, largely by the work of Masao Ito and his colleagues, has since shown that the cerebellar afferents excite the nuclei by collaterals on their way to the similarly excited Purkinje cells. The latter in their turn inhibit the nuclear discharge set up in this manner (summarized in Eccles *et al* 1967). The nuclear efferent activity is thus counteracted from the same original sources which inhibit it across the Purkinje cells. The balanced net effect in the resting animal emerges in the irregular 'spontaneous' discharge from the nuclei (cf. Thach 1972). If this organization were designed for symmetry, input and output would cancel out and the nuclear discharge would remain constant. Nothing seems less likely. It was pointed out above that the rostral and caudal portions of the cat's *n. fastigii* control tone on the ipsi- and contralateral sides respectively and thus are played out against each other in asymmetrical postures forced on the animal by gravity.

Considering such facts it indeed seems most likely that a cerebellar nuclear organization operates like a pair of scales balancing out peripheral, cerebral and olivary input messages. The modulating inhibition shaping the nuclear efferent (output) message would come from the Purkinje cells. Since in monkey and man the lateral lobes, and hence the dentate nucleus, are preponderant in the symptom of hypotonia, cerebellar regulation of tone has a dominating cerebral component across the thalamic path to the motor cortex. This may be regarded as but another example of the increased encephalization of function that accompanies the extension of the cerebral cortex upwards in the phylum.

As to the motor cortex itself, recent evidence from single-cell work on the monkey by Evarts (1967), since confirmed by Takahashi (1965) and by Kostiuk and Vasilenko (1968), has shown that there are two types of cell: small ones which discharge tonically with but slight modulation in movement, larger ones which fire at high rates in advance of, and in conjunction with, the phasic movements for which the monkeys were trained. The small cells may well be the ones that under cerebellar facilitation produce the tonic discharge in the pyramidal tract that long ago was noted by Adrian and Moruzzi (1939); it was also shown by Tower (1940) that pyramidotomy and cerebellectomy produced similar types of hypotonia and this theme has since been developed by Gilman (see below), in whose papers the historical development of this subject will be found. All recent work confirms the statement by Sarah Tower, that the pyramidal tract 'is organized in complexity to match virtually the full range of activity, from simple tonic functions wherein it merely assists, to complicated performance which are primarily its responsibility' (Tower, p. 88).

Switches in alpha-gamma linkages

In our early work on supraspinal gamma control (Granit & Kaada 1952) it excited us greatly to find in the cat that the well-known inhibition of decerebrate rigidity to stimulation of the anterior lobe was accompanied by a corresponding silence of the gastrocnemius extensor spindles that had been isolated in thin dorsal root filaments. The relaxation of the main muscle ought really to have excited the spindle by pulling upon it, the way it does in the relaxation phase of the knee jerk, discussed above. Such remote effects of cooperation were new and striking at that time. When in our later work (Granit et al 1955) this portion of the cerebellum was cooled or destroyed, there often ensued the great increase in rigidity, described by Pollock and Davis (1930). However, in these animals the spindle, so far from being coactivated, was selectively suppressed, that is, rendered passive because of removal of gamma support. The idea of some kind of a 'switch' capable of throwing the motor organization into either the alpha or the gamma path was suggested to explain the failure of a coactivation that already at the time seemed to be the most likely normal kind of spindle behaviour. No attempt was made to elaborate this notion into a finished hypothesis.

In the last twenty years much work has been devoted to the interneurons biasing neural responses in opposite or similar directions, and we can now think of such 'switches' in more realistic terms. The best known ones in the spinal cord are those centred around reciprocally innervated limb muscles which, alternatively, also have to be able to act conjointly. The proprioceptive and supraspinal influences make use of the Ia inhibitory interneuron and the Renshaw cell of the recurrent path from alpha motoneurons (Hultborn *et al* 1971a, b, c) to switch from reciprocal to synergetic action or to modulate either or both these modes of behaviour. A number of reliable wiring diagrams explain these 'switchings'. Other examples show that in the spinal cat the static fusimotor gamma fibres are 'switched' off while the dynamic ones keep on firing (Alnaes *et al* 1965). It has long been known that there is no clasp-knife effect in the Davis–Pollock type of alpha cat. This is good evidence for the conclusion that the spindle mechanism is selectively suppressed as we had found it to be (Granit *et al* 1955).

The mechanisms in the spinal cord employ postsynaptic inhibition, but, fundamentally, processes such as presynaptic inhibition should not be excluded. The term 'switch' itself has rightly gone out of fashion wherever it is known by what means a path is closed or opened. It can be used only in a figurative sense to describe unexplained observations.

Some findings by Gilman and his co-workers from experiments on monkeys are of interest in this connexion (Gilman 1969, Gilman & Marco 1971, Gilman *et al* 1971a, b, Gilman 1975). These authors have taken the trouble of studying individual spindle afferents from the gastrocnemius before and after cerebellectomy (sometimes unilateral) and after pyramidotomy and generally found their responsiveness to stretching depressed. Studies were conducted also on the hypotonia following unilateral ablation of areas 4 and 6 in the monkey (Gilman *et al* 1974). Again the result was a diminished spindle response to stretch. Once diminution of a spindle response had been established by interference with the motor areas or by pyramidal section, bilateral removal of the cerebellar hemispheres and the dentate nucleus 'did not alter substantially the responses of these units' (Gilman *et al* 1971a).

The final result of these laborious experiments thus supported the idea that the cerebellar depression of spindle sensitivity originates in the motor cortex whose normal tonic activity is dependent on an intact cerebello-thalamo-cortical path. This is the path that, beginning in the lateral lobes, chiefly engages the dentate nucleus, to a lesser extent the others (Jansen & Brodal 1954, Evarts & Thach 1969). By cooling the VL nucleus of the thalamus to about $-20°$, a depression of spindle activity was found similar to that obtained by the other operations mentioned above. The loss of spindle sensitivity in all these experiments was not complete, as suggested by subsequent deafferentations.

All these results imply that the alphas and gammas are linked in the motor area which for normal function requires cerebellar facilitation. The linkage itself could be explained by the simple model in Fig. 12.1 showing a thalamic fibre branching to alpha and gamma neurons in the cortex. However, it is too simple for our purpose, which is to include in the circuit an explanation of those alpha rigidities which are combined with heavy spindle suppression (Granit *et al* 1955). The diagram also fails to account for the

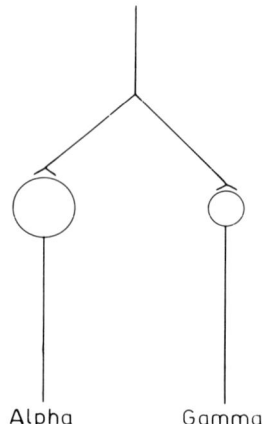

Fig. 12.1   Basic circuit of coactivation by alpha-gamma linkage.

hypertonia that Gilman's group noted after a couple of months of recovery in their monkeys, because in these cases there was no accompanying supernormal spindle activity. Whatever the nature of the compensatory process responsible for this hypertonic state, one would, naturally, prefer to explain similar asymmetries of alpha-gamma co-activation by a diagram capable of taking care of all of them.

Since recurrent fibres are known from the motor area (Ramón y Cajal 1911) and cortical recurrent inhibition has been many times described, ever since it was first seen by Phillips (1959), there is every reason to design our circuit on the principles known from extensive work on the spinal cord. There would then be a recurrent interneuron, corresponding to the Renshaw cell, it would have at its disposal some 70% of the motor cells, the rest would be free. The gamma neurons would lack recurrent fibres of their own as would also some of the alphas. These postulates are incorporated in the diagrams a, b and c of Fig. 12.2. By a and b alone, alpha hypertonia and an alpha type of rigidity would occur in response to an abnormal facilitation by release of the cerebello-thalamic input. Adding c to the circuits would emphasize this effect. A diminished facilitation would clearly cause linked hypotonia.

We have good reasons for thinking of alpha and gamma activities being linked in several sites but my interpretation has been designed to take care of the experiments referring to the related clinical symptoms of hypotonia and asthenia. It would not be difficult to devise explanations based on wholly independent alpha and gamma paths but present experience of microrecording from afferents in man would not support it. Vallbo (1971) found co-activation even in the fast, voluntary twitches of the finger muscles and it is preserved in the tremor of patients with Parkinsonism (Hagbarth *et al* 1975b). One of the rare exceptions refers to clonus in spastic patients

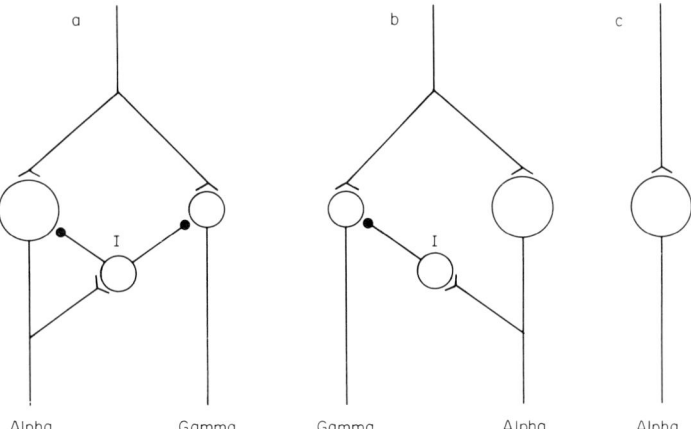

Fig. 12.2 Complex circuits, based on properties of motoneurons of limb muscles, to explain the observations mentioned in text. A, B and C all supposed to operate in parallel.

(Hagbarth *et al* 1975b, Szumski *et al* 1974); the spindles responded passively to stretch in the phase of relaxation. It was thus an alpha clonus similar to the one seen in precollicular cats (Granit 1959). In Fig. 12.2—as stated—the asymmetry of the alpha-gamma linkage would favour alpha dominance as a consequence of a high degree of facilitation. The opposite effect, such as the strong gamma-spindle activity in the decerebrate cat, has not yet been found in man.

Significance of diminished spindle output

By microrecording in man Hagbarth *et al* (1970) showed that lidocaine infiltration of the nerve in order to block the fusimotor gamma fibres produced a very marked reduction of contractile force that could be restored to normal by vibratory stimulation of the spindles. This is a good imitation of the symptom of asthenia. Yet only the gamma component of the link was removed! A diminution of spindle activity would also reduce load compensation by the stretch reflex, the more so, as in cerebellar hypotonia the small alpha motoneurons sustaining it likewise would be depressed. In recent years, the significance of the large spindle afferents for the co-operating Ia inhibitory and recurrent circuits has become greatly clarified (for a simplified presentation, see Granit 1975). These inter-dependent circuits serve stabilization of both flexor and extensor contractions and act to coordinate central and peripheral influences governing reciprocal action and its opposite, sc. joint action. In this system, too there are likely to be segmental repercussions from spindle depressions.

In addition the spindles feed back information to higher centres, particularly to the cerebellum, and there their dynamic sensitivity may be important in timing. However, we do not possess the information required for interpreting any of these feedback functions.

All this should not be interpreted as a plea for the spindle as a Jack-of-all-trades in cerebellar symptomatology. Indeed, on the notion of alpha-gamma linkage, this seems excluded (cf. also Gilman 1972). Rather is it my intention to emphasize the difficulty in interpreting all its roles in the complex circuits connecting the cerebellum with the rest of the nervous system. 'Coordination is the function of the whole and of every part of the nervous system', said Holmes (1939) quoting Hughlings Jackson and, if this can be accepted, the spindle must be held to add its particular contribution at several sites. But at the moment it is only possible to make sense of its role in a hypotonia and an asthenia based on alpha-gamma linkage.

It has not been possible to discuss the interesting work of Vernon Brooks and his colleagues (summary by Brooks 1975) on cooling the dentate nucleus nor that of Carlo Terzuolo's group (e.g. Terzuolo *et al* 1973) on a kind of 'brake' function lacking in cerebellar patients and including flexor–extensor coordination. I can only mention them briefly as important approaches to the role of the cerebellum in the initiation of motor acts and in controlling their speed.

Summary

The clinical symptoms of hypotonia and asthenia have been considered from the point of view of present-day physiology. Experimental support has been sought for the following statements:

(i) The finding by Holmes that small unilateral lesions produce extensive ipsilateral hypotonia has been explained by the hypothesis of a right side–left side equilibrium centre in the dentate nucleus. The evidence is based on the discovery of such a centre in the *n. fastigii* of the cat.

(ii) Hypotonia and asthenia have here been regarded as essentially identical deficiencies of a cerebellar facilitation operating an alpha-gamma linked site in the motor cortex. The early recruiting small, tonic motoneurons and slow motor units are held to be dominant in hypotonia; to the larger phasic motoneurons, naturally incapable of sustained action, has been ascribed the symptom of asthenia. Thus the differentiation of these two symptoms produced by a loss of cerebellar facilitation is regarded as postcerebellar and dependent on the properties of the segmental and peripheral executives.

(iii) A wiring diagram (Fig. 12.2) has been designed to take care of alpha-gamma linked effects in cerebellar symptomatology.

References

ADRIAN E.D. & MORUZZI G. (1939) Impulses in the pyramidal tract. *J. Physiol.* **67**, 153–99.

ALNAES E., JANSEN J.K.S. & RUDJORD T. (1965) Fusimotor activity in the spinal cat. *Acta physiol. scand.* **63**, 197–212.

BATINI C. & POMPEIANO O. (1957) Chronic fastigial lesions and their compensation in the cat. *Arch. ital. Biol.* **95**, 147–65.

BROOKS V.B. (1975) Roles of cerebellum and basal ganglia in initiation and control of movement. *J. Canad. Sci. Neurobiol.* August No., 265–77.

BURG D., SZUMSKI A.J., STRUPPLER A. & VELHO F. (1974) Assessment of fusimotor contribution to reflex reinforcement in humans. *J. Neurol. Neurosurg. Psychiat.* **37**, 1012–21.

CHAMBERS W.W. & SPRAGUE J.M. (1955) Functional localization in the cerebellum. II. Somatotopic organization in cortex and nuclei. *Arch. Neurol. Psychiat.* (Chicago) **74**, 653–80.

DOW R.S. & MORUZZI G. (1958) *The Physiology and Pathology of the Cerebellum.* University of Minnesota Press, Minneapolis.

ECCLES J.C., ITO M. & SZENTÁGOTHAI J. (1967) *The Cerebellum as a Neuronal Machine.* Springer-Verlag, Berlin.

EVARTS E.V. (1967) Representation of movements and muscles by pyramidal tract neurons of the precentral motor cortex. In: Yahr M.D. & Purpura D. (Eds) *Neurophysiological Basis of Normal and Abnormal Motor Activities,* pp. 215–51. Raven Press, New York.

EVARTS E.V. & THACH W.T. (1969) Motor mechanisms of the CNS: Cerebrocerebellar interrelations. *Ann. Rev. Physiol.* **31**, 451–98.

GILMAN S. (1969) The mechanism of cerebellar hypotonia. *Brain* **92**, 621–38.

GILMAN S. (1972) The nature of cerebellar dyssynergia. In: Williams D. (Ed.) *Modern Trends in Neurology,* Ch. 4 pp. 60–79. Butterworths, London.

GILMAN S. (1975) Primate models of postural disorders. In: Meldrun B.S. & Marsden C.D. (Eds) *Advances in Neurology,* pp. 55–76. Raven Press, New York.

GILMAN S., LIEBERMAN J.S. & MARCO L.A. (1974) Spinal mechanisms underlying the effects of unilateral ablation of areas 4 and 6 in monkeys. *Brain* **97**, 49–64.

GILMAN S. & MARCO L.A. (1971) Effects of medullary pyramidotomy in the monkey. I. *Brain* **94**, 495–514.

GILMAN S., MARCO L.A. & EBEL H.C. (1971a) Effects of medullary pyramidotomy in the monkey. II. *Brain* **94**, 515–30.

GILMAN S., MARCO L.A. & LIEBERMAN J.S. (1971b) Experimental hypertonia in the monkey: Interruption of pyramidal-extrapyramidal cortical projections. *Trans. Amer. Neurol. Assn.* **96**, 162–8.

GRANIT R. (1959) Observations on clonus in the cat's soleus muscle. *Ann. Facult. Med. Montevideo* **44**, 305–10.

GRANIT R. (1970) *The Basis of Motor Control.* Academic Press, London & New York.

GRANIT R. (1972) *Mechanisms Regulating the Discharge of Motoneurons.* Liverpool University Press, Liverpool.

GRANIT R. (1975) The functional role of the muscle spindles—facts and hypotheses. Hughlings Jackson Lecture. *Brain* **98**, 531–536.

GRANIT R. & KAADA B.R. (1952) Influence of stimulation of central nervous structures on muscle spindles in cat. *Acta physiol. scand.* **27**, 130–60.

GRANIT R., HOLMGREN B. & MERTON P.A. (1955) The two routes for excitation of muscle and their subservience to the cerebellum. *J. Physiol.* **130**, 213–24.

GRANIT R., KELLERTH J.O. & SZUMSKI A.J. (1966) Intracellular autogenetic effects of muscular contraction on extensor motoneurones. The silent period. *J. Physiol.* **182**, 484–503.

GYDIKOV A. & KOSAROV D. (1973) Physiological characteristics of the tonic and phasic motor units in human muscles. In: Gydikov A.A., Tankov N.T.

& Kosarov D.S. (Eds) *Motor Control,* pp. 75–94. Plenum Press, New York.

HAGBARTH K.-E., HONGELL A. & WALLIN B.G. (1970) The effect of gamma fibre block on afferent muscle nerve activity during voluntary contractions. *Acta physiol. scand.* **79,** 27A–28A.

HAGBARTH K.-E. & VALLBO Å.B. (1967) Mechanoreceptor activity recorded percutaneously with semi-microelectrodes in human peripheral nerves. *Acta physiol. scand.* **69,** 121–2.

HAGBARTH K.-E. & VALLBO Å.B. (1968) Discharge characteristics of human muscular afferents during muscle stretch and contraction. *Exp. Neurol.* **22,** 674–94.

HAGBARTH K.-E., WALLIN G., BURKE D. & LÖFSTEDT L. (1975a) Effects of Jendrassik manoeuvre on muscle spindle activity in man. *J. Neurol. Neurosurg. Psychiat.* **38,** 1143–53.

HAGBARTH K.-E., WALLIN G., LÖFSTEDT L. & AQUILONIUS S.-M. (1975) Muscle spindle activity in alternating tremor of Parkinsonism and in clonus. *J. Neurol. Neurosurg. Psychiat.* **38,** 636–41.

HOLMES G. (1922) The Croonian lectures on the clinical symptoms of cerebellar disease. *Lancet* **202,** 1177–82; 1231–7.

HOLMES G. (1922) The Croonian lectures on the clinical symptoms of cerebellar disease. *Lancet* **203,** 59–65; 111–15.

HOLMES G. (1939) The cerebellum of man. *Brain* **62,** 1–30.

HULTBORN H., JANKOWSKA E. & LINDSTRÖM S. (1971a) Recurrent inhibition from motor axon collaterals of transmission in the Ia inhibiting pathway to motoneurons. *J. Physiol.* **215,** 591–612.

HULTBORN H., JANOWSKA I. & LINDSTRÖM S. (1971b) Recurrent inhibition of interneurones monosynaptically activated from group I afferents. *J. Physiol.* **215,** 613–36.

HULTBORN H., JANOWSKA E. & LINDSTRÖM S. (1971c) Relative contribution from different nerves to recurrent depression of Ia IPSPs in motoneurones. *J. Physiol.* **215,** 637–64.

JANSEN J. & BRODAL A. (1954) *Aspects of Cerebellar Anatomy.* J. G. Tanum, Oslo.

JOHNSON M.A., POLGAR J., WEIGHTMAN D.

& APPLETON D. (1973) Data on the distribution of fibre types in thirty-six human muscles. *J. neurol. Sci.* **18,** 111–29.

KERNELL D. (1966) Input resistance, electrical excitability, and size of ventral horn cells in the cat spinal cord. *Science* **152,** 1637–40.

KOSTIUK P.G. & VASILENKO D.A. (1968) Transformation of cortical motor signals in spinal cord. *Proc. IEEE* **56,** 1049–58.

MORUZZI G. & POMPEIANO O. (1956) Crossed fastigal influences on decerebrate rigidity. *J. comp. Neurol.* **106,** 371–92.

MORUZZI G. & POMPEIANO O. (1957) Inhibitory mechanisms underlying the collapse of decerebrate rigidity after unilateral fastigal lesions. *J. comp. Neurol.* **107,** 1–25.

PHILLIPS C.G. (1959) Actions of antidromic pyramidal volleys on single Betz cells in the cat. *Quart. J. exp. Physiol.* **44,** 1–25.

POLLOCK L.J. & DAVIS L. (1930) The reflex activities of a decerebrate animal. *J. comp. Neurol.* **50,** 377–411.

RAMÓN Y CAJAL S. (1911) *Histologie du système nerveux.* Vols. I & II. Trans. L. Azoulay. Instituto Ramón y Cajal, Madrid.

STELLA G., ZATTI P. & SPERTI L. (1955) Decerebrate rigidity in forelegs after deafferentation and spinal transection in dogs with chronic lesions in different parts of the cerebellum. *Am. J. Physiol.* **181,** 230–4.

SZUMSKI A.J., BURG D., STRUPPLER A. & VELHO F. (1974) Activity of muscle spindles during muscle twitch and clonus in normal and spastic human subjects. *EEG Clin. Neurophysiol.* **37,** 589–97.

TAKAHASHI K. (1965) Slow and fast groups of pyramidal tract cells and their respective membrane properties. *J. Neurophysiol.* **28,** 908–24.

TERZUOLO C.A., SOECHTING J.F. & VIVIANI P. (1973) Studies on the control of some simple motor tasks. I. Relations between parameters of movement on EMG activities. *Brain Res.* **58,** 212–16.

THACH W.T. (1972) Cerebellar output: properties, synthesis and uses. *Brain Res.* **40,** 89–97.

TOWER S.S. (1940) Pyramidal lesions in the monkey. *Brain* **63,** 36–90.

VALLBO Å.B. (1971) Muscle spindle reponse at the onset of isometric voluntary contractions in man. Time difference between fusimotor and skeletomotor effects. *J. Physiol.* **318,** 405–31.

PERSISTENCE OF STRETCH REFLEXES FOLLOWING CEREBELLAR ABLATION
—AND—
A RESONANCE THEORY OF CEREBELLAR FUNCTION

E. GEOFFREY WALSH

Introduction

In the human being, lesions of the cerebellum commonly give rise to hypotonia. Recently, some neurosurgeons have been undertaking the operation of dentatotomy for spastic and dystonia states. The results, recently reviewed by Hitchcock (1973), show that the predominant result here too is a reduction of tone. In some animals, however, the effects of damage to the cerebellum is to increase pre-existing rigidity caused by decerebration (as shown by Bremer & Ley (1972) in the pigeon). Furthermore, the anaemic method of decerebration, where the basilar artery is ligated in the cat, gives rise to a very stiff animal, evidently because there is infarction of the anterior part of the cerebellum (Pollock & Davis 1930). The rigidity of the decerebrate animal is caused by excessive action of stretch reflexes, but what is the cause of the rigidity of the decerebrate–decerebellate animal? It has been hitherto generally accepted that this is an alpha rigidity. The cerebellar lesion is regarded as inactivating the stretch reflex at the same time as it increases the drive to the motor neurones (vide Pollock & Davis 1931, Granit *et al* 1955). I wish to describe experiments undertaken with Professor W. E. Watson which show that this explanation of the phenomena needs radical review.

Method

Sheep were anaesthetized with halothane and ether and decerebrated using a trephine technique with division of the midbrain, the forebrain and later the cerebellum, being removed by suction. At the end of the experiment the brain stem was taken from the carcass and inspected macroscopically. In the animals discussed in this report the removal of the cerebellum had been almost complete.

The carpal joint of the animal was arranged to be concentric with the spindle of a printed motor (G9M4). This is a device which I have used for studying the biomechanics of the wrist joint (Walsh 1975). According to the

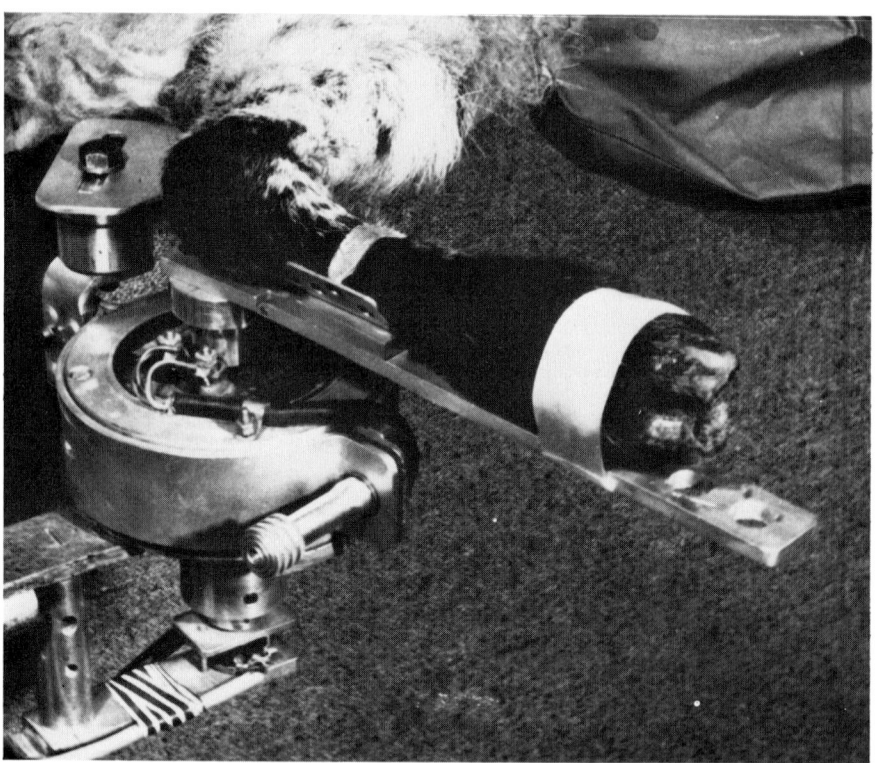

Fig. 13.1 Arrangements for testing biomechanics of carpal joint of foreleg of sheep. Printed motor concentric with axis of motion can apply force to the limb. Motion in horizontal plane. It often happens that as the joint flexes and extends there is also a rise and fall of the hoof. The lever is accordingly hinged to allow for this motion.

current through the motor so a corresponding torque is set up. The current changes are derived from a waveform generator and may take a wide range of alternatives. I have been principally concerned with the response to slow square waves giving abrupt alternations of torque from flexor to extensor and vice versa, but have also used sinusoidal fluctuations, the rate of which can be fixed or arranged to increase logarithmically. The spindle of the motor is double ended; to one end is attached a lever to which the hoof of the animal is fixed with adhesive plaster (Fig. 13.1). A metal plate is fixed to the bone of the shank proximal to the joint by self-tapping screws to stabilize the limb. To the other end of the spindle is fixed a conductive plastic potentiometer that records the position of the joint and, by differentiation, velocity is obtained. Electromyographs are obtained from the flexor and extensor musculature by the use of a pair of fine silver wires intramuscularly. The wire is enamel insulated; the covering was removed by flaming from the terminal mm or so and from a greater distance at the ends of the wires connected to the terminals of the recorder. The recorder also registered the torque applied by the motor; the voltage drop along the return lead gave an appropriate signal.

Results

Sinusoidal torques

The data to be presented relate to six animals which developed rigidity. When rhythmic forces were used the phenomenon of resonance was seen. The motion was greatest at a certain rate, the resonant frequency, which rose as the limb became stiffer. Results with one of the sheep are shown in Fig. 13.2. In the decerebrate state there was in this animal no stiffness for with full doses of a relaxant drug there was no drop of resonant frequency. After decerebellation the animal became stiff and this is shown in the records by the substantially increased resonant frequency for forces at each of the five levels shown in the figure. This increase of stiffness corresponded with the effects of decerebellation recorded in other animal species. It is with the neurophysiological mechanism of this increase that the first part of this paper is concerned.

Low frequency abruptly alternating torques

The waveform generator could be arranged to provide a slow square wave so that the torque changed abruptly from being extensor to being flexor every few seconds. The limb moved in the direction of the force until a plateau was recorded with a little overshoot. By studying the electromyogram with this system it was possible to ascertain whether or not a stretch reflex was operative. The responses of one animal are seen in Fig. 13.3. In the decerebrate state there was only a phasic stretch reflex in the extensor—a minimal discharge was seen just as flexion occurred. After decerebellation, the extensor stretch activity was clearly brought out and was then continued throughout flexion; a lesser degree of stretch activity was seen in the flexor muscle. An example where the flexor stretch activity is more clearly seen is

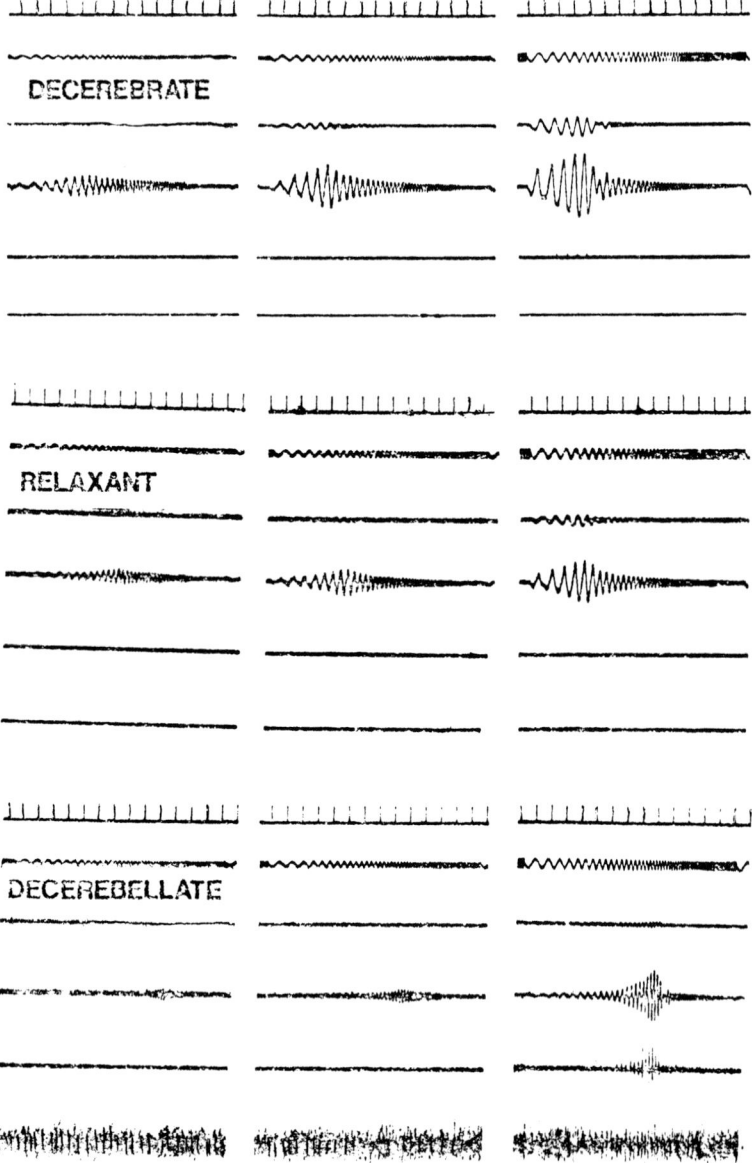

Fig. 13.2 Sinusoidal torques of logarithmically increasing frequency are applied to the limb of the sheep. Motion is greatest at a certain rate, the resonant frequency which varies according to muscle tone. Five levels of torque are used in the three states, decerebrate, under a relaxant, and decerebrate–decerebellate. Animal is stiff

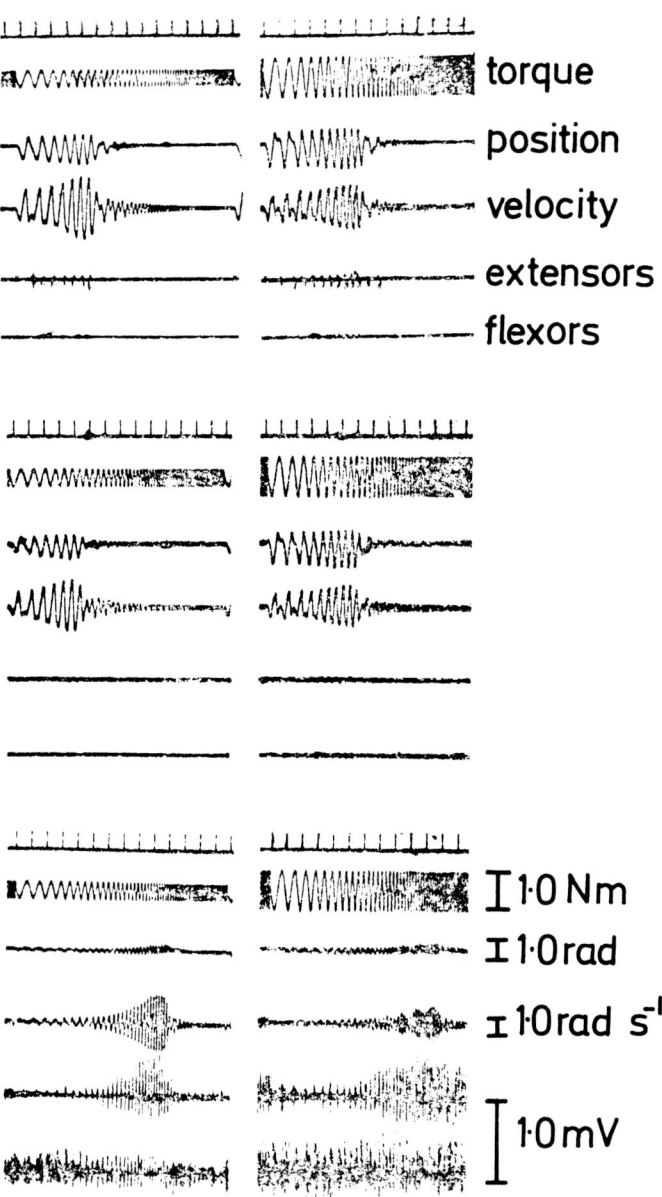

torque

position

velocity

extensors

flexors

$\mathbf{I}\,1{\cdot}0\,\text{Nm}$

$\mathbf{I}\,1{\cdot}0\,\text{rad}$

$\mathbf{I}\,1{\cdot}0\,\text{rad s}^{-1}$

$\mathbf{I}\,1{\cdot}0\,\text{mV}$

when decerebrate–decerebellate as is shown by elevated resonant frequency and shows concomitant activity in the flexor, and, to a lesser extent, extensor electromyogram. Time seconds.

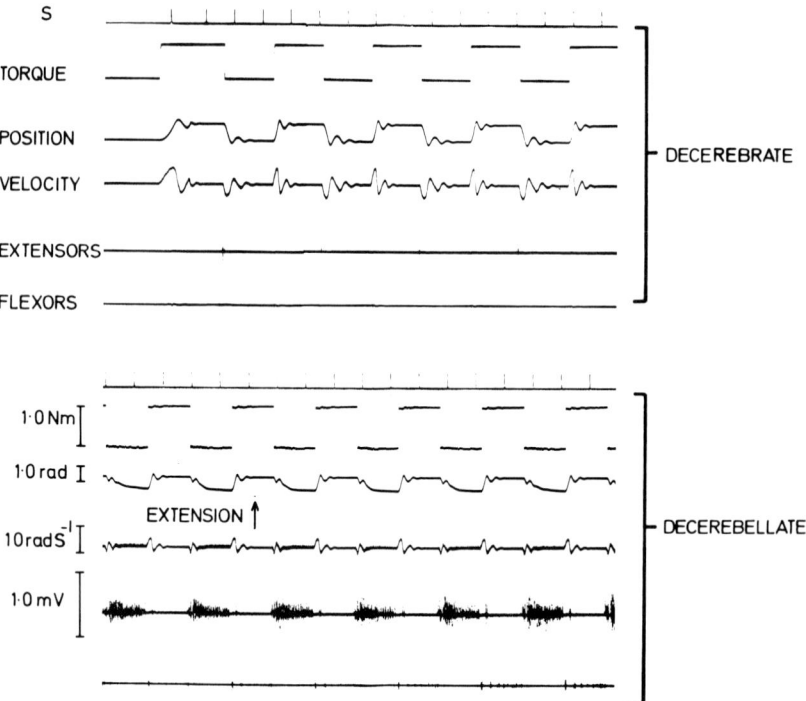

Fig. 13.3   Effect of abruptly alternating torque. Limb moves in direction of applied force until equilibrium is reached after about two cycles of oscillation. This animal showed no definite stiffness in the decerebrate state and the electromyogram was almost silent. Following decerebellation the limb moved less for the same force. In the electromyogram stretch activity was seen in the extensor and to a lesser extent in the flexor musculature.

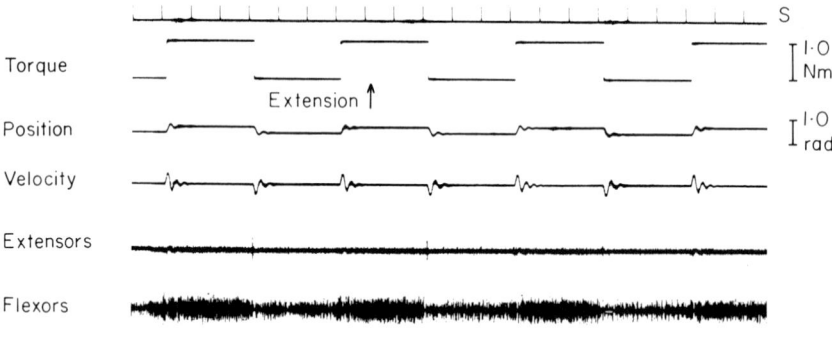

21.11.73   Decerebrate – decerebellate sheep

Fig. 13.4   Continuous electromyographic activity in the flexor musculature, but showing clear accentuation during extension, another example of a stretch response.

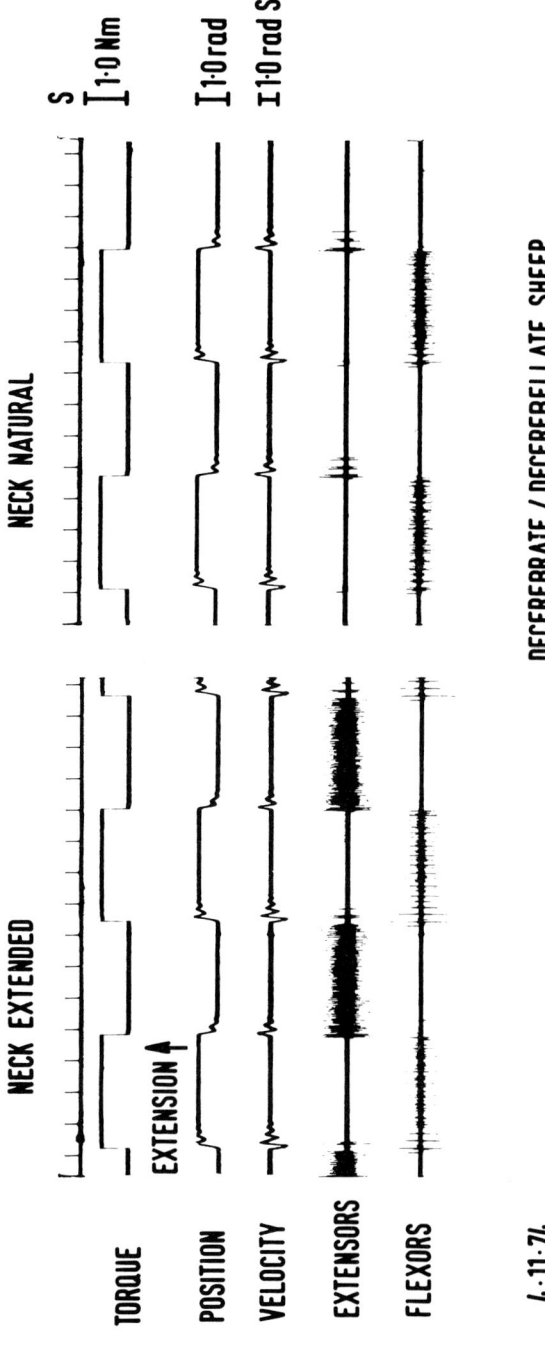

Fig. 13.5 Effect of neck reflexes on stretch activity in flexor and extensor musculature in decerebrate-decerebellate sheep. Animal is on its side with the neck extended. Both the extensor and, to a lesser extent, the flexor musculature showed stretch activity. With the neck straight the predominant stretch responses were in the flexors.

Fig. 13.4; there is continuous activity but this is clearly more prominent during the phases of extension.

It was sometimes possible to see clear effects from changing the position of the head. An example of the effects of neck reflexes on the responses is shown in Fig. 13.5; with the neck extended there is sustained stretch activity in both the extensors and flexors but more particularly in the former. With the neck in the natural position, the flexor stretch activity is seen more prominently whilst that of the extensors is reduced to three small phasic bursts related to the mechanical ringing of the limb at the end of the motion.

Discussion

Stretch reflexes

The results show clearly that stretch reflexes may persist and indeed be enhanced following extensive resection of the cerebellum. The author has observed in human beings that the responses to applied force at the wrist varies according to the stiffness with which the part is held. Thus when the subject is relaxed, shortening reactions are seen: stretch reflexes come up when the hand is partially stiff but are less prominent when held as stiff as possible. The decerebrate–decerebellate animals in the present study were stiff but usually the stiffness did not appear maximal. It is possible that had they been stiffer then the stretch reflexes would have been less prominent. Whatever role the cerebellum may play in modifying stretch reflexes, it is not essential for the reflex. Denny-Brown and Liddell (1927) showed that stretch reflexes could be obtained in the chronic spinal dog.

A resonance theory of cerebellar function

I have recently been studying certain problems in biomechanics where I have used a printed motor as a source of torque coupled to a human limb in a manner similar to that of the sheep. When, at the wrist, rhythmic forces of about 0·75 Nm are used with the subject relaxed, the oscillation which results is greatest at a certain rate, 2 to $2\frac{1}{2}$ Hz, the 'resonant frequency', and reduced if the frequency is below or above this value. The measurements are usually made in the horizontal plane to get rid of the complexities introduced by the action of gravity.

Some observations have been made during surgical anaesthesia; the resonance at the wrist persists even when the person has been anaesthetized and curarized. Resonances are present at the elbow, knee, foot and elsewhere but the jaw, however, shows no definite resonance (Walsh 1970).

The normal relaxed subject can reach a basal level of muscle tone mechanically equal to that of the anaesthetized curarized subject. He commonly shows for the low frequency movements shortening reactions electromyographically; the muscle from which tension is being removed takes up the slack (Sherrington 1908, Walsh 1976). From this basal level the person may voluntarily stiffen and as he does so the resonant frequency rises. With maximal stiffening this has been seen to reach 16 Hz, although 10 Hz is more usual. The true figure may be higher still as with this degree of stiffening there is some vibration in the apparatus itself which it has not so far been possible to eliminate. For a linear system an increase of resonant frequency from 2 to 16 Hz represents an increase in tension of 8^2 or 64 times.

All this can be done at a moment's notice by somebody with healthy muscles and a normal nervous system. People with rigidity have resting resonant frequencies which are elevated as compared to normal.

In making a movement we use systems which are resonant. Given an impulse there will be overshoot and oscillation at the end of the travel unless some action is arranged to take away these effects. In programming a muscle to act appropriately it may be necessary for the excitation to take place briefly and abruptly at the correct interval, and for the prime mover to become active after the movement is completed to prevent the limb springing back.

My theory is that in everyday life the resonant frequency of the joints must be continually adapted to the needs of the movement. Furthermore, the excitation of muscle must be arranged according to information available as to the resonant characteristics of the system involved.

Most movements include more than a single joint. The body is resonant at a series of junctions and unless appropriate control systems were available unpleasant oscillations could built up between one segment and another.

Although the cerebellum has been likened to a computer, it is not always clear what is being computed. I propose that the cerebellum is concerned with evaluating limb resonances, adjusting limb resonances and preparing muscle patterns to minimize the deficiencies inherent in operating movements with systems of this type. The cerebellum would thus be an adaptive control system computing information about limb resonances and the best way of achieving motion with minimal wobble. The inherent damping of the muscles is non-linear. It is less for higher velocities (allowing for a fast response) than for those which are lower, where, towards the end of a movement, the demands of stability are predominant. For data on resonant frequency it would need information about muscle tension; presumably the Golgi endings would be vitally concerned here. The resonant frequency varies a great deal with the amplitude of motion, being substantially higher for small forces than for those which are large. The system is much stiffer for small movements as compared with those which are more substantial (Walsh 1973). Finally with motion which is so large that the anatomical limits are reached, it becomes again stiff. The resonant system is thus highly non-linear: furthermore it is asymmetrically non-linear, the change of properties with extension differs quantitatively from that with flexion.

The C.N.S. computations needed must take into account these various factors, and the effects of varying load as when something is carried in the hand. Furthermore, when the inertia is increased the resonant frequency falls. As the limb stiffens the resonant frequency rises but the Q, or sharpness of tuning, is quite low. Occasionally I seem to have obtained some information that, by appropriate setting of neural pathways, the Q of the system may be increased so that it 'rings' with several oscillations. Finally, the behaviour of the system will depend on its orientation with regard to the vertical and, here, labyrinthine information, from the otolith, may provide an important datum. The ataxia of cerebellar disease is, I suggest, the result of a failure to match muscle action to the resonant properties of the joints.

Acknowledgments

The apparatus was purchased with the aid of (government) grants from the Royal Society. Technical assistance was provided by Mr G. Wright.

References

BREMER F. & LEY R. (1927) Recherches sur la physiologie du cervelet chez le pigeon. *Archs int. Physiol.* **28**, 58–95.

DENNY-BROWN D.E. & LIDDELL E.G. (1927) The stretch reflex as a spinal process. *J. Physiol.* **63**, 144–50.

GRANIT R., HOLMGREN B. & MERTON P.A. (1955) The two routes for excitation of muscle and their subservience to the cerebellum. *J. Physiol.* **130**, 213–24.

HITCHCOCK E. (1973) Dentate lesions for involuntary movements. *Proc. R. Soc. Med.* **66**, 877–9.

POLLOCK L.J. & DAVIS L. (1930) The reflex activities of a decerebrate animal. *J. comp. Neurol.* **50**, 377–411.

POLLOCK L.J. & DAVIS L. (1931) Studies in decerebration. VI. The effect of deafferentation upon decerebrate rigidity. *Am. J. Physiol.* **98**, 47–49.

WALSH E.G. (1970) Movements of the jaw resulting from the application of external forces. *J. Physiol.* **210**, 179–80P.

WALSH E.G. (1973) Motion at the wrist induced by rhythmic forces. *J. Physiol.* **230**, 44–5P.

WALSH E.G. (1975) A torque induced motion analyser. *J. Physiol.* **244**, 14–15P.

FAMILIAL DEGENERATION OF THE CEREBELLUM

W. B. MATTHEWS

In 1907, Gordon Holmes published a paper in *Brain* entitled, 'A form of familial degeneration of the cerebellum' (Holmes 1907a). His personal clinical observations seem to have been limited to examining one of the four affected members of the family on a single occasion, and also an unaffected member who was able to provide important information on the family history. As he acknowledged, Holmes owed a great deal to the careful notes of Dr Lunn of the staff of the St Marylebone Infirmary. What must, by modern standards, be regarded as somewhat meagre involvement in the clinical field, was redeemed by a meticulous neuropathological description of the findings in the case on whom an autopsy was performed. These observations were naturally those of Holmes himself, exceptional even for his own period, and far beyond the capacity of all but a handful of modern clinical neurologists.

Nearly 70 years later it is not easy to appreciate the contemporary significance of this communication. The detailed classification and minute subdivision of the forms of degenerative disease of the nervous system are no longer burning topics, and indeed are now relatively neglected. We are, however, considering an era in which descriptive neurology and, in particular, the relation of clinical observations to the findings at autopsy, reigned supreme. This was an entirely necessary stage of development of the specialty and the task of identifying specific entities from among the mass of chronic neurological disorders is by no means complete, even today. Around the turn of the century the process of classification still had far to go. It was, for example, still possible to publish a heterogeneous collection of cases and label them 'pseudosclerosis' on the basis of some fancied resemblance to disseminated or diffuse cerebral sclerosis. In no field did controversy rage so fiercely as in that of the cerebellar degenerations and Holmes' paper was a welcome flash of clarity in this obscure field.

Friedreich had drawn attention to a familial form of ataxia, distinct from tabes dorsalis, as early as 1861, and first wrote of hereditary ataxia in his definitive paper of 1876. The initial emphasis was on the affection of the spinal cord, but subsequently forms were identified in which cerebellar symptomatology, in so far as it was understood at the time, and cerebellar pathology, predominated. In 1893, Pierre Marie wrote a most influential paper in which he claimed to identify a condition of hereditary cerebellar ataxia distinct from Friedreich's disease. Few papers can have aroused such a prolonged storm of criticism, and Gordon Holmes (1907b), in the same issue of *Brain*, took Marie severely to task. It was certainly unfortunate for Marie that he could not contribute any personal observations to his new category, and relied entirely on evidence published by others, including only two post-mortem examinations. Holmes described the justification for Marie's hereditary cerebellar ataxia as being 'completely shattered' by the post-mortem reports on members of the families reviewed by Marie but published subsequently. Some showed prominent spinal cord pathology and others an abnormally small cerebellum without signs of acquired disease. Only in Fraser's (1880) case did disease appear to be confined to the cerebellum. Holmes (1907b) stated that Fraser examined the spinal cord by naked eye alone, but this is not correct, although the olivary nuclei were not sectioned. Kinnier Wilson (1940) pointed out that Marie scarcely deserved all the execration he received, as he clearly stated an opinion in conformity with many modern views, that transitional forms existed between classical Friedreich's disease and other forms of hereditary ataxia. Moreover, the family described by Holmes may fairly be accepted as confirming the existence of hereditary cerebellar ataxia. The pattern of transmission in recessively inherited disorders is now better understood, and the objection raised by Holmes, that only members of one generation were affected, now carries little weight.

Greenfield (1954) regarded Holmes' family as the prototype of hereditary cerebello-olivary degeneration, in which both the pontine nuclei and the spinal cord are spared. Whether it is indeed possible to isolate such an entity must be regarded as problematical. It is well known that the ataxias can seldom be differentiated in life, but even the morbid anatomy is not conclusive, and authors did not always agree with the categories in which Greenfield (1954) so authoritatively placed their published cases.

It would be easy to dismiss such controversy as sterile, but there is a purpose beyond that of mere taxonomy. The concept that the somatic expression of genetically determined disease is through biochemical disorder has led to dramatic therapeutic success in hepato-lenticular degeneration. The hope has often been expressed that similar success might be achieved in other genetic degenerations of the nervous system. So far the search for biochemical disorders has been disappointing, particularly in disease transmitted by dominant inheritance. In hepato-lenticular degeneration an important clue lay in the association of systemic and nervous disease, and a similar association is present in such conditions as the lipidoses, where knowledge of the biochemical disorder has not yet led to effective treatment. Any link between hereditary cerebellar ataxia and systemic disease should therefore be closely examined.

The family described by Holmes consisted of 4 affected and 3 unaffected sibs, an 8th sib having died young. The 3 affected males were all noted to have abnormally small genitalia and scanty body and facial hair. They were of small stature and one was described as 'cretinoid' in appearance. There is no information on the gonadal function of the affected female except that she was married but childless. She is said to have had symptoms of myxoedema. The post-mortem examination appears to have been confined to the nervous system and the histology of the testes was not described. There is, however, no doubt that hypogonadism was present in the three affected males. It is interesting to find that Fraser in 1880, still under the influence of phrenology, expected that destruction of the cerebellum would lead to hypergonadism, and stated that he could not ascertain whether there was any undue sexual appetite; in his opinion there was not.

Developmental hypogonadism occurs in two distinct forms—primary gonadal dysgenesis and hypogonadotrophic hypogonadism, and both have been described in association with cerebellar disease. Hecht and Ruskin (1960) described an example of the former, a case of Klinefelter's syndrome with female sex chromatin, tremor, ataxia, and low intelligence. Two siblings were also ataxic, but the endocrine disorder was not familial. Boudin *et al* (1960) described non-familial progressive ataxia in a patient with Klinefelter's syndrome but without female chromatin. Indemini and Amman (1963) described the occurrence of Klinefelter's syndrome in two brothers in a family in which a mild form of spino-cerebellar ataxia occurred in three generations.

The association with hypogonadotrophic hypogonadism is more clearly established, probable examples being described by Cooper *et al* (1950, case 1), Spota and Novizki (1954) and Altschul and Kotlowski (1956). The family reported by Richards and Rundle (1959), in which 5 out of 13 children suffered from hypogonadism and severe progressive ataxia, was eventually found to have the pathological changes of the Roussy–Levy syndrome (Sylvester 1972). A definite association of failure of gonadotrophin secretion associated with progressive cerebellar or spino-cerebellar ataxia has been described in 4 families. Volpé *et al* (1963) reported 2 brothers in whom puberty did not occur, who developed relatively minor ataxic symptoms. Boucher and Gibberd (1969) reported 2 sisters with spino-cerebellar ataxia and retinal degeneration. They had primary amenorrhoea and low gonadotrophin excretion. Two brothers, one with signs of spino-cerebellar ataxia and the other with more restricted cerebellar signs were reported by Boitelle *et al* (1956), Vignalou *et al* (1959) and Bernard-Weil and Endtz (1962). Puberty did not occur and eunuchoid features were marked.

In the family I was able to study (Matthews & Rundle 1964, Howell & Matthews 1975), the endocrine aspects were particularly striking as hypogonadism was established before the age of puberty. The propositus,

Willy, first attended hospital at the age of 30 with the recent onset of ataxia. He lived in a small isolated farm overshadowed by the dirt tip from a neighbouring colliery in a typical Derbyshire landscape. Minor symptoms would pass unnoticed in this environment, but he had experienced no difficulty during military service between the ages of 18 and 20. He appeared much younger than his age, and he had eunuchoid proportions. His voice had never broken and there was no facial hair. The genitalia were underdeveloped and pubic hair scanty and of female distribution. When first seen he had moderately severe symmetrical cerebellar ataxia, without nystagmus. Over the next 10 years the ataxia worsened, he developed bilateral nerve deafness and became mildly demented, but the plantar reflexes remained flexor and tendon reflexes were preserved, and no sensory loss was ever found. He died at the age of 40.

His brother, a year older, had precisely the same endocrine and neurological syndrome, although initially in a milder form, in that although he was obviously ataxic at the age of 31, he had no complaints. The disease was, however, progressive, and he died at the age of 43. No post-mortem was performed. One younger sister was also affected by ataxia and eventually became helpless and died at the age of 41. In contrast, she showed no endocrine abnormality and menstruated regularly, although she suffered from a fixed delusion that she was pregnant. There were 2 unaffected sisters and the parents were normal and were not related.

Autopsy on the propositus showed cerebello-olivary degeneration, the complete loss of inferior olivary nuclei being particularly striking. The pontine nuclei were spared. Despite the absence of physical signs of spinal cord disease, the fasciculus gracilis was severely demyelinated in the cervical region, although intact in the lower regions of the cord. The dorsal spino-cerebellar tract was also involved. There was some diffuse loss of myelinated fibres in the cerebrum and thalamus. No systematized abnormality was found in the hypothalamus and the pituitary gland was histologically normal.

In this family, the hypogonadism was secondary to failure of gonadotrophin excretion and the histology of the testis was in conformity with this. No other endocrine abnormality was detected in life or at autopsy. Sex chromatin was male and the chromosome structure was normal.

As in other families, the association of hypogonadism and ataxia, while definite enough, was not complete, in that one ataxic patient had normal gonadal function. This immediately disposes of hypogonadism as an essential element of the syndrome and of any causal role for hypogonadism in the production of cerebellar degeneration. A common cause for both conditions remains a possibility, but attempts to demonstrate a specific metabolic abnormality have failed. The association is probably more closely analogous to that between diabetes and Friedreich's ataxia and is an expression of genetic linkage.

Since the era in which Holmes' paper was published, it has been recognized that hereditary ataxia in many forms can occur in combination with a wide variety of other anomalies, some confined to a single family. It is accepted without question that progressive primary disease can affect the cerebellum, although perhaps seldom in complete isolation. The goal of strict classification has not, however, been achieved, and may well not be attainable. A valid classification would imply not only pathological characteristics, to be determined after death, but genetic and prognostic indications. The hope that a series of distinctive clinical and pathological forms of hereditary ataxia could be defined, each caused by a genetically determined and possibly treatable metabolic defect, has not been fulfilled, the only advance being the discovery of immunoglobulin deficiency in ataxia telangiectasia. Holmes was almost certainly describing hypogonadotrophic hypogonadism associated with cerebello-olivary degeneration, but restriction of the central nervous disease to the cerebellum has not proved to be an essential feature. Holmes was, however, undoubtedly and regrettably correct in not considering a causal role for the hypogonadism and in believing that in his patients it represented merely further evidence that the cerebellar disease was 'primarily due to an hereditary defective vital endurance' of this tissue. In the field of the hereditary ataxias, we have so far failed to substantiate any more hopeful concept than that of primary degeneration of the nervous system. It is, perhaps, salutory to find that Fraser (1880) wrote that his patient 'at the end, appreciated much his mother's remark that there would be "nae cripples in the next war"'.

References

ALTSCHUL R. & KOTLOWSKI K. (1956) Pallidocerebello-olivary degeneration and eunuchoidism. *J. nerv. ment. Dis.* **123**, 112–16.

BERNARD-WEIL E. & ENDTZ L.-J. (1962) Sur un cas familial de dégénération spino-cérébelleuse avec eunuchoidisme hypogonadotrophique. *Presse méd.* **70**, 524–6.

BOITELLE G., DELTEIL P., NOEL P. & FONCIN J.F. (1956) Dégénération spino-cérébelleuse, type Friedreich, avec infantilisme hypogonadotrophique et sénilité précoce. *Ann. méd-psychol.* **114**, 839–44.

BOUCHER B.J. & GIBBERD F.B. (1969) Familial ataxia, hypogonadism and retinal degeneration. *Acta neurol. scand.* **45**, 507–10.

BOUDIN G., BARBIZET J., PEPIN B. & WIART J.-P. (1960) Observation d'une hérédo-ataxie cérébelleuse de Pierre Marie associée à un syndrome dysmorphique et à un hypogonadisme. *Bull. Soc. méd. Hôp. Paris* **76**, 908–12.

COOPER I.S., RYNEARSON, E.M., BAILEY, A.A. & MacCARTY, C.S. (1950) Relation of spinal cord disease to gynaecomastia and testicular atrophy. *Proc. Mayo Clin.* **25**, 320–6.

FRASER D. (1880) Defect of the cerebellum in a brother and sister. *Glasgow med. J.* **13**, 199–210.

FRIEDREICH N. (1876) Ueber Ataxie mit besonderer Berucksichtigung der hereditären Form. *Virchov's Arch.* **68**, 145–245.

GREENFIELD J.G. (1954) *The Spino-cerebellar Degenerations*. Blackwell Scientific Publications, Oxford.

HECHT A. & RUSKIN H. (1960) Seminiferous tubule dysgenesis (Klinefelter's syndrome) (associated with familiar cerebellar ataxia. *J. clin. Endocr.* **20,** 1184–90.

HOLMES G.M. (1907a) A form of familial degeneration of the cerebellum. *Brain* **30,** 466–89.

HOLMES G.M. (1907b) An attempt to classify cerebellar disease, with a note on Marie's hereditary cerebellar ataxia. *Brain* **30,** 545–67.

HOWELL D.A. & MATTHEWS W.B. (1975) Cerebellar ataxia and hypogonadism. In: Vinken P.J. & Bruyn G.W. (Eds) *Handbook of Clinical Neurology*, pp. 467–76. North-Holland Publishing Company, Amsterdam.

INDEMINI M. & AMMAN F. (1963) Hérédo-dégénérescence spino-cérébelleuse (HDSC) associée au syndrome de Klinefelter. *Confin. neurol.* **23,** 155–64.

MARIE P. (1893) Sur l'hérédo-ataxie cérébelleuse. *La Semaine médicale* **13,** 444–7.

MATTHEWS W.B. & RUNDLE A.T. (1964) Familial cerebellar ataxia and hypogonadism. *Brain* **87,** 463–8.

RICHARDS B.W. & RUNDLE A.T. (1959) A familial hormonal disorder associated with mental deficiency, deaf-mutism and ataxia. *J. ment. Defic. Res.* **3,** 33–5.

SPOTA B.B. & NOVIZKI I. (1954) Sindrome adiposa genital en el Freidreich. *Prensa méd, argent.* **41,** 1223–6.

SYLVESTER P.E. (1972) Spino-cerebellar degeneration, hormonal disorder, hypogonadism, deaf mutism and mental deficiency. *J. ment. Defic. Res.* **16,** 203–14.

VIGNALOU J. BERTHAUX P., GOUYGOU Q., COLAS BELCOUR J.F., LEMARCHAL A. & HAMMEL A. (1959) Hypogonadisme hypogonadotrophique associé à une maladie de Friedreich. *Ann. Endocr. (Paris)* **20,** 172–7.

VOLPÉ R., METZLER W.S. & JOHNSON M.W. (1963) Familial hypogonadotrophic eunuchoidism with cerebellar ataxia. *J. clin. Endocr.* **23,** 107–15.

WILSON S.A.K. (1940) *Neurology*. Butterworth, London.

HYPOXIC MYOCLONUS: CLINICAL AND PATHOLOGICAL OBSERVATIONS

J., C. RICHARDSON, N. B. REWCASTLE AND J. DE LÉAN

When the human brain survives a period of sudden severe anoxia and ischaemia there often persist certain symptoms of neuronal damage such as dementia, visual defect, dysphasia and ataxia. An especially rare cerebral derangement is hypoxic action myoclonus, first clarified as unique by Lance and Adams in 1963. Recent evidence of a serotonin transmitter fault gives special importance to this hypoxic motor system disorder. In this past two years at the Toronto General Hospital we were able to study clinically two patients suffering this condition. One did not survive and the brain was subjected to careful neuropathological examination. Drug trials have been made in these two instances, and in three other patients with non-hypoxic myoclonus.

Anoxic encephalopathy

But to begin let us first look briefly at the general spectrum of anoxic brain dysfunction as we have reviewed it through a series of patients with late neurological sequelae and from autopsy reports of fatal cases. Fifteen patients with residential neurological symptoms of cerebral anoxia and ischaemia resulting from industrial accidents were assessed at the Hospital and Rehabilitation Centre of the Ontario Workmen's Compensation Board. These were men from 19 to 63 years of age, seen from six months to fifteen years after their industrial accident. Causes and symptoms are tabulated (Table 15.1).

There was an initial period of coma in all cases, with a graded recovery of consciousness, in periods of one hour to three weeks. Early symptoms such as convulsions, tremor, rigidity and myoclonic jerking were usually transient. Much the most common residual symptoms suggested cerebral cortical damage with dementia, spasticity and parietal lobe effects. Versions of ataxia and intention tremor were fairly common, implicating the cerebellum as the second most prominent site of damage.

Autopsy reports from the Division of Neuropathology at the Banting

Table 15.1

Anoxic Encephalopathy—15 Cases

Cause		Early symptoms		Residual symptoms		Affected regions	
Cardiac Arrest		Coma	15	Mental impairment	9	Cerebral cortex	13
Surgery anaesthesia	3	Convulsions	5	Paresis	5	Cerebellum	5
Electrocution	1	Paresis	4	Ataxia	5	Basal ganglia	2
Curare	1	Chorea	1	Dysarthria	3	Thalamus	1
Cardiac disease	1	Rigidity	1	Sensory loss	2	Brain stem	1
Heart Chest Injury	4	Myoclonus	1	Tremor	3		
CO.	3	Tremor	1	Dyslexia	1		
Buried	2			Dyscalculia	1		

Institute of Toronto provide examples of frequent cardiac and respiratory arrest of varied cause and duration. Forty-five examples from a recent five-year period were reviewed. Each one revealed obvious neuronal damage and often glial changes in a varying but rather stereotyped pattern. Commonly involved were deeper layers of cerebral cortex, hippocampus and Purkinje cells of the cerebellum. The essential point to mention would perhaps be that post-mortem examination seemed to expose regularly a neuronal damage that would be expected to explain the general and focal cerebral symptoms noted in life. (Such usual clinical and pathological effects of cerebral anoxia, as well as hypoglycaemia, was the basis of a paper from Toronto by Richardson, Chambers and Heywood in 1959. Myoclonus was not even mentioned!)

Hypoxic myoclonus

Viewed against this background, hypoxic myoclonus presents a striking picture. Our two Toronto patients with this syndrome were studied pharmacologically at the General Hospital (De Lean, Richardson and Hornykiewicz 1976).

The first of these two patients whose disorder was caused by an industrial accident was seen, as were the fifteen patients mentioned above, at the rehabilitation centre.

Case history

A 62-year-old Hungarian machinist suffered an accidental compression and fixation of his chest when caught between an iron brace and the descending arm of a barrel lift on 1 February 1974. He was liberated unconscious and blue from mid chest upwards after being held with little or no respiration for a period of about ten minutes. He was intubated and transferred on a respirator to a neurological unit. He remained comatose with repeated general seizures for four days. On the sixth day he started to have jerking movements of trunk and limbs. His mentality seemed normal after several weeks. He went home after four months but was sent to a rehabilitation centre because of severe and disabling muscular jerking. He was transferred to the Toronto General Hospital in October 1974.

Examination prior to his special drug trials showed striking motor neurological abnormalities. His speech was halting and interrupted at times. There was some coarse twitching of the left lower facial muscles. At rest there was no involuntary movement of limbs or trunk and myoclonus was not produced by visual or auditory stimuli. There was a striking violent coarse myoclonic jerking of limb and trunk muscles provoked by voluntary movement. He could not stand or walk without strong support because of violent myoclonic jerks of trunk muscles and transient collapse of supporting muscles. The limb jerking was chiefly in proximal muscles occurring chiefly in the left arm and in both legs.

As well as myoclonus, there was an intention tremor and some incoordination of the left arm and of both legs shown in finger–nose and heel–knee testing. There was no paresis or dystonia and reflexes and sensation remained normal. EEG normal. CSF total protein 30 mg%.

For this patient extensive pharmacological investigation was pursued. Methysergide, 2 mg t.i.d. brought marked improvement. After a few days it was withdrawn and when again repeated he failed to improve. When the dosage of methysergide was increased to 12 mg per day, the myoclonus was clearly aggravated. There was a moderate but definite improvement with L-tryptophan, 10 g per day, an improvement which did not increase with the addition of an MAO inhibitor phenelezine, 45 mg per day. Strikingly good results came from an intravenous injection of 100 mg of 5 hydroxytryptophan, and a continuing pronounced benefit was maintained by oral 5 HTP, 1·5 g per day, along with carbidopa, 125 mg daily.

Case history

A 72-year-old woman was seen in a hospital emergency department on 9 September 1972 in a comatose cyanosed pulseless state. She had taken 25 capsules of tuinal, 200 mg, in a suicidal attempt. She was resuscitated from a cardiac arrest of uncertain duration. On regaining consciousness thirty-six hours later, violent jerking movements of her trunk and limbs were noted. These myoclonic jerks persisted and were activated by voluntary activity, and by auditory or tactile stimuli. Moderate improvement was obtained by oral diazepam, 100 mg per day. After several weeks she could walk with help. She was then sent to a convalescent hospital. After two months the jerking became worse and eventually she was transferred to a chronic care hospital where she remained bedridden for two years. Several years earlier this patient had suffered repeated depressive states requiring electroshock treatment on three occasions.

She was transferred to the Toronto General Hospital in December 1974 for further investigation and drug trials. Her intellect and speech were normal. She was depressed and resigned to a state of helpless invalidism which hampered our therapeutic efforts. On finger–nose testing there was bilateral action myoclonus, as well as some intention tremor. Heel–knee–shin tests showed similar myoclonus and intention tremor of the lower limbs. Attempts to sit, stand and walk initiated such uncontrollable myoclonic movements that she was confined to bed. The limb stretch reflexes and plantar reflexes were normal. The EEG failed to show any spike activity.

Pharmacological study of this elderly woman patient reflected the results of our experiments with Case No. 1. Methysergide, 12 mg per day aggravated the myoclonus and L-dopa, 2 g daily, again worsened her condition. L-tryptophan gave mild aid. PCPA (parachlorophenylalanine) 4 g daily over a nine-day period, failed to change the myoclonus and indeed caused fatigue and a slurring of speech.

When this same patient was given 200 mg of 1–5 HTP (1–5 hydroxytryptophan) intravenously, there was marked cessation of myoclonus for a five-hour period, but not without vomiting and diarrhoea from peripheral serotonin. She was later given orally 1–5 HTP, combined with carbidopa as preventitive of side effects. On a regime of 1 g of 5 HTP and 75 mg of carbidopa daily, there was complete disappearance of myoclonus and some reduction of intention tremor. The patient became able to feed herself, and to walk short distances unassisted. Sad to relate, this improvement was not lasting and our patient returned to a deeply depressed, totally uncooperative state, getting little assistance from an antidepressant, amitriptyline. It seemed futile here to continue with active treatment of a neurological motor disorder. The effective drug 5 HTP was therefore discontinued and the patient was sent back to the chronic hospital to continue previous medication. Her physical condition continued much as before, with severe myoclonus confining her to bed and wheelchair, and her mental state one of resigned helplessness and dependency along with moderate depression. Suddenly, during dinner on 11 June 1975, she was found unconscious and cyanosed. Resuscitation efforts failed. Autopsy showed death as caused by choking on food. Unfortunately for our study, the brain of this patient was fixed in formalin, and fresh tissue for chemical assay was not available. However, after fixation the brain was extensively studied, histologically.

Neuropathology

Post-mortem examination: Mrs S.J. Age 74 years. The fixed brain weighed 1450 g and no abnormalities were detected on the surface or following sectioning (Fig. 15.1). Microscopic examination was in some detail using haematoxylin and eosin—Luxol fast blue, cresyl violet, phosphotungstic acid haematoxylin, Holzer and oil red 0 staining techniques. The basal ganglia, thalamus and related structures were studied in sections cut at 1 mm intervals at right angles to the anterior commissure–posterior commissure axis for comparison with the Schaltenbrand Atlas, while transverse sections of the brain stem from upper midbrain to lower medulla were cut at similar 1 mm

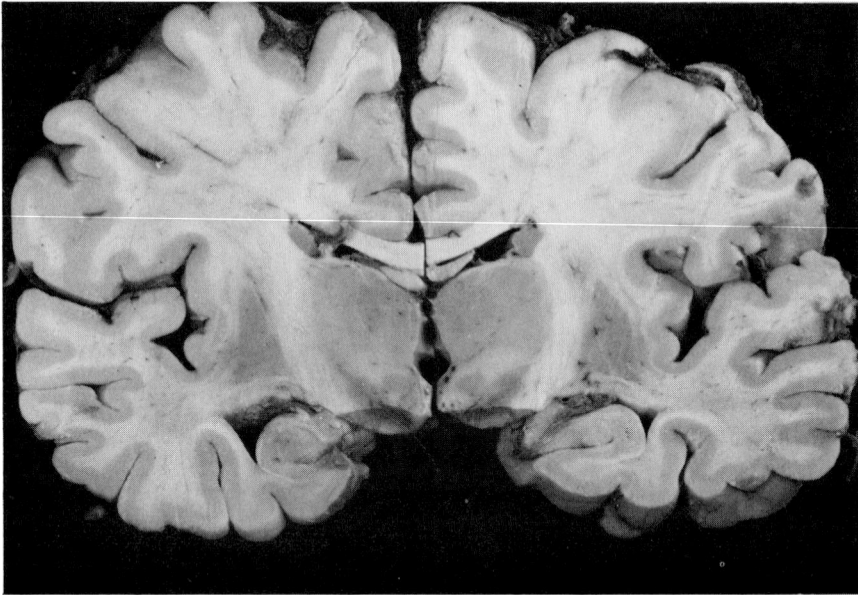

Fig. 15.1 Coronal view of the brain 7 mm anterior to the posterior commissure
shows a normal architecture throughout all areas.

intervals for comparison with the Olszewski-Baxter Atlas. Superficial and
deep midline and lateral areas of the cerebellum and representative areas of
the cerebral hemispheres completed the study.

There was a surprising paucity of structural changes. A prominent
astrocytic reaction of some duration, indicated by scattered hypertrophied
cells and tight clusters of two or three such cells, was present in the lateral
parts of the supratrochlear nucleus, the lateral subnucleus of the
mesencephalic grey and the immediately adjacent cuneiform and
subcuneiform nuclei of the caudal half of the midbrain. Actual neuronal loss
was more difficult to assess, but sites of presumed nerve cell disintegration
were indicated by tight clusters of macrophages distended by lipochrome
pigment (Fig. 15.2). Otherwise neuronal populations throughout the brain
stem were well maintained for a patient of this age (Fig. 15.3). No neuronal
loss or gliosis was evident in the basal ganglia, subthalamic nuclei, thalami,
midbrain tectum, pons or medulla. In the many areas of cerebral cortex
studied, laminar type damage was not found, nor were lipid containing
macrophages present in the cortical parenchyma on oil red 0 stained frozen
sections. The hippocampal formation was undamaged. Likewise, the
cerebellar cortex and deep cerebellar nuclei were normal; even Bielchowsky
silver staining techniques demonstrated only a few collapsed basket
arrangements denoting sites of rare Purkinje cell loss. Incidental findings

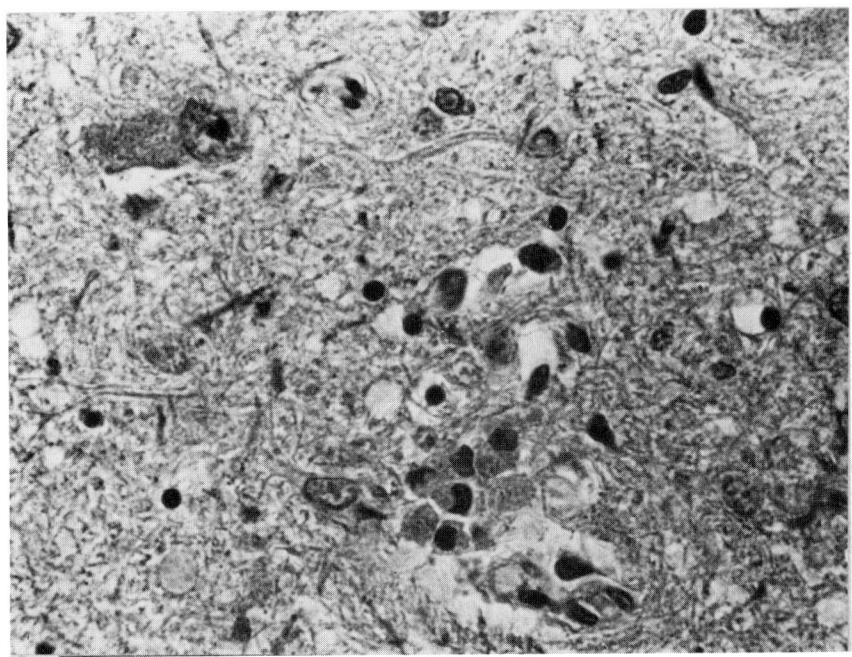

Fig. 15.2 Astrocytic hypertrophy of some duration and tight clusters of macrophages indicate damage in the lateral part of the supratrochlear nucleus that lies dorsal to the medial longitudinal fasciculus. Haematoxylin and eosin/Luxol fast blue stain. (×595.)

included the occasional midline brain stem neurone containing an intracytoplasmic neurofibrillary tangle and a small focus of mononuclear cell infiltration in the pontine tegmentum.

Fibrillary astrocytes in the midbrain periaqueductal grey matter are often a little prominent in patients of advanced years, but after comparison with age matched controls, we believe that the astrocytic prominence in this area in our patient, together with sites of presumed neuronal loss, represent change in excess of age, though this change is by no means marked.

It is of interest then to compare our autopsy case with the only other one detailed in the literature, that of Castaigne, Cambier and Escourolle (1964) which is mentioned in more detail later in the discussion. Though their study showed, relatively speaking, much more widespread damage, both studies demonstrated astrocytic prominence and some degree of neuronal loss in the midbrain periaqueductal grey and dorsolateral grey matter of the tegmentum.

Biochemical and topographical studies have suggested the localization of serotonin activity to the neurones of the brain stem raphe areas (Lloyd *et al* 1974, Nobin & Bjorklund 1973). The most oral of these areas, the Nucleus

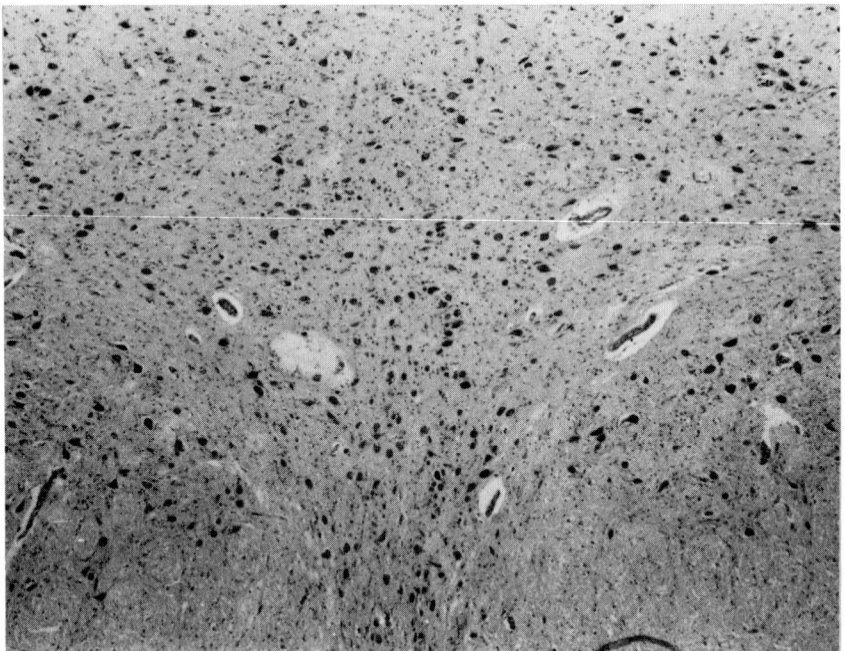

Fig. 15.3 The supratrochlear nucleus contains abundant neurones; here it is seen lying between and dorsal to the medial longitudinal fasciculi and the motor nuclei of the fourth cranial nerve. Cresyl violet stain. (×33.)

raphae dorsalis, corresponds to the supratrochlear nuclear which in our patient, and possibly the one described by Castaigne *et al*, was associated with some neuronal loss and astrocytic reaction. Even so, the overall neuronal populations of this nucleus and the other raphe nuclei, centralis, linearis, magnus, pallidus and obscurus, were well maintained though cell counting techniques were not performed. The locus coeruleus was also well populated with neurones allowing for the age of the patient. No alterations in individual cell structure were encountered that might have indicated distal damage in the axon.

Thus, it is difficult to correlate in any meaningful fashion the presumptive 5HT-serotonin deficiency in the patient, the presently known localization of serotonin in the human brain stem and the minor structural changes evident in the caudal midbrain of our patient. Perhaps, as is discussed later, the degree of cardiac arrest suffered by the patient resulted in a lasting functional derangement of the neurone rather than absolute cell death with significant reduction in the neuronal populations.

Biochemical and pharmacology findings

Both of these patients showed a low level of cerebrospinal fluid 5 hydroxyindolacetic acid (5 HIAA) which increased significantly after the successful therapy. These results are shown in the two graphs, Figs. 15.4 and 15.5.

Recently we have studied three patients with myoclonus of non-hypoxic cause.

Case history

One was a 51-year-old Italian woman with a thirty-year history of myoclonus and epilepsy. She had not developed dementia or other progressive brain symptoms, though she showed a severe action myoclonus and some intention tremor of the hands. Detailed investigation has not revealed the cause of a chronic myoclonic epilepsy. The cerebrospinal fluid 5 hydroxyindolacetic acid was normal (10·6 ng/ml—normal 9–16). She has experienced a quite pronounced reduction in myoclonus while taking 1·8 g of 5 hydroxytryptophan and 150 mg of carbidopa daily. Though responding

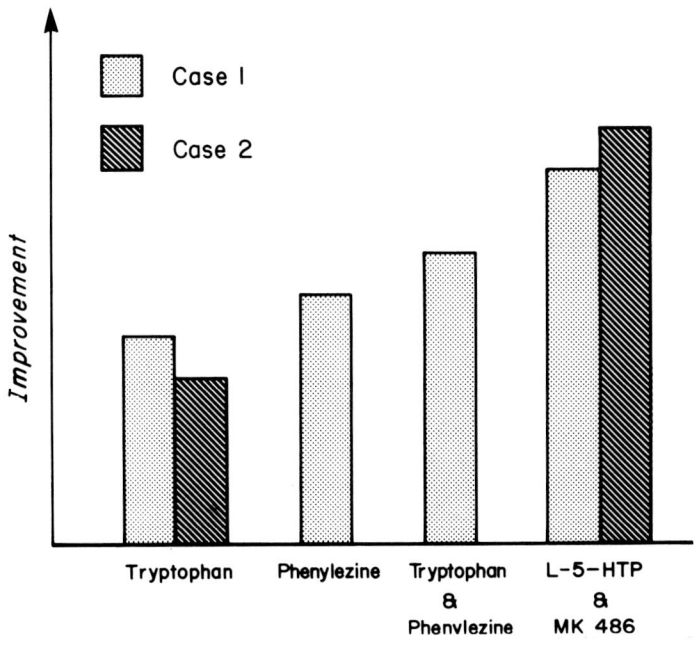

Fig. 15.4 Drug trial no. 1

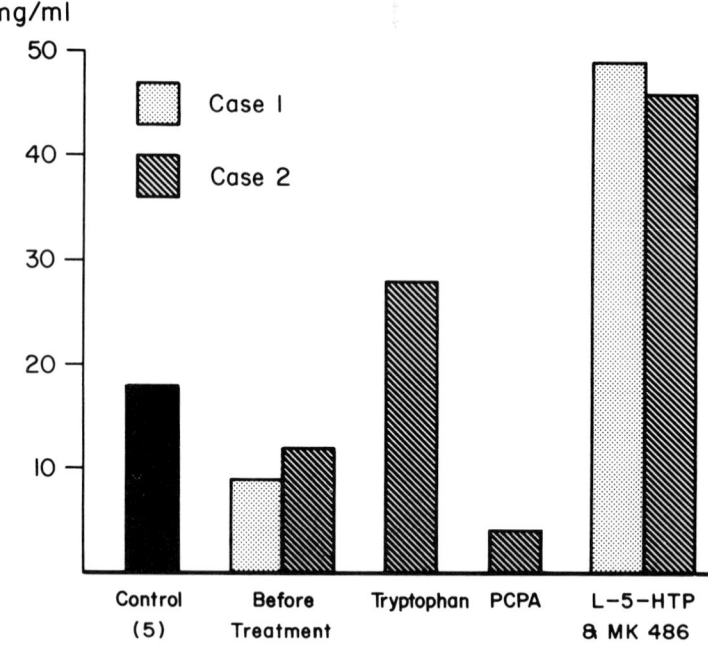

Fig. 15.5   CSF 5HIAA

less dramatically than the two hypoxic cases, she is assessed as about 50% improved.

Case history

A fourth patient in this series, a 28-year-old woman, has recently been treated with clonazepam, with excellent improvement. She has been suffering grand mal epilepsy for three years, and for a shorter period of one year a severe widespread myoclonus of limbs and trunk. There was no history of any known anoxic accident. She has become mildly demented and it is thought that she may have a lipid storage disease. Her CSF 5 HIAA was found to be 18·9 ng/ml—normal control 17·6. Treatment by 5 HTP was considered but the surprisingly good response to clonazepam has led to postponing other drug trials.

There is considerable evidence that clonazepam is effective through increasing cerebral serotonin activity.

Case history

Currently under study is a fifth patient, a 28-year-old woman with quite disabling severe action myoclonus, very similar to that presented by our two hypoxic cases. She has suffered mild dementia and has a cerebellar intention tremor of the arms. She is one of a well-known family of Huntington's chorea. The other afflicted members of the family showed the more typical severe chorea and dementia. This young woman with her unusual myoclonic variety of Huntington's disease presents interesting problems regarding cerebral serotonin. The CSF 5 HIAA measured 18·9 ng/ml—normal control 17·6. A preliminary intravenous 5 HTP test has been done and there was a striking reduction of myoclonus, almost complete clearing for four hours after the injection of 200 mg of 5 HTP. She has responded to oral 5 HTP (and carbidopa) with moderate improvement, but this therapy was started only recently and full dosage has not been reached as yet.

Discussion

This clinical and pharmacological experience with two patients suffering hypoxic myoclonus, along with the autopsy examination of one of these, allow some limited conclusions. It is a striking extra-pyramidal motor disorder, occurring as a rare effect of cerebral anoxia, without the more common anoxic cerebral symptoms. Pharmacological results strongly implicate an underlying fault of serotonin neurotransmission. Detailed microscopic examination of the brain in the fatal case showed after nearly three years of hypoxic myoclonus, very minimal changes in only one small area of central midbrain. The paucity of visible pathological change is perhaps in keeping with a chemical neurotransmitter disturbance, rather than related to neuronal damage of the more usual anoxic encephalopathy. The moderate improvement of one patient with chronic myoclonic epilepsy vaguely suggests a possible less important transmitter disorder in non-hypoxic myoclonus.

Before Lance and Adams' important paper of 1963, myoclonus persisting after an episode of cerebral anoxia was only mentioned by Courville (1939), Gastaut and Remond (1952) and Hassler (1959). More recently there have been many writings about hypoxic myoclonus and a few important papers will be mentioned.

In 1964 Castaigne, Cambier *et al* presented the post-mortem findings of an 80-year-old woman who suffered typical Lance–Adams hypoxic myoclonus following a period of cardiac and respiratory arrest during anaesthesia. This is the one single pathological study of the condition prior to our own. The autopsy was done three weeks after the anoxic incident. The cerebral cortex here showed only minimal discrete glial changes in deeper frontal layers, with no significant nerve-cell lesions. Neuronal loss and astrocyte proliferation were noted in pontine nuclei, subthalamic nucleus and mildly in tegmental neurones. Moderate damage was found in both ventrolateral and ventromedian thalamic nuclei. And, strikingly, there was a notable lack of the more usual anoxic changes such as laminar cerebral cortical degeneration and cerebellar nerve-cell damage. The authors discuss the possible pathophysiology of the disorder giving support to the Lance–Adams suggestion of repetitive or synchronous discharge of neurones of the ventrolateral thalamic nucleus, the main relay station between cerebellum and cerebral motor cortex. The need for further anatomical clinical studies was stressed in this French study, and so it is especially disappointing that our second autopsy study fails to clarify the physiological derangement. Castraigne and his colleagues, in a second paper of 1968, consider further the clinical features and physiological studies of reported cases and their own single study.

A paper of 1971 by Lhermitte *et al* reported stereotactic investigation in a patient with hypoxic myoclonus. Their work supporting the view that myoclonus was related to discharges along the cortico-spinal tract added the finding that discharges from V.L. followed and never preceded the cortical discharge. They suggested a likely involvement of other subcortical mechanisms.

At a meeting in London, Ontario, in June 1975, Irving Cooper described cerebellar biopsy and stimulation in a patient with hypoxic action myoclonus. He reported some pathology in the dentate and nucleus and showed, in a film, some relief of the myoclonus by cerebellar stimulation. The search continues for the actual physiological fault in myoclonus. The conception of an interruption of cerebellar inhibition of thalamus and other basal ganglia, remains attractive.

A landmark in the study of this unique motor disorder was the discovery by Lhermitte *et al* (1971) of the beneficial effect of the serotonin precursor 5 hydroxytryptophan. These important findings have been confirmed by Van Woert and Sethy (1975), by Chadwick *et al* (1974), and by others. There are now approximately twelve described patients with hypoxic myoclonus for whom excellent responses have been obtained by 5 HTP, and there is a smaller number with a lesser but still beneficial response to the precursor L-tryptophan. These therapeutic observations, and our own, along with the suggestive correlation of drug response with cerebrospinal fluid 5 HIAA levels, provide strong evidence of a serotonin neurotransmitter fault. Much can be expected and hoped from continuing this pharmacological approach to motor system problems.

The human victim of brain anoxia with motor system derangement is an imperfect and rather crude research model. Perhaps we should turn to the neuroscientist pursuing basic research for some answers and, in fact, there has been a tremendous amount of recent animal research dealing with energy metabolism and ultrastructural tissue changes from cerebral anoxia and ischaemia. Traditional conceptions of an hierarchical system of relative vulnerability to anoxia in different brain areas, has been challenged by studies in the rat by MacMillan *et al* (1974). These workers and others, moreover, have shown that the animal brain tolerates, without damage, surprisingly low levels of blood oxygen if blood flow persists. The importance of arterial perfusion is accordingly emphasized. (In our own patients with accidental respiratory arrest, it is probable that there is present a factor of ischaemia and seldom a pure anoxic anoxia. Though accepting that we are usually dealing with anoxia plus ischaemia, for simplicity and brevity the single adjective 'hypoxic' or 'anoxic' has been perpetuated.) Biochemical research on brain anoxia in the rat suggests that the transmitter serotonin is markedly depleted in the acute stage of anoxia-ischaemia, but that it is later restored. There is evidence that anoxia may cause an arrest of transmitter synthesis (MacMillan, personal communication).

Conclusion

This disease, hypoxic action myoclonus, is a rare effect of brain anoxia with only twenty-five to thirty reported cases since it was first clearly identified in 1963.

The myoclonic disorder tends to emerge early after an initial few days of coma, during which time convulsions frequently occur. Once established the action myoclonus continues indefinitely, with little change unless modified by treatment. The myoclonus tends to appear in rather pure form without other hypoxic cerebral cortical or striatal signs. In most patients there has been a mild cerebellar deficit, chiefly as an intention tremor.

This uncommon and unusual effect of cerebral anoxia-ischaemia must be explained by some special variant or site of the disturbed cerebral chemistry and energy metabolism. That remains to be explained. In the reported cases the causative cardiac or respiratory arrest seems of moderate severity and not obviously different from other patients with more usual types of anoxic encephalopathy. Patients with residual severe dementia and paralysis from severe hypoxia rarely present any concomitant persistent myoclonus. We have not heard of any case of hypoxic myoclonus persisting after carbon monoxide asphyxia, though that is one of the commonest causes of cerebral anoxia.

There is strong presumptive evidence of an underlying disturbance of serotonin neurotransmission, perhaps either a faulty synthesis of the transmitter or a disturbance of serotonin facilitating neuronal pathways, or both.

It is possible that cell counts or other special histological techniques might reveal neuronal loss or changes which we did not see by ordinary light microscopy. Yet the absence of obvious pathology in this myoclonic syndrome (from our one autopsy), does contrast with the changes seen in cerebral cortex and cerebellum in other more usual anoxic encephalopathies.

We are left groping for answers about the pathogenesis, as well as the exact physiological derangement, in hypoxic myoclonus. Perhaps, tentatively, it may be concluded that the defective serotonin neurotransmission must have been due to a biochemical lesion which brought almost no visible damage. The abnormal movement disorder is not explained by demonstrable neuronal loss in motor structures such as cerebellum or thalamus.

At this time, the often quoted phrase of Haldane—'anoxaemia not only stops the machine but wrecks the machinery'—might be supplemented by a line from Shakespeare—'and like this insubstantial pageant faded, leave not a rack behind'.

References

AIGNER B.R. & MULDER D.W. (1960) Myoclonus; clinical significance and an approach to classification. *AMA Arch. Neur.* **2**, 600.

CASTAIGNE P., CAMBIER J., ESCOUROLLE R., CATHALA H.P. & LECASBLE R. (1964) Observation anatomo-clinique d'un syndrome myoclonique post-anoxique. *Société Française de Neurologie, Séance du 4 Juillet 1964*, 60–73.

CHADWICK D., REYNOLDS E.H. & MARSDEN C.D. (1974) Relief of action myoclonus by 5 hydroxytryptophan. *Lancet* **ii** 111–12.

COURVILLE C.B. (1939) *Untoward Effects of Nitrous Oxide Anaesthesia.* Pacific Press Publishing Association, Mountain View, California.

DE LÉAN J., RICHARDSON J.C. & HORNYKIEWICZ O. (1976) Beneficial effects of serotonin precursors in post anoxic action myoclonus. *Neurology* **26**, 863–868.

GASTAUT H. & REMOND A. (1952) Etude electroencephalographique des myoclonies. *Rev. Neurol.* **85**, 596.

HASSLER R. (1959) Clinical and anatomical findings in stereotactic pain operations on the thalamus. *Arch. Psychiat. & Nervenkr.* **200**, 93–122.

LANCE JAMES W. & ADAMS RAYMOND D. (1963) The syndrome of intention or action myoclonus as a sequel to hypoxic encephalopathy. *Brain* **86**, 111–36.

LHERMITTE F., TALAIRACH J., BUSER P., GAUTHIER J.C., BANCAUD J., GRAS R. & TRUELLE J.L. (1971) Myoclonies d'intention et d'action post-anoxiques étude stereotoxique et destruction du noyau ventral lateral du thalamus. *Rev. Neurol.* **124**, 5–20.

LHERMITTE P., PETERFALVI M., MARTEAU R., GAZENGEL J. & SERDARU M. (1971) Analyse pharmacologique d'un cas de myoclonies d'intention et d'action post-anoxiques. *Rev. Neurol.* **124**, 21–31.

LLOYD K.G., FARLEY I.J., DECK J.H.N. & HORNYKIEWICZ O. (1974) Serotinin and 5-hydroxyindoleacetic acid in discrete areas of the brainstem of suicide victims and control patients. *Advances in Biochemical Psychopharmacology*, **11**, 387–97.

MACMILLAN V., SALFORD G. & SJESJO B.K. (1974) Metabolic state and blood flow in rat cerebral cortex, cerebellum and brainstem in hypoxic hypoxia. *Acta. Physiol. Scand.* **92**, 103–13.

NOBIN A. & BJORKLUND A. (1973) Topography of the monoamine neurone systems in the human brain as revealed in fetuses. *Acta Physiol. Scand. (Suppl.)* **388,** 1–40.

RICHARDSON J.C., CHAMBERS R.A. & HEYWOOD P.M. (1959) Encephalopathies of anoxia and hypoglycaemia. *AMA Arch. Neur.* **1,** 178–90.

VAN WOERT M.H. & SETHY V.H. (1975) Therapy of intention myoclonus with 1–5 hydroxytryptophan and a peripheral decarboxylase inhibitor MK 486. *Neurology* **25,** 135–40.

THE PYRAMIDAL TRACT AND THE NEURAL MECHANISM CONTROLLING VOLUNTARY MOVEMENT

A TRIBUTE TO ANTONIO Y. LOPEZ

PAUL C. BUCY

This paper is written as a tribute to a remarkable man without whose cooperation our knowledge of the pyramidal tract and of the neural control of the skeletal musculature would have been retarded for years. Mr Lopez was a Mexican workman. Although he had little formal education, he was an intelligent, well-read man. What we subsequently learned about the pyramidal tract was dependent upon his willingness to undergo the operation in which the pyramidal tract in the right cerebral peduncle was destroyed, his personal participation in his rehabilitation, his willing cooperation in repeated examinations and recording of his condition in motion pictures, and his insistence to his disinterested family that after his death an autopsy should be performed.

On this occasion we shall be concerned entirely with the neural control of voluntary movements. The matter of reflex activity of the skeletal musculature, although of great importance, will not be dealt with.

When the idea that the destruction of the pyramidal tract might not give rise to the so-called 'pyramidal syndrome' was first tentatively proposed to a group of neuroscientists, it met with harsh criticism from one of the world's most outstanding physiologists, A. V. Carlson of the University of Chicago. At that meeting the suggestion was made on purely theoretical grounds. It was not until some time later that actual evidence appeared which established the facts, not only that destruction of the pyramidal tract did not give rise to the 'pyramidal syndrome', but that the pyramidal tract was not the sole descending pathway from the cerebral cortex giving rise to voluntary movements.

Later, the central half of the cerebral peduncle, the portion containing the cortico-spinal pathway, was divided in three patients without producing a complete paralysis of the contralateral extremities. All of these patients had voluntary movement, some of them 'nearly normal muscular activity' with 'delicately controlled, well-coordinated, strong movements, even of the individual digits'. These observations were reported in a paper entitled, 'Is there a pyramidal tract?' (Bucy 1957). However, although I was convinced that I had divided the pyramidal tract in these patients there was no anatomical proof—an important deficiency.

Finally, the opportunity came for the development of positive proof. We were confronted with a patient with severe left-sided hemiballismus which had been resistant to many forms of medical therapy, which had persisted for 77 days and which was rapidly exhausting this 70-year-old man (Antonio Y. Lopez). On 19 December 1958 his right cerebral peduncle was exposed and the central one-half was divided. The lateral and medial quarters of the peduncle were left intact. The incision was 10 mm long, lying transversely in the peduncle, and 7 mm deep. Immediately following the operation he had a total left flaccid hemiplegia involving his face, arm and leg. Within 24 hours, slight movement in the paralysed extremities, particularly in the fingers and the foot and toes, began to return. Thereafter there was a continuous slow recovery of the paralysed parts until by eight months after the operation the face had recovered completely and the recovery in the upper and lower extremities could be conservatively evaluated as 85% of normal. He could move all digits. He had good use of his arm and hand. He could walk well, although favouring the left leg slightly. He could hop on either foot alone. (As the patient said, 'Doc, you damn near paralysed me!')

For the next year and a half his neurological condition remained about the same. The abnormal involuntary movements of hemiballismus had disappeared immediately after the operation and had never returned.

A little over two years after the operation Mr Lopez developed increasing cardiac failure and evidence of a malignant disseminated lymphosarcoma. These resulted in his death on 3 July 1961, a little more than two and a half years after the operation.

Examination of the brain and spinal cord revealed the lesion in the cerebral peduncle and the degeneration of 83% of the fibres in the cortico-spinal tract from the right cerebral hemisphere, as established by counting the fibres in the normal left medullary pyramid and in the degenerated right one. It was believed that most of the remaining 17% of the fibres in the pyramidal tract were parieto-spinal fibres from the post-central area which lie in the lateral part of the central half of the cerebral peduncle (Bucy 1964).

As there were some cortico-spinal fibres still intact in this man, even though we did not believe them to be from the precentral motor cortex and thought that they were concerned with the modulation of sensation, we could not on the basis of this case exclude the possibility that these few fibres were responsible for the voluntary movements which he had. Furthermore, he still had the innervation from his left precentral motor cortex. How much ipsilateral innervation might there be? Another opportunity such as that presented by Mr Lopez was not likely to come in the immediate future, and in fact has never again come to me. Accordingly, we turned to subhuman primates for further information.

A series of monkeys were operated upon. At first an operation similar to that in Mr Lopez was performed. The animals appeared to recover completely with no motor dysfunction except that they moved somewhat less quickly than a normal monkey. Unfortunately these animals, like Mr Lopez, still retained a few cortico-spinal fibres after operation so that it was necessary to become more destructive and we endeavoured to section the entire cerebral peduncle to ensure complete section of the pyramidal tract and to do it on both sides. A series of monkeys was produced that subsequent study of their brain demonstrated to have complete bilateral destruction of the pyramidal tract. None of them was totally paralysed. All could sit, stand and walk and use their hands although somewhat awkwardly (Bucy 1966).

Mr Lopez and this series of monkeys had clearly shown that the pyramidal tract is not necessary in either man or monkey for well coordinated, strong, discrete, useful voluntary movements. They also showed that destruction of the pyramidal tract does not produce the so-called 'pyramidal syndrome'—paralysis, spasticity, hyperactive tendon reflexes, absent abdominal reflexes, and the sign of Babinski. Of these, only the sign of Babinski results from destruction of the pyramidal tract.

Although these facts have now been known for a number of years and have been confirmed by others, we have made no further progress. Obviously there are some very important questions still to be settled. Until they are settled we will not understand the neural mechanism which controls the skeletal musculature and which is responsible for voluntary movements.

As voluntary movements are possible in the absence of the pyramidal tract, it is obvious that some other pathway or pathways must be responsible for them. There are a few things which can be said about that pathway. (1) As decortication of the cerebral hemisphere in the monkey results in the degeneration of only one descending pathway in the spinal cord (the pyramidal tract), it is obvious that the 'other' pathway must be a multi-synaptic one. (2) As these movements are present even though the entire cerebral peduncle has been destroyed, it is obvious that this pathway from the cerebral cortex to the spinal cord must descend through the tegmentum of the midbrain. It appears unlikely to me that Brodal's suggestion, that the other pathway concerned is the rubro-spinal pathway, is correct. The rubro-spinal pathway in man is so insignificant, so much smaller than it is in the carnivores. Nevertheless, at this time that possibility cannot be completely denied. It appears far more likely that the pathway concerned is a reticulo-spinal pathway but for this there is no evidence and further investigation is required.

There is still another important question. Both man and monkey require from eight to twelve months to recover after the pyramidal tract is divided.

Why? Obviously this delayed recovery is not due to regeneration of the pyramidal tract as that tract did not regenerate in either man or monkey. It also seems obvious that the 'other' pathway concerned with the production of voluntary movement existed at the time the pyramidal tract was destroyed. If so, why did it not function immediately? Various possibilities suggest themselves. Does destruction of the pyramidal tract result in such serious derangement within the cells of the spinal cord, either structural, electrical or chemical, that the anterior horn cells can not respond adequately to impulses descending from the cerebral cortex? (They can, within a few days, respond to the monosynaptic reflex responsible for the stretch reflexes.) Or with the degeneration of the pyramidal tract and of its terminal boutons must the axons of the 'other' descending pathway sprout and send new connections to the cells of the spinal cord? Or does this degeneration produce changes in the cell membranes in the spinal cord which require months to recover? Obviously we do not know, but again, if we are ever to understand the neurophysiology of voluntary movement we must find out.

References

BUCY P.C. (1957) Is there a pyramidal tract? *Brain* **80,** 376.

BUCY P.C. KEPLINIEN J.E. & SIQUEIRA E.B. (1964) Destruction of the pyramidal tract in man. *J. Neurosurg.* **21,** 285.

BUCY P.C. LADPLI R. & EHRLICH A. (1966) Destruction of the pyramidal tract in the monkey. The effects of bilateral section of the cerebral peduncles. *J. Neurosurg.* **25,** 1.

PATHOPHYSIOLOGY OF THE PARKINSONIAN TREMOR

P. RONDOT

The lesion which provokes the tremor associated with Parkinson's disease cannot at present be differentiated from that which causes other symptoms of the condition. Whether the predominant feature is tremor or rigidity, neuropathologists have observed the same depigmentation of the 'substantia nigra' when compared with other pigmented brain-stem areas. Although it is well established that parkinsonian tremor is related to the moderating influence of the substantia nigra and its efferent pathways, the actual site of origin of the rhythmic activity is still controversial.

Is it caused by a higher centre freed from the inhibition of the substantia nigra and which, in the same way as a pacemaker, periodically activates motor neurons? Or is the tremor elaborated at spinal level following loss of central control over the descending tracts in the spinal cord? The following discussion considers these two hypotheses.

A. Central control of the tremor

The operating probe during stereotactic operations designed to improve parkinsonian tremor is able to monitor the activity from various thalamic nuclei traversed before arriving at the chosen target (Albe-Fessard et al 1963). By this means, it is possible to identify rhythmic activities in certain thalamic structures, the frequency of which was close to that of the tremor (Albe-Fessard et al 1963, 1966, Jasper & Bertrand 1966). These thalamic rhythms were probably not simply induced since, according to Albe-Fessard et al (1963), they appeared before any rhythmic activity was registered on the electromyogram and subsequently disappeared during a voluntary movement, before the tremor ceased. According to these authors, the cells of these thalamic nuclei were the site of origin of the tremor.

Early observations from de-afferentation of a limb give conflicting results; after cervical radicotomy, Leriche in 1914 observed a lessening of the resting tremor but Pollock and Davies (1930) and Altenburger (1937) did not. Experimental tremors induced by Ohye et al (1950) were modified, but not stopped, by posterior radicotomy.

Is it possible to conclude from these variable results that the tremor is produced by rhythmic activity of certain thalamic nucleii? The answer appears to be no, for several reasons. In the first place, the units registered in the thalamus are not synchronous in the resting phase, afferent inputs being necessary to bring about this synchronization. Secondly, destruction of the thalamic zones, where the rhythms are recorded, does not always stop the tremor, whereas the introduction of a second lesion close by is often more effective. Finally, it has been shown that radicotomy *does* disorganize the tremor, emphasizing the importance of peripheral mechanisms in its elaboration. For those who still defend the hypothesis that the tremor has cerebral origins, the movement induced by the tremor is necessary to maintain the rhythm of certain thalamic cells (Albe-Fessard 1971).

B. Peripheral mechanisms modulating parkinsonian tremor

Parkinsonian tremor can be modified by the action of various peripheral factors, the study of which has helped to elucidate the nature of the peripheral pathways which modulate tremor.

Since the work of Jung in 1941, which emphasized the role of these peripheral factors, several studies have been concerned with the modification of tremor using the action of ischaemia on vibration applied to the tendon (Halliday and Redfearn 1954). Studies have been taken up again on the basis of recording, either by multi-electrodes or coaxial electrodes, the tremor being recorded by an accelerometer or strain gauge (Fig. 17.1) (Renou, Rondot & Metral 1970, Rondot & Bathien 1975, Rondot, Bathien & Ribadeau Dumas 1975). Motor unit discharges were as distinct as the intervals which separated them. With this method, it was possible to select the phases during which motor unit discharges were very regular, while the tremor remained steady. The experimental conditions were varied in several ways, viz. ischaemia, vibration applied to tendons, noxious nervous stimuli, blocking the nerve by local anaesthetic, alteration of the H-reflex action by various stimuli including injection of an L-dopa agonist.

(1) Ischaemia

Ischaemia first diminishes the amplitude of the tremor which, after 5 to 10 minutes, ceases. Motor units which, before induction of ischaemia, frequently discharged twice during each cycle of tremor, only discharged once before stopping. Before finally stopping, it occasionally missed one burst and re-appeared in the next; the time interval between each of the discharges increased from 200 to 400 msec (Fig. 17.2). Before stopping, the tremor is not disorganized in the strict sense, because its rhythm persists, but the time

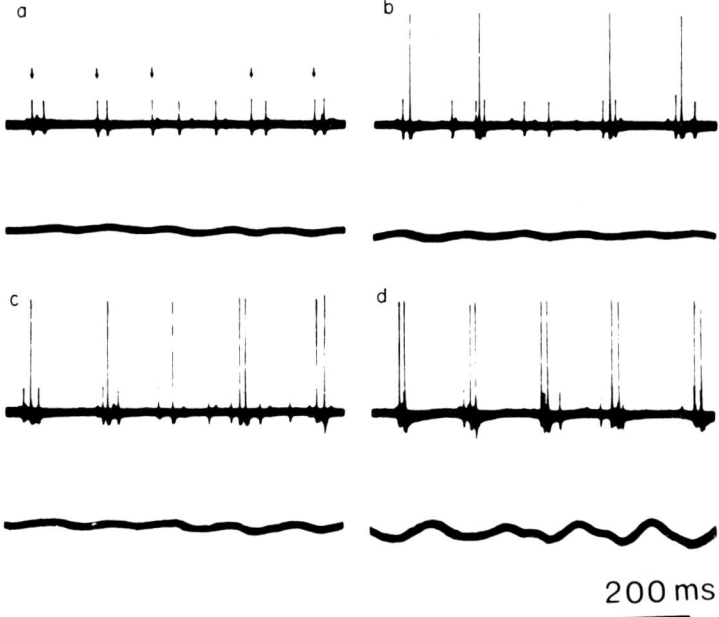

Fig. 17.1 Recording of the tremor with the aid of a multi-electrode. The double discharges are easily distinguished with rising amplitude of tremor.

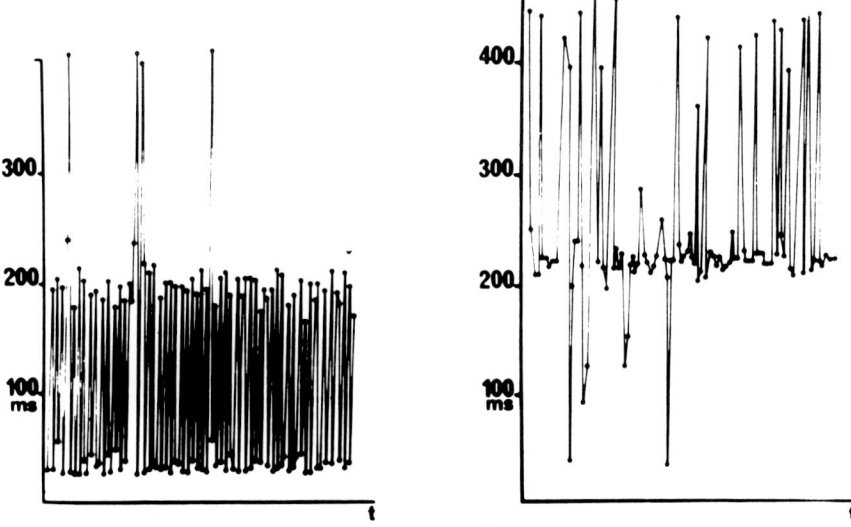

Fig. 17.2 Unit activity (a) before and (b) after 10 min ischaemia. The ordinate represents the time interval between successive discharges of the same motor unit.

interval separating each motor unit discharge remains constant, or may double or treble before stopping.

(2) Vibration

Vibration at 100 Hertz and an amplitude of 1 to 3 mn applied to the extensor tendon have an effect opposite to that of ischaemia (Fig. 17.3). The double-discharges of a motor unit during a tremor become more numerous, and new motor units are recruited during each cycle of tremor. The amplitude of the tremor is augmented, but its rhythm is only slightly modified; the duration of intervals between motor unit discharges is identical before, and during, the stimulation by vibration.

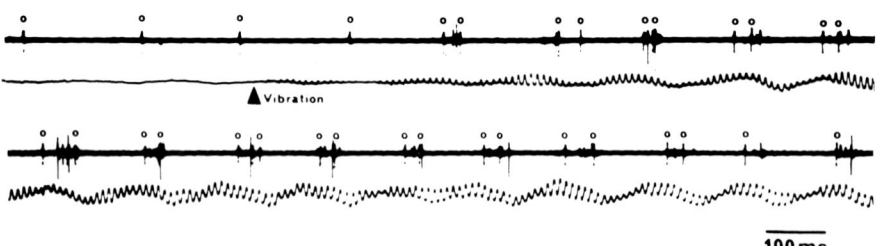

100 ms

Fig. 17.3 Effects of vibration applied on extensor indicis tendon. A and B, upper trace E.M.G. of extensor indicis, lower trace accelerometer recording tremor and vibrations. Increase in number of motor units and double-discharges (rev. *EEG Neurophysiol.* 1971, **1**, 121).

(3) Noxious nervous stimuli

Noxious nervous stimuli (Fig. 17.4) were obtained by shocks lasting 1 msec, applied to the sural nerve, while their intensity was measured by obtaining a response from the biceps after a latency period of 80 to 100 msec. Unlike other cutaneous stimuli, this nociceptive stimulus diminished the amplitude of the rhythmic bursts, temporarily arresting the double-discharges and

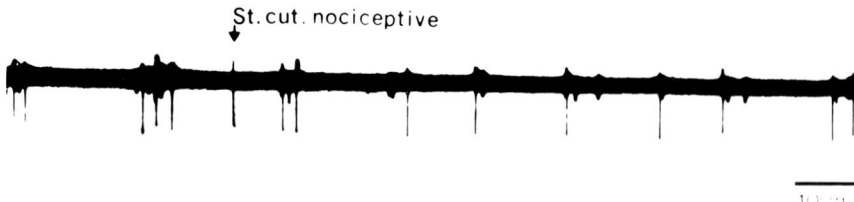

Fig. 17.4 Nociceptive cutaneous stimulation. This provokes a decrease in number of motor units and alters the rhythm.

disorganizing the tremor, while the time intervals between discharges became irregular.

(4) Lidocaine nerve block

Anaesthetic nerve block diminished the amplitude of the tremor and then disorganized its rhythm (Fig. 17.5). The double-discharges disappeared and, simultaneously, the intervals between discharges became irregular and shorter. The tremor then ceased altogether, before the isometric muscular force was diminished, the anaesthetic having acted secondarily on extrafusal motor fibres.

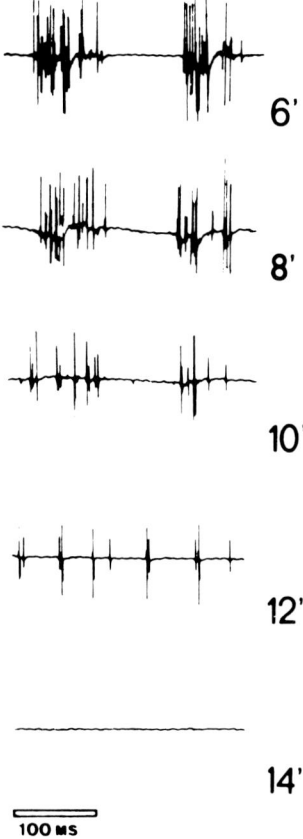

6'

8'

10'

12'

14'

100 ᴍs

Fig. 17.5 Anaesthetic block (lidocaine) showing a decrease in tremor amplitude, the rhythm being modified before disappearing.

(5) H-Reflex

With a constant stimulus, the H-reflex varied considerably in amplitude during the tremor cycle. The response was greatest if the stimulus was given at the beginning of a burst, but then decreased rapidly as the stimulus was progressively delayed. The response was very small between beats and increased rapidly at the beginning of the next (Fig. 17.6).

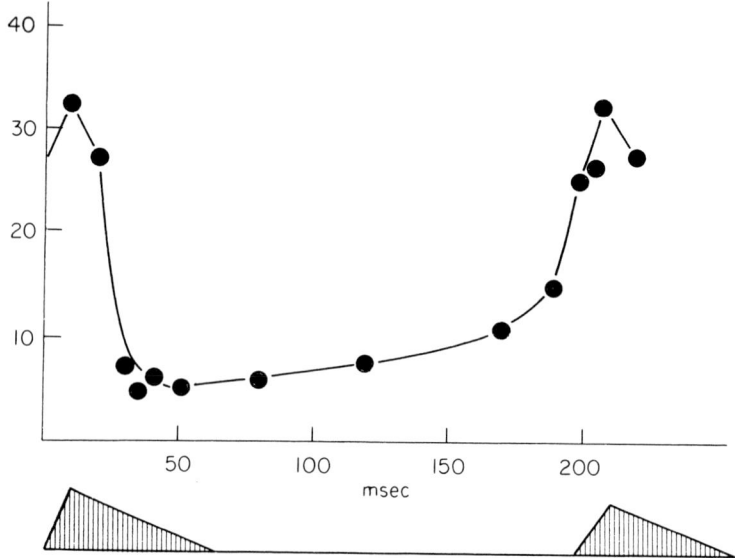

Fig. 17.6 Amplitude variation of monosynaptic reflex plotted against tremor cycle. Abscissa: on the lower line the beats of tremor are drawn diagrammatically in grey. Ordinate: the amplitude of the H response as a percentage of the direct motor M. response.

Different effects on the tremor were observed, depending on the intensity of the stimulus:

—Weak stimuli, provoking $\frac{1}{2}$ or $\frac{1}{3}$ of the maximum H-reflex, had no effect on the tremor.

—as the intensity was increased, the H-reflex (or the M response) was followed by a prolonged period, without electrical activity (Fig. 17.7), a further burst of tremor appearing after 250 msec. A greater number of motor unit potentials discharged in this burst than in those preceding the stimulus; the succeeding cyclic discharges were at the same frequency as the tremor. An injection of L-dopa did not stop the tremor. When piribedil, an L-dopa agonist (Corrodi *et al* 1971) was used, an intravenous injection of 1 to 3 mg

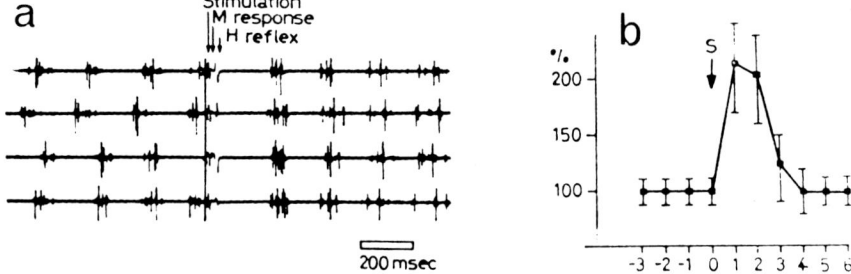

Fig. 17.7 a. Silent phase after stimulation. Note the constancy of duration of the silent phase irrespective of time of stimulation. Note also that the first beat after the silent phase contains more motor unit potentials than the preceding beats. b. Amplitude of beats in relation to their rank before and after stimulation. Ordinate: planimetric measures of integrated E.M.G. activity expressed as a percentage of control values preceding the stimulus. (These are mean values obtained from several patients: the vertical lines indicate the range of value and not standard deviations.) Abscissa: rank of beats of tremor before and after stimulation.

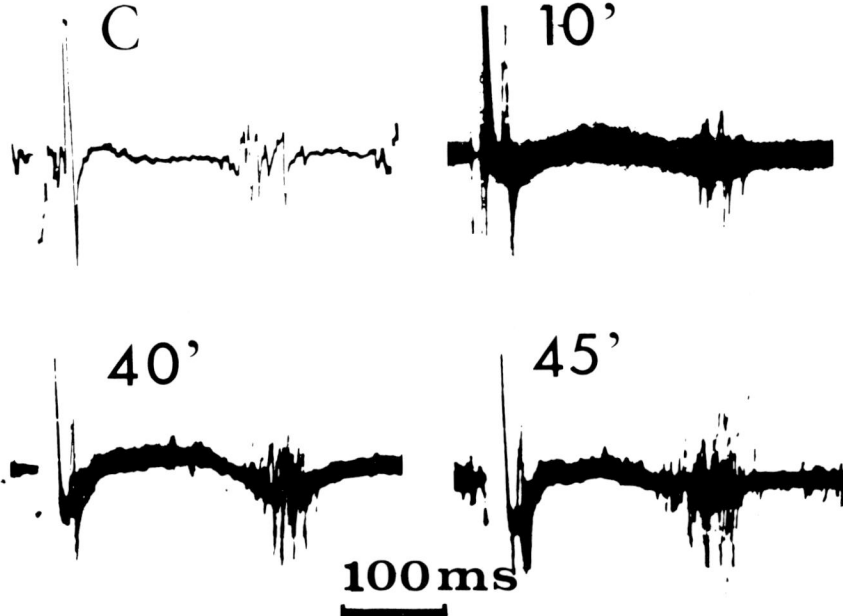

Fig. 17.8 Top left: stimulation followed by an H response, a silent phase of 200 msec and then a new phase of activity. Top right: summation of 10 responses 10 min after injection of piribedil. The silent phase persists, and the following burst of activity is weak. Bottom: summation of 10 responses at 40 min (left) and at 45 min (right) after injection of piribedil. The same silent phase is seen again, and the following phase of activity regains its initial activity.

arrested the parkinsonian tremor in 10 to 15 minutes (Rondot *et al* 1975). After injection of piribedil, stimulation provoked the reflex motor response, as before (Fig. 17.8); this motor response was followed by a period without electrical activity, of the same duration as before the injection, viz. 200 to 250 msec. On the other hand, the first burst of tremor did not show reinforcement, as it had done previously but, on the contrary, was weaker than preceding bursts. The effects of this L-dopa agonist can be summarized by saying that, although it does not modify the time interval following stimulation, it nevertheless suppresses reinforcement of the first burst of tremor which follows the reflex response so that these effects have been dissociated.

The main conclusion drawn from these studies is that tremor is made up of two distinct elements which evolve differently, according to modifications used under trial conditions, viz.:

1. *the rhythmic cycle*, characterized by the presence of several motor units which have a tendency to discharge in synchronized fashion, the same unit pulsating once or twice in each rhythmic cycle.

2. *the silent phase* between two cycles, lasting between 200 to 300 msec. This is characterized, not only by the absence of any activity, but also by a diminution of excitability of the motor neurons, as evidenced by diminution in the amplitude of the H-reflex provoked during this phase of the tremor. Ischaemia or vibration do not modify the duration of this silent phase, but they diminish or augment the amplitude of tremor by reducing or augmenting, respectively, the number of motor units by modifying the frequency of their discharges within each rhythmic cycle. Furthermore, ischaemia acts upon the large, rapidly conducting fibres (Magladery *et al* 1950); vibration stimulates the annulo-spiral receptors of muscle spindles, and augments the afferent inputs passing through large Ia fibres (Hagbarth & Bertrand 1966). It is probable that afferent fibres transmit inputs which facilitate tremor, without modifying its rhythm.

Noxious impulses transmitted by the sural nerve have an inhibiting action on the rhythmic bursts and on the intervals separating them. They, therefore, have an inhibiting effect on the first phase of activity and a disinhibitory effect on the second phase. It is a non-selective effect; the motor neurons are modulated by the long latency flexion reflex afferents both in the excitatory and inhibitory phases. Local anaesthetic injected into the trunk of the nerve produces similar action by causing disorganization of tremor, modifying the intervals between motor unit discharges, before acting on the motor fibres themselves. It has been shown that lidocaine acts first on the small fibres (Matthews & Rushworth 1957) and, by paralysing gamma fibres, diminishes intrafusal discharges. Hagbarth *et al* (1975) have shown that Ia discharges disappear after the introduction of lidocaine but this suppression is not sufficient to explain the simultaneous modification of time interval separating the discharges of a motor unit. Another factor must be present, and this will probably be determined by study of the H-reflex.

This study emphasizes an important point: when stimulation is applied immediately before, or during, a rhythmic cycle, its amplitude is augmented. This is probably due to facilitation transmitted by Ia afferents, as discussed above. There is a second phenomenon worthy of consideration: the reflex response which follows a stimulus of great intensity is followed by an interval of silence which lasts between 200 and 250 msec, a period identical to that following application of a stimulus during tremor or a tonic contraction. In the latter case, this interval can be compared to a resting phase which has been abnormally prolonged until its duration is double that of a normal resting phase. This abnormally prolonged duration could be due to a short pause in the intrafusal discharges which suddenly stop activating the motor neurones. Such an interpretation would not explain why this pause should be twice as long in a parkinsonian patient compared to a normal subject; furthermore, if the silent phase is studied in a parkinsonian patient using the unloading test, its duration returns to normal (Angel *et al* 1966).

The difference between the resting period obtained by this manoeuvre and that due to stimulation of muscle in a state of contraction, depends on the fact that the former exclusively provokes arrest of intrafusal discharges while, in the latter, the arrest of the intrafusal discharges acts as a quick stimulus on the tendon organ. It seems likely that the different duration of the resting phase in these two particular circumstances is due either to unusual sensitivity of the tendon spindles, or to a reinforcement of their action at the

Table 17.1 Peripheral mechanisms modulating parkinsonian tremor

EFFECTS	Ischemia	Vibrations	Noc. Stim.	Lidocaïne	H Reflex
Burst	−	+	−	−	+
Silent interval	0	0	−	−	+
Pathway	Ia	Ia	FRA	γ, II,III	Ia, Ib
RESULTS					

spinal level. It is almost certain that this resting phase and the resting phase of tremor is very probably induced by afferents acting via the Ib fibres.

This data can be summarized in the following way (see also Table 17.1):

Parkinson tremor depends on two principal mechanisms.

The first, the activator, is responsible for the rhythmic burst; large afferent fibres transmit impulses increasing the amplitude, but not the frequency, of the tremor.

The other, the inhibitor, manifests itself during the silent phase of the tremor; small, sensitive fibres transmit inhibitory impulses during the resting phase.

The hypothesis that a central pacemaker is the origin of parkinsonian tremor becomes difficult to support, taking into consideration the importance of peripheral factors which modulate tremor. Apparently, the supraspinal influences exert themselves in two ways.

First, there is the activation which, while exerting itself on the gamma motor neurons, also probably augments the afferent impulses transmitted to Ia fibres. The second influence, of an inhibitory nature, is probably due to lack of control exercised on the afferents, probably at spinal level.

References

ALBE-FESSARD D. (1971) Tentative d'explication neurophysiologique de la pathologie due Parkinson. In: de Ajuriaguerra J. & Gauthier G. (Eds) *Monoamines, noyaux cris centraux et syndrome de Parkinson*, p. 243. Georg. Genève; Masson, Paris.

ALBE-FESSARD D., ARFEL G. & GUIOT G. (1963) Activités caractéristiques de quelques structures cérébrales chez l'homme. *Ann. Chir.* **17**, 1185–1214.

ALBE-FESSARD D., GUIOT G., LAMARRE Y. & ARFEL G. (1966) Activation of thalamo-cortical projections related to tremorogenic processes. In: Purpura D.P. & Year M.D. (Eds) *The Thalamus*, p. 237. Columbia University Press, New York.

ALTENBURGER H. (1937) In: Bumke-Foersters (Ed.) *Handbuch der Neurologie*, vol. 3, p. 749. Springer, Berlin.

ANGEL R.W., HOFMANN W.W. & EPPLER W. (1966) Silent period in patients with parkinsonian rigidity. *Neurology* **16**, 529–32.

CORRODI H., FUXE K. & UNGERSTEDT U. (1971) Evidence for a new type of dopamine receptor stimulating agent. *J. Pharmacol.* **23**, 989–91.

HAGBARTH K.E. & EKLUND G. (1968) The effects of muscle vibration in spasticity, rigidity and cerebellar disorders. *J. Neurol. Neurosurg. Psychiat.* **31**, 207–13.

HAGBARTH K.E., WALLIN G. & LÖFSTEDT L. (1975) Muscle spindle activity in man during voluntary fast alternating movements. *J. Neurol. Neurosurg. Psychiat.* **38**, 625–35.

HALLIDAY A.M. & REDFEARN J.W.T. (1954) The effects of ischemia on finger tremor. *J. Physiol. (London)* **123**, 23–4.

JASPER H.H. & BERTRAND G. (1966) Thalamic units involved in somatic sensation and voluntary and involuntary movements in man. In: Purpura D.P. & Year M.D. (Eds) *The Thalamus*, p. 365. Columbia University Press, New York.

JUNG R. (1941) Physiologische Untersuchungen über den Parkinson tremor und andere Zitterformen bein Menschen. *Zeitsch. Ges. Neurol. Psych.* **173**, 263–332.

LERICHE R. (1914) Radicotomie cervicale pour un tremblement parkinsonien. *Lyon*

Med. **122,** 1075–6.

MAGLADERY J.W., MCDOUGAL, D.B. & STOLL J. (1950) Electrophysiological studies of nerve and reflex activity in normal man. II. The effects of peripheral ischemia. *Bull. Johns Hopkins Hospital.* **86,** 290–321.

MATTHEWS P.B.C. & RUSHWORTH G. (1957) The relative sensitivity of muscle nerve fibres to procaine. *J. Physiol. (London)* **135,** 263–9.

OHYE C., BOUCHARD R., LAROCHELLE K., BEDARD P., BOUCHER R., RAPHY B. & POIRIER L.J. (1970) Effect of dorsal rhizotomy on postural tremor in the monkey. *Exp. Brain Res.* **10,** 140–50.

POLLOCK L.J. & DAVIS L. (1930) Muscle tone in Parkinsonian states. *Arch. Neurol. Psychiat.* **23,** 303–19.

RENOU G., RONDOT P. & METRAL S. (1970) Analyse de décharges itératives d'une même unité motrice dans les bouffées de tremblement. *Rev. Neurol.* **122,** 420–3.

RONDOT P. & BATHIEN N. (unpublished) Peripheral mechanisms modulating Parkinsonian's tremor. *Vth International Symposium on Parkinson's disease. Vienne 17–19 September 1975.*

RONDOT P., BATHIEN N. & RIBADEAU DUMAS J.L. (1975) Indications of piribedil in L-DOPA treated Parkinsonian patients. Physiopathological implications. In: Calne D, Chase T.N. & Barbeau A. (Eds) *Advances in Neurology*, Vol. 9, p. 373. Raven Press, New York.

RONDOT P. & RENOU G. (1971) Analyse E.M.G unitaire du tremblement parkinsonien de repos et d'attitude. *Rev. E.E.G. Neurophysiol.* **1,** 121–4.

PART III
MISCELLANEOUS

MUSCLE PAIN: WHICH RECEPTORS ARE
RESPONSIBLE FOR THE
TRANSMISSION OF NOXIOUS STIMULI?

S. MENSE AND R. F. SCHMIDT

Introduction

At the turn of this century, Sherrington, in one of his brilliant contributions to Schäfer's *Textbook of Physiology* (1900), saw no reason to assume that there are specific afferent muscle nerve fibres for the transmission of noxious stimuli. In his opinion, the adequate stimulus for muscle spindles and tendon organs 'seems under certain circumstances . . . to elicit pain from the muscular sense' and 'a specific set of nerve fibres and end organs, devoted solely to production of pain, . . . , does not appear a warrantable postulate for muscle'.

Within the next thirty to forty years it became increasingly clear that Group Ia and II fibres coming, respectively, from primary and secondary endings of muscle spindles, as well as Group Ib fibres stemming from tendon organs, are not involved in transmission of painful sensations from muscle, but indicated the thin myelinated (Group III) and unmyelinated fibres (Group IV or C-fibres) as the appropriate pathway, as in the skin. Several monographs and textbooks give detailed accounts of this development (Creed *et al* 1932, Lewis 1942, Fulton 1943, Bishop 1960, Knighton & Dumke 1966).

In the second third of this century, despite the introduction of new methods in neuroanatomy and neurophysiology, very little evidence has been added to the now generally held view that the afferent fibres of muscular nociceptive units belong to the Groups III and IV. An electronmicroscopical study by Stacey (1969) revealed that the freely branching, unencapsulated endings of these fibres are found throughout the muscle in association with all types of tissue, with particularly dense projections to the regions of tendons, aponeuroses and fascial sheaths, and in the adventitia of blood vessels (with the exception of the capillary network). By recording impulses from isolated Group III (Paintal 1960, Bessou & Laporte 1961) and Group IV fibres (Iggo 1961) it was shown that the application of pressure, and the intramuscular injection of 0·5 ml or less of 5–6% NaCl, will fire their terminal receptors,

265

while stretching or contracting muscle during ischaemia will not do so. Paintal (1960) suggested that the receptors stimulated by pressure may also be excited by chemical nociception to evoke pain, although he admitted that other receptors might be involved. Bessou and Laporte (1958), using Douglas and Ritchie's (1957) method of 'antidromic collision', have demonstrated that the unmyelinated afferent fibres from the gastrocnemius–soleus muscle of the cat are stimulated when the muscle is made to contract for one minute under conditions of ischaemia.

In view of Stacey's (1969) finding that the unmyelinated afferent fibres outnumber the myelinated ones by a factor of two (but even this is probably an under-estimation: von Düring, personal communication), more detailed data on the receptor characteristics of these afferents are highly desirable, particularly since other work suggests that impulses in Group IV (and Group III) fibres not only inform the central nervous system of painful events occurring in muscle, but that these impulses participate in the induction of circulatory and respiratory reflexes during muscular work (McCloskey & Mitchell 1972, Kalia *et al* 1972).

Our own approach to the analysis of the receptor characteristics of Group IV fibres has been to assume that there exist at least two major types or classes of unmyelinated afferent units in skeletal muscle which may tentatively be called nociceptors and metaboceptors respectively; the former are excited by nociceptive stimuli, and the latter by mechanical and/or chemical changes occurring in their environment during muscular work. In regard to the nociceptors, the major topic of this presentation, the additional assumption has been made that they should not only be responsive to strong mechanical stimuli, but even more so to chemicals which elicit pain when applied to living tissue. The most prominent of these pain-producing substances or 'algesic agents' are the nonapeptide bradykinin, 5-hydroxytryptamine (5-HT = serotonin), histamine and potassium ions. These substances evoke pseudaffective responses in animals (vocalization, blood pressure and respiratory changes) when injected intra-arterially to various organs (Guzman *et al* 1962, Lim *et al* 1962), and they give rise to pain in humans when administered on the exposed base of an artificial blister (Keele & Armstrong 1964) or when given by intradermal, intra-peritoneal, or intra-arterial injection (Harpman & Allen 1959, Lim *et al* 1967, Burch & DePasquale 1962).

Experimental methods

All experiments in this series were performed on cats anaesthetized with chloralose, paralysed with Flaxedil and artificially respired. All details regarding the general handling of the animal and the routine operating and

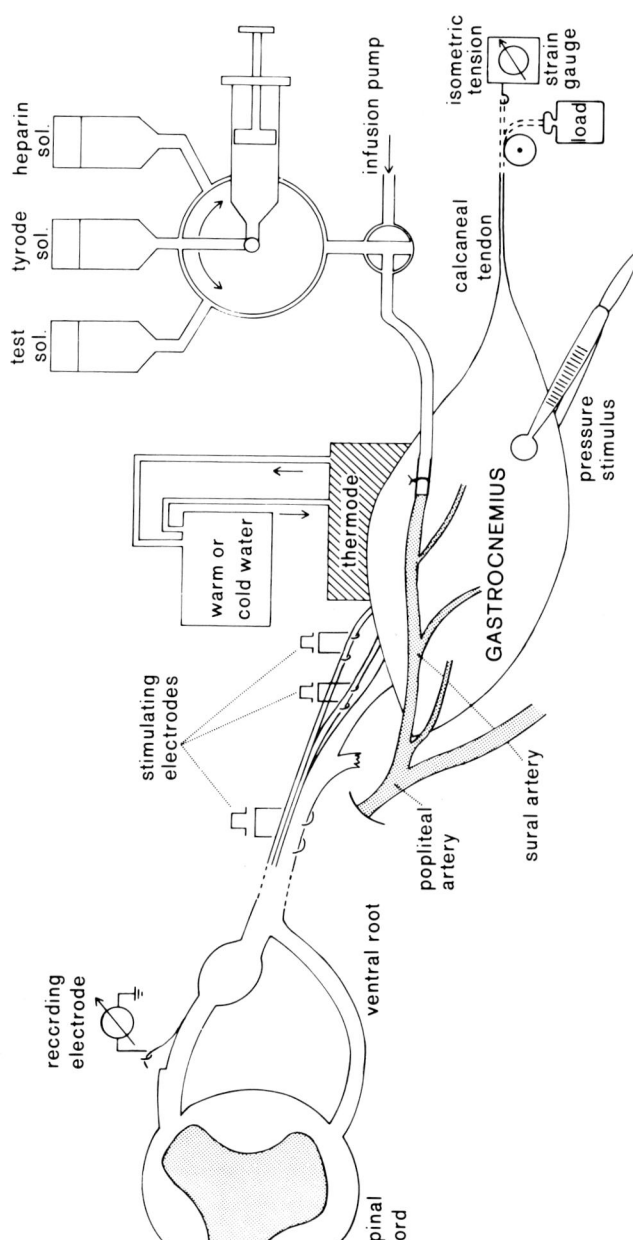

Fig. 18.1 Experimental set-up showing schematically various types of stimulating procedures used (explanation in text).

maintaining procedures are described in previous publications (cf. Franz &
Mense 1975, Kniffki *et al* 1976, Mense 1977).

Afferent nerve fibres from the gastrocnemius–soleus muscle were
dissected from fine strands of dorsal rootlets or the sciatic nerve. They were
identified by their conduction velocity, determined by electrical stimulation
of the muscle nerve at the popliteal fossa. Fibres conducting with less than
2·5 msec were classified as Group IV fibres, those from 30 to 2·5 msec as
Group III, those from 72–30 msec as Group II and those above 72 msec (at
normal body temperature) as Group I fibres. In the Groups I and II this
classification was supplemented by other criteria, particularly the responses
of the receptors to mechanical events (for details, see Mense 1977).

Figure 18.1 is an assemblage showing the different methods of
stimulation. For technical reasons only a few are used with any given
experiment. The two basic procedures practically always employed are (a)
the testing of local mechanical sensitivity by means of a forceps with round
plates and (b) testing chemical sensitivity by intra-arterial injection of algesic
or other agents up-stream into the sural artery (for details see Franz & Mense
1975). Other procedures are (c) stretching of muscle by weights attached to
the calcaneal tendon, (d) recording of isometric tension following single or
repetitive stimulation of ventral roots or peripheral motor nerves (see Kniffki
et al 1976) and (e) warming or cooling the medial head of the gastrocnemius
muscle by thermodes placed alongside (see Hertel *et al* 1976).

Neurohumoral mediators and muscle pain

Squeezing any muscle firmly between finger and thumb gives rise to pain, as
does a needle prick or knife cut. Ever since the work, some 40 years ago, of
Lewis and others, who showed that severe pain can be elicited by injecting
small amounts of hypertonic saline or other irritant substances or by
performing muscle activity under ischaemic conditions (cf. Lewis 1942), it
has been assumed that certain forms of muscle pain may be due to chemical
substances released, or activated by, cellular injury and exciting nociceptive
units. In the course of time, the field of candidates has been narrowed down
considerably, and it now includes, in particular, those substances which have
been termed algesic agents (see above) and which in Fig. 18.2 are shown to
excite a Group IV afferent fibre.

All algesic agents used as stimulants in Fig. 18.2 are endogenous
substances which reach particularly high levels of concentration in the course
of painful tissue affections. Examples have recently been quoted and
discussed by Mense and Schmidt (1974), Franz and Mense (1975), and Fock
and Mense (1976) and need not be repeated here. It may be pointed out,
however, that only about 50% of the muscular Group IV afferents, sensitive

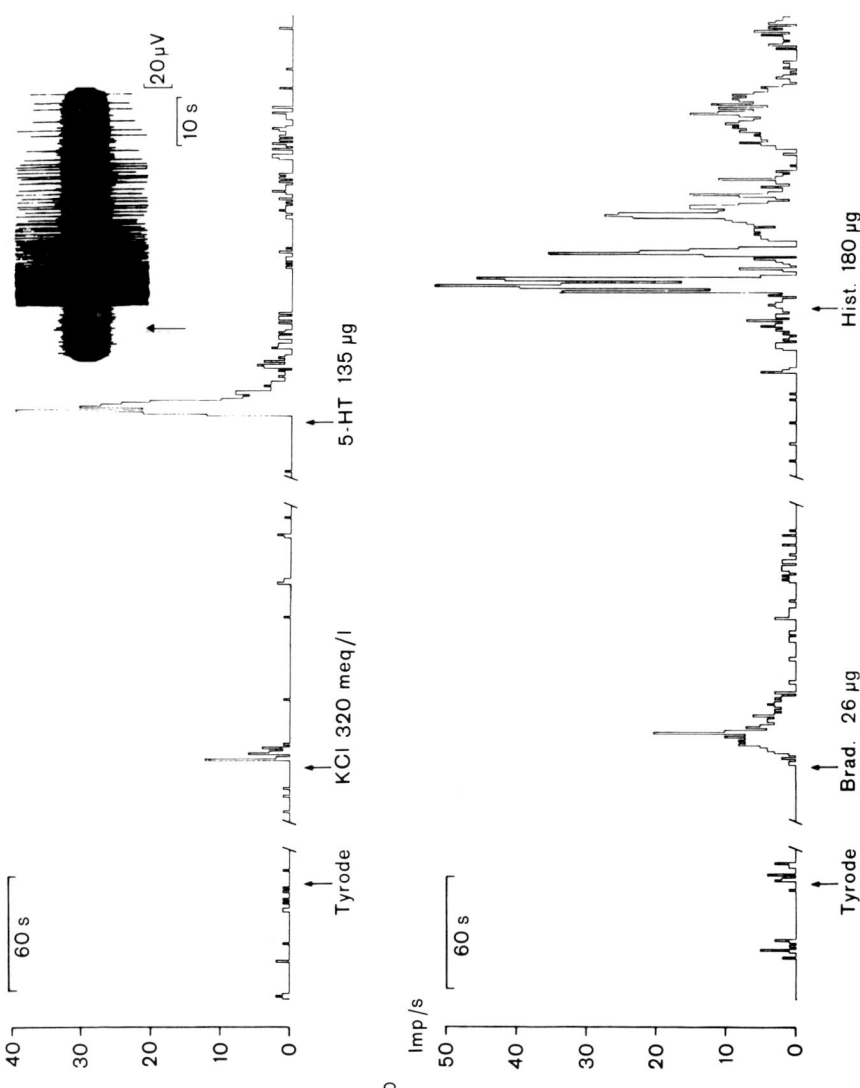

Fig. 18.2 Activity in a single Group IV afferent unit in response to the intra-arterial injection of various algesic agents. Recording from gastrocnemius part of the sciatic nerve at the upper part of thigh. Conduction velocity of the fibre was 1·27 msec. The fibre was sensitive to strong pressure exerted on the distal third of the lateral head of the gastrocnemius muscle. The poststimulus time histograms in this (and the following Figs. 18.3 and 18.5) were plotted from computer records using a dwell time of 1 second for each address. The start of the intra-arterial injections is marked by an arrow; they are completed within a few seconds. The inset in the upper right-hand corner shows the receptor discharge following the injection of 135 μg 5-HT. Before each injection a rest period of at least 3 min elapsed. (Modified from Mense & Schmidt 1974.)

to one of the algesic agents, are also sensitive to the other three substances. The rest of the units display various combinations of differential sensitivity, that of bradykinin plus KCl being more frequent (about 25% of all units) than any other (Fock & Mense 1976). Whether this unexpected finding is due simply to the methods employed or whether it signals that the various units do have specific sets of pharmacological receptors at their sensory endings has to remain open at present. We tend to favour the second possibility for reasons which will be discussed below.

A major point related to this question has been illuminated by observing the responses to repetitive application of the various substances. Whereas the sensitivity to bradykinin did not decrease even at injection intervals as close as one per minute, that to 5-HT decreased dramatically in the course of repetitive applications (Fig. 18.3); recovery took about 10 to 15 min. This tachyphylactic response to 5-HT was not associated with a decrease in sensitivity to bradykinin (Fig. 18.3). Such a lack of cross-tachyphylaxis seems also to apply to the effects of histamine on one side and bradykinin or 5-HT on the other, though this has not yet been fully documented (Hiss & Mense 1976). The most simple and obvious assumption derived from this finding is that different receptor sites for bradykinin, 5-HT and histamine exist at the sensory nerve endings of these Group IV afferent units (the responses to KCl probably are a consequence of the direct depolarizing action of this substance), some units having one type of receptor only, others various combinations, most often all three (see preceding paragraph). Certainly, more indirect modes of action of the algesic drugs appear possible. Some of them have been made unlikely by direct experimental evidence (Hiss & Mense 1976), others need not be considered as long as the hypothesis of direct action gives a satisfactory explanation of the results.

Therapeutic consequences

Pharmacological suppression of afferent activity induced by noxious stimuli can be exerted at any place in the centripetal pathways, but it appears most economical to do it at the earliest possible sites, even before the unwanted afferent activity has produced any appreciable effects in the central nervous system. This strategy being accepted, the prime target for such a therapeutic attack, obviously, should be the pharmacological receptor at the peripheral sensory endings of the nociceptors. This simple concept has, of course, stimulated considerable experimental efforts but, so far, success has been limited. This is not surprising in view of the results just reported, namely, the existence of nociceptors with various types of pharmacological receptors (and there are probably more receptor types than revealed by our testing procedures). Nevertheless, it seems worthwhile to continue the search for

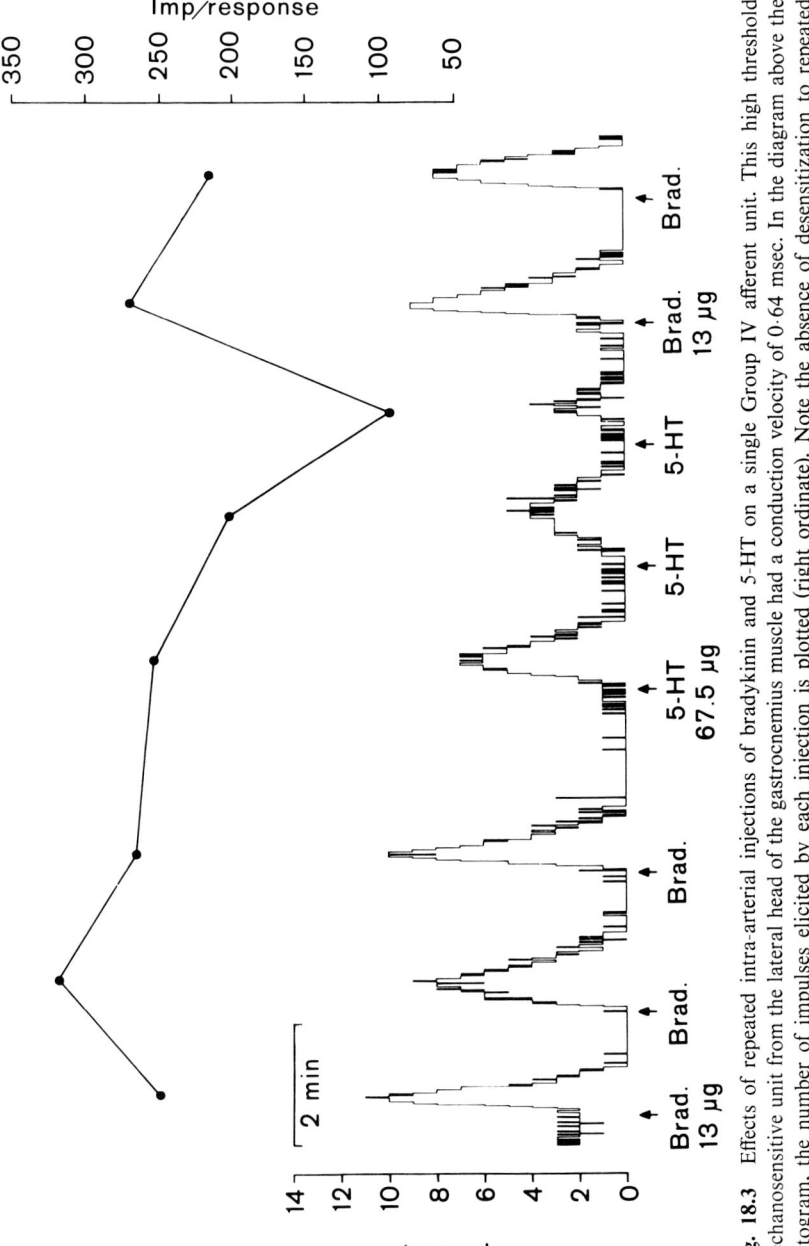

Fig. 18.3 Effects of repeated intra-arterial injections of bradykinin and 5-HT on a single Group IV afferent unit. This high threshold mechanosensitive unit from the lateral head of the gastrocnemius muscle had a conduction velocity of 0·64 msec. In the diagram above the histogram, the number of impulses elicited by each injection is plotted (right ordinate). Note the absence of desensitization to repeated bradykinin injections and the lack of cross-tachyphylaxis between bradykinin and 5-Ht. (From Hiss & Mense 1976.)

analgesic agents which act preferentially on peripheral receptors and have little or no action on the central nervous system itself.

In animal and man, bradykinin-evoked pseudaffective responses or pain sensations, respectively, can effectively be blocked by acetylsalicylic acid. Various types of experiments, including those using animals with crossed circulation to prevent central actions of the drug, have shown that this algesic effect is mainly due to aspirin reducing at the periphery the action of bradykinin on sensory nerve endings (Guzman *et al* 1964, Lim *et al* 1964, 1967, Coffman 1966, Lim 1966, Taira *et al* 1968).

The antagonistic effect of aspirin on the action of bradykinin at the periphery has recently been demonstrated by Mense (1976) who was able to show that the bradykinin-induced responses of muscle Group IV afferents can be effectively blocked by aspirin, whereas the responses to 5-HT seem to remain unchanged (Fig. 18.4). Again it is not possible to say, at present, whether this interaction is taking place at the pharmacological receptor of the terminal itself (the most simple explanation with no evidence to the contrary) or whether it reflects the interference of both substances at a preceding step at present unknown (such a step could be the suppression of prostaglandin formation by aspirin, Vane 1971, Ferreira *et al* 1973). The advantage of the direct recording of drug effects on the discharges of nociceptive afferents as compared to more indirect testing procedures (such as the registration of pseudaffective responses) is obvious. It is to be expected that in the future the screening procedures for potentially analgesic drugs will be supplemented by the observation of their effects on the response characteristics of cutaneous, visceral and muscular nociceptive afferent units.

Nociception by Group IV units only?

There is ample evidence that cutaneous pain is transmitted by two specific sets of nerve fibres which are differentially nociceptive in function, namely, certain Group III or A delta-fibres, subserving the short-latency pricking pain, and certain Group IV or C-fibres, subserving the long-latency burning pain. Thus the dual quality of cutaneous pain depends in the first instance upon the existence of these two sets of fibres.

In comparison, muscular pain is more of a single quality (aching, burning). It may be asked, therefore, whether it is subserved by Group IV fibres only and whether the other candidates, namely the Group III fibres (which are much smaller in number, cf. Stacey 1969), subserve different functions, for instance as metaboceptors. Against such a view is the evidence of Paintal (1960) and Bessou and Laporte (1961) quoted above that Group III units often have to be classified as 'pressure-pain receptors' according to their mechanical and chemical sensitivity.

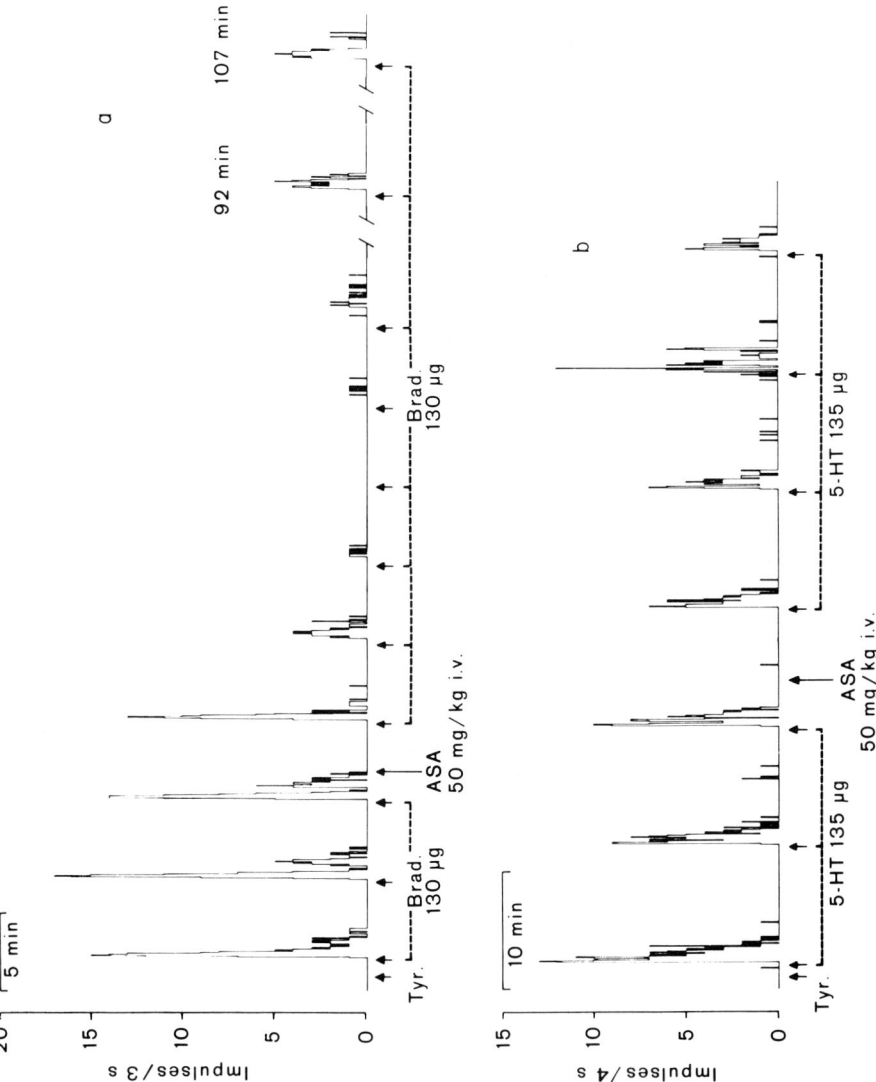

Fig. 18.4 Effects of acetylsalicylic acid (ASA) on the responses of two Group IV afferent units to bradykinin (a) and 5-Ht (b). The unit in a was a Group IV afferent fibre from the lateral head of the gastrocnemius muscle. It was not sensitive to mechanical stimulation. Conduction velocity: 2·1 msec. Dwell time of the histogram 3 sec. The histogram showing the last two injections of bradykinin start 92 min and 107 min respectively after the beginning of the continuous histogram to the left. The unit in b was also mechano-insensitive; it came from the medial head, and its conduction velocity was 0·85 msec. Dwell time of the histogram 4 sec. Note, in spite of the long injection intervals (10 min), slight tachyphylaxis to 5-HT is still present. The injection of ASA does not seem to interfere with the progressive decrease in the response to 5-HT. (Mense, unpublished.)

A more detailed re-investigation of the receptive properties of Group III afferents from muscle has revealed that the responsiveness of these units to chemical noxious stimulation is quite similar to that of Group IV afferents (Fig. 18.5 Mense 1977). This similarity includes the fact that the responses to bradykinin are also not tachyphylactic (Fig. 18.5 d). However, within the Group III sample there is quite a high proportion of fibres (35%) which have rather low thresholds to local mechanical stimulation. Group IV fibres of this type are rare (4%).

Group I and Group II fibres from muscle spindles and tendon organs do not take part in the transmission of noxious stimuli from skeletal muscle. This is already borne out by the everyday experience in neurological examination that transcutaneous electrical stimulation of Group I fibres to elicit the H-reflex is not accompanied by painful sensations. It is well in line with this finding that intra-arterial algesic agents, such as bradykinin, do not excite Group I and II afferent units from muscle (Mense 1977).

Thus, as in the skin, certain sets of Group III and Group IV afferent fibres seem to be responsible for the reception and transmission of noxious events in skeletal muscle. Their chemical sensitivity seems to be similar, as appears to be the quality of the sensations induced. On the whole Group III fibres have a lower threshold to pressure stimuli, which makes them the preferential candidates to register potentially harmful mechanical events.

Metabo- versus Noci-ceptors

Of the total sample of Group IV afferent units from gastrocnemius–soleus muscle, only about 50% can be classified as nociceptors, according to their response to local pressure stimuli and chemical irritants. It is tempting to assume, as has been done at the outset of this study, that the others are metaboceptors participating in the circulatory and respiratory adjustments to muscular work (McCloskey & Mitchell 1972, Kalia *et al* 1972). In an effort to substantiate this assumption it has been shown that there is, indeed, a group of fibres which can be excited by muscle contractions (and/or muscle stretch), and that some of these fibres also show responses to chemical changes in their environment, such as increases in phosphate, lactate or H^+-ion concentrations, which are supposed to occur during muscular activity (Kniffki *et al* 1976).

It has to be admitted, however, that rather high concentrations of these chemicals were required to obtain the excitatory effects. Thus parameters other than changes in the chemical composition of the extracellular fluid, which were induced in these experiments, may be responsible for the activation of metaboceptors during exercise. Such a parameter could be the increase in temperature that occurs in a working muscle. Evidence is just

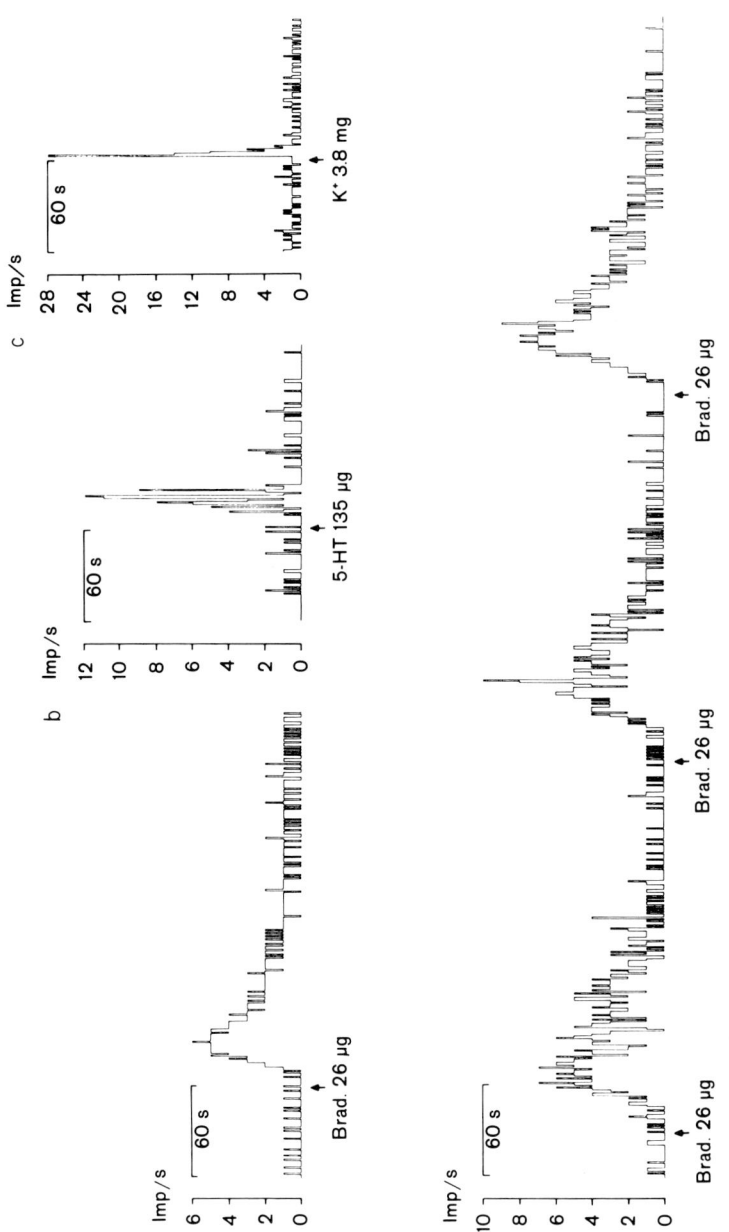

Fig. 18.5 Activation of four different (a–d) muscle Group III afferent units by pain-producing substances. In a, b and c single intra-arterial injections of the indicated agents were administered. In d the injection of bradykinin was repeated at intervals of 4 min in order to show that no tachyphylaxis is present in the responses to this substance. (From Mense 1977.)

coming foward that temperature changes of a few centigrade below and above body core temperature effectively modify the discharge frequency of muscle Group IV units (Kumazawa & Mizumura 1976, Hertel *et al* 1976).

Conclusions

All lines of evidence point to a certain proportion of Group III and IV afferent units in muscle as those responsible for the reception of noxious chemical and mechanical stimuli. (There is also evidence for the existence of receptors responding to presumably noxious heat, i.e. temperatures above 43°C, cf. Iggo 1961, Kumazawa & Mizumura 1976.)

Some 50% of all Group III and IV afferent units belong to this nociceptive category so that their absolute number exceeds that of all other myelinated afferents.

The data presently available suggest that the nociceptive units are a very heterogeneous group with diverse receptive properties. The sensitivity of an individual unit may be restricted to a single chemical substance only, whereas other receptors respond to a great variety of chemical, mechanical and probably thermal stimuli. Further experimental results are required before a more detailed specification of the various types of units may be attempted.

The sensitivity to chemical stimuli is probably due to the existence of specific pharmacological receptors at the sensory nerve terminals of afferent units. These receptors seem to operate independently of each other, some displaying considerable tachyphylaxis, others not. It is undecided whether the responses to pressure stimuli are due to release of a neurohumoral substance from damaged tissue.

The excitatory effect of bradykinin on muscular nociceptors is effectively blocked by acetylsalicylic acid. In the future, the topical application of analgesics with a peripheral site of action may develop into a powerful therapeutic tool in the management of cutaneous, visceral and muscle pain.

It is postulated that the central connections of nociceptive afferent units differ from that of other Group III and IV fibres, the former ones activating spinal structures related to the centripetal transmission of pain. This assumption is presently being tested in our laboratory making use of the specific activation of nociceptive units by the intra-arterial injection of algesic substances.

Acknowledgment

Work reported from this laboratory has been supported by the Deutsche Forschungsgemeinschaft.

References

BESSOU P. & LAPORTE Y. (1958) Activation des fibres afférentes amyéliniques d'origine musculaire. *C.R. Soc. Biol. (Paris)* **152**, 1587–90.

BESSOU P. & LAPORTE Y. (1961) Some observations on receptors of the soleus muscle innervated by Group III afferent fibers. *J. Physiol.* **155**, 19P.

BISHOP G.H. (1960) The relation of nerve fibre size to modality of sensation. In: W. Montagna (Ed.) *Cutaneous Innervation.* 88–98 Pergamon Press, Oxford.

BURCH G.E. & DePASQUALE N.P. (1962) Bradykinin, digital blood flow, and the arteriovenous anastomoses. *Circulat. Res.* **10**, 105–115.

COFFMAN J.D. (1966) The effect of aspirin on pain and hand blood flow responses to intra-arterial injection of bradykinin in man. *Clin. Pharmacol. Ther.* **7**, 26–37.

CREED R.S., DENNY-BROWN D., ECCLES J.C., LIDDELL E.G.T. & SHERRINGTON C.S. (1932) *Reflex Activity of the Spinal Cord*, pp. 1–183. Oxford University Press, London.

DOUGLAS W.W. & RITCHIE J.M. (1957) Non-medullated fibres in the saphenous nerve which signal touch. *J. Physiol.* **139**, 385–99.

FERREIRA S.H., MONCADA S. & VANE J.R. (1973) Further experiments to establish that the analgesic action of aspirin-like drugs depends on the inhibition of prostaglandin biosynthesis. *Br. J. Pharmac.* **47**, 629P.

FOCK S. & MENSE S. (1976) Excitatory effects of 5-hydroxytryptamine, histamine and potassium on muscular Group IV afferent units: a comparison with bradykinin. *Brain Res.* **105**, 459–69.

FRANZ M. & MENSE S. (1975) Muscle receptors with Group IV afferent fibres responding to application of bradykinin. *Brain Res.* **92**, 369–83.

FULTON J.F. (1943) *Physiology of the Nervous System.* Oxford University Press, London, New York, Toronto.

GUZMAN F., BRAUN C. & LIM R.K.S. (1962) Visceral pain and the pseudaffective response to intra-arterial injection of bradykinin and other algesic agents. *Arch. int. Pharmacodyn.* **136**, 353–84.

GUZMAN F., BRAUN C., LIM R.K.S., POTTER, G.D. & RODGERS D.W. (1964) Narcotic and non-narcotic analgesics which block visceral pain evoked by intra-arterial injection of bradykinin and other algesic agents. *Arch. int. Pharmacodyn.* **149**, 571–88.

HARPMAN J.A. & ALLEN R.T.J. (1959) Neural activity and polypeptides. *Brit. med. J.* **1**, 1043.

HERTEL H.-C., HOWALDT B. & MENSE S. (1976) Responses of Group IV and Group III muscle afferents to thermal stimuli. *Brain Res.* **113**, 201–5.

HISS E. & MENSE S. (1976) Evidence for the existence of different receptor sites for algesic agents at the endings of muscular Group IV afferent units. *Pflügers Arch.* **362**, 141–6.

IGGO A. (1961) Non-myelinated afferent fibres from mammalian skeletal muscle. *J. Physiol.* **155**, 52–53P.

KALIA M., SENAPATI J.M., PARIDA B. & PANDA A. (1972) Reflex increase in ventilation by muscle receptors with non-medullated fibers (C fibers). *J. appl. Physiol.* **32**, 189–93.

KEELE C.A. & ARMSTRONG D. (1964) *Substances Producing Pain and Itch.* Arnold, London.

KNIFFKI K.-D., MENSE S. & SCHMIDT R.F. (1976) Chemo- and mechanosensivity of possible metabo- and nociceptors in skeletal muscle. *Pflügers Arch.* **362**, R32.

KNIGHTON R.S. & DUMKE P.R. (Eds) (1966) *Pain.* Little, Brown & Co., Boston.

KUMAZAWA T. & MIZUMURA K. (1976) The polymodal C-fiber receptor in the muscle of the dog. *Brain Res.* **101**, 589–93.

LEWIS T. (1942) *Pain.* Macmillan, New York.

LIM R.K.S. (1966) Salicylate analgesia. In: Smith M.J.H. & Smith P.K. (Eds) *The Salicylates: A Critical Bibliographic Review.* John Wiley & Sons, Inc., New York.

LIM R.K.S., GUZMAN F., RODGERS D.W.,

GOTO K., BRAUN C., DICKERSON G.D. & ENGLE R.J. (1964) Site of action of narcotic and non-narcotic analgesics determined by blocking bradykinin-evoked visceral pain. *Arch. int. Pharmacodyn.* **152**, 25–58.

LIM R.K.S., LIU CH.N., GUZMAN F. & BRAUN CH. (1962) Visceral receptors concerned in visceral pain and the pseud-affective response to intra-arterial injection of bradykinin and other algesic agents. *J. comp. Neurol.* **118**, 264–77.

LIM R.K.S., MILLER D.G., GUZMAN F., RODGERS D.W., ROGERS R.W., WANG S.K., CHAO P.Y. & SHIH T.Y. (1967) Pain and analgesia evaluated by the intraperitoneal bradykinin-evoked pain method in man. *Clin. Pharmacol. Ther.* **8**, 521–42.

McCLOSKEY D.I. & MITCHELL J.H. (1972) Reflex cardiovascular and respiratory responses originating in exercising muscle. *J. Physiol.* **224**, 173–86.

MENSE S. (1976) Reduction of the bradykinin induced activation of muscular nociceptors by acetylsalicylic acid. *Pflügers Arch.* **362** (Suppl.), R 32.

MENSE S. (1977) Nervous outflow from skeletal muscle following chemical noxious stimulation. *J. Physiol.* (accepted for publication).

MENSE S. & SCHMIDT R.F. (1974) Activation of Group IV afferent units from muscle by algesic agents. *Brain Res.* **72**, 305–10.

PAINTAL A.S. (1960) Functional analysis of Group III afferent fibres of mammalian muscle. *J. Physiol.* **152**, 250–70.

SHERRINGTON C.S. (1900) Cutaneous Sensations. In: *Schäfer's Textbook of Physiology*, Vol. 2, pp. 920–1001. Y. J. Pentland, London and Edinburgh.

STACEY M.J. (1969) Free nerve endings in skeletal muscle of the cat. *J. Anat.*, **105**, 231–54.

TAIRA N., NAKAYAMA K. & HASHIMOTO K. (1968) Vocalization response of puppies to intra-arterial administration of bradykinin and other algesic agents, and mode of actions of blocking agents. *Tohoku J. exp. Med.* **96**, 365–77.

VANE J.R. (1971) Inhibition of prostaglandin synthesis as a mechanism of action for aspirin-like drugs. *Nature, New Biol.* **231**, 232–5.

INNERVATION OF INTRACRANIAL STRUCTURES:
A REAPPRAISAL

F. L. MCNAUGHTON AND W. H. FEINDEL

Our interest in the nerve supply of intracranial structures was stimulated in the 1930s by the observations of Wilder Penfield and Bronson Ray on the pain sensitive intracranial structures in man, as well as by the work of Stanley Cobb, Henry Forbes and their co-workers in Boston, on the neural control of the cerebral circulation. Their findings were of obvious importance for the basic understanding of headache, epilepsy and cerebral vascular disorders, and led us to undertake a thorough review of the nerve supply of intracranial structures (McNaughton 1937, Penfield & McNaughton 1940, Feindel, *et al* 1960).

In view of the many new developments in the study of cerebral circulation in recent years (Purves 1972), a re-appraisal of the earlier anatomical studies seems appropriate.

The contributions of Thomas Willis

As we meet to commemorate the life and work of Gordon Holmes, eminent British neurologist, investigator and teacher, it is fitting to quote from one of his distinguished predecessors, Thomas Willis, who has been rightly called the founder of Neurology (Feindel 1962) (Fig. 19.1).

In the Preface to his famous book on the *Anatomy of the Brain*, Willis described how he found it necessary because of the lack of precise studies on the brain before his time, to devote himself 'wholly to the study of Anatomy', so that, he continued, 'a firm and stable Basis might be laid, on which not only a more certain Physiologie than I had gained in the Schools, but what I had long thought upon, might be built' (Feindel 1965). One can see similarities to the approach which Willis made, in the work of Gordon Holmes, whose classical studies of the visual cortex and the cerebellum in particular, combined anatomical and pathological findings to elucidate disturbances in physiology.

Willis is, of course, best known for his description of the Arterial Circle at the base of the brain, which is called after his name. The beautiful drawing

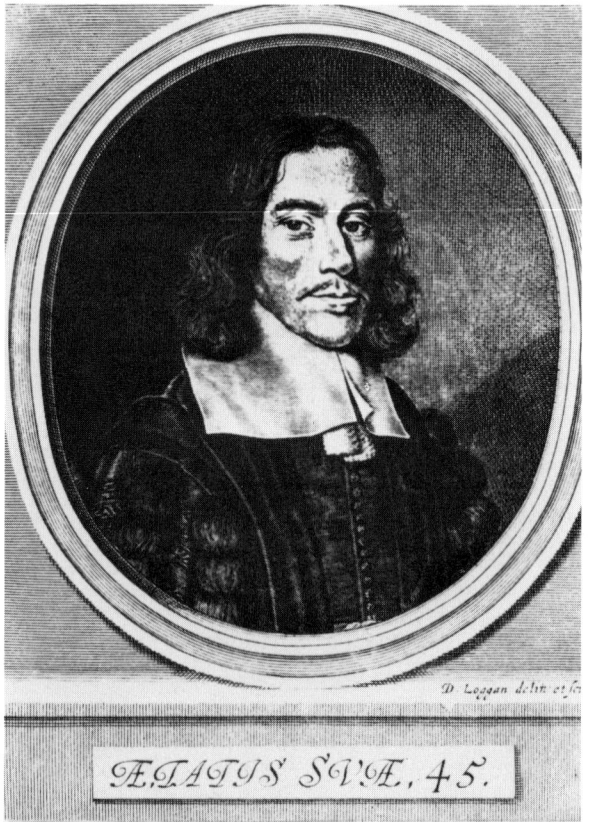

Fig. 19.1 Portrait of Thomas Willis at the age of 45 (engraved by David Loggan in 1666).

of the Circle by his friend Christopher Wren, which appears in Willis' *Anatomy of the Brain*, us justly famous. Close scrutiny of the drawing fails to reveal any trace of a nerve plexus on the arteries at the base of the brain. However, Willis describes in his book the close anatomical relationship of nerves to the arteries supplying the head, and indicates clearly his view that the circulation is under direct nervous control. He writes (Feindel 1965, Vol. 2, p. 151) 'Moreover, that the thick fibres and shoots of the nerves are inserted both into the Veins and Arteries, and bind both those kind of Vessels, and variously compass them about, we may lawfully suppose, that these nerves, as it were Reins put upon these blood-carrying Vessels, do sometimes dilate, and sometimes bind them hard together for the determining the motion of the Blood according to the various force of the Passions, or to deduce it here and there after a manifold manner; for by this means it comes

to pass, that in fear the excursion of the blood is hindered, and in other
Affections its motion is respectively altered.'

Willis seems to have had a wide experience with the clinical problem of
headaches, and as a Physician-Scientist he took great care to correlate his
clinical experience with normal and pathological anatomy. Let us hear his
views on headache mechanisms. 'As to the differences of the headache, the
common distinction is, that the pain of the head is either without the skull, or
within its cavity; the former is a more rare and a more gentle disease, because
the parts above the skull are not so sensible as the interior meninges, nor are
they watered with so plentiful a flood of blood, that by its sudden and
vehement incursion, they may be easily distended, or inflamed above
measure. Secondly, the other kind of headache, to wit, within the skull, is
more frequent, and much more cruel, because the membranes, clothing the
brain, are very sensible, and the blood is poured upon them by a manifold
passage, and by many and greater arteries.' He adds that the brain itself, and
the skull are *not* a source of head pain, because 'they want sensible Fibres,
apt to be wrinkled and distended' (Willis 1683).

Referring later to the dura mater, Willis wrote, 'And as to sense, 'tis not
to be doubted, but that it hath it exquisitely,' and further noted that 'the pains
of the Head often proceed from the breach of unity excited in this Membrane'
(Feindel 1965, Vol. 2, p. 79). He considered that the pia-arachnoid, as well as
the dura, was pain sensitive.

We suspect that Willis found opportunities to demonstrate the sensitivity
of the meninges during some of his animal experiments, though he does not
seem to have recorded such observations.

Although written more than three centuries ago, his views on headache
have a distinctly modern ring. Note how he stresses the sensitivity of the
meninges, and the abundant intracranial blood circulation as major factors in
the production of headaches. Let us see how far his view has been confirmed
by modern neurosurgical studies of intracranial pain, and by our present
knowledge of the sensory innervation of intracranial structures.

Innervation of the dura and intracranial arteries and veins

The first detailed observations on the sensitivity of intracranial structures and
their pain references in conscious man were reported in the 1930s by Penfield
(1935) and by Ray and Wolff (1940). These observations were made during
intracranial operations carried out under local anaesthesia.

Some of Penfield's findings are summarized in Fig. 19.2. Pain or pressure
was the only sensation experienced, whether the stimulus used was traction,
pressure, or a mild faradic current. The most sensitive structures were the
middle meningeal arteries and the adjacent dura, the tentorium, falx, the

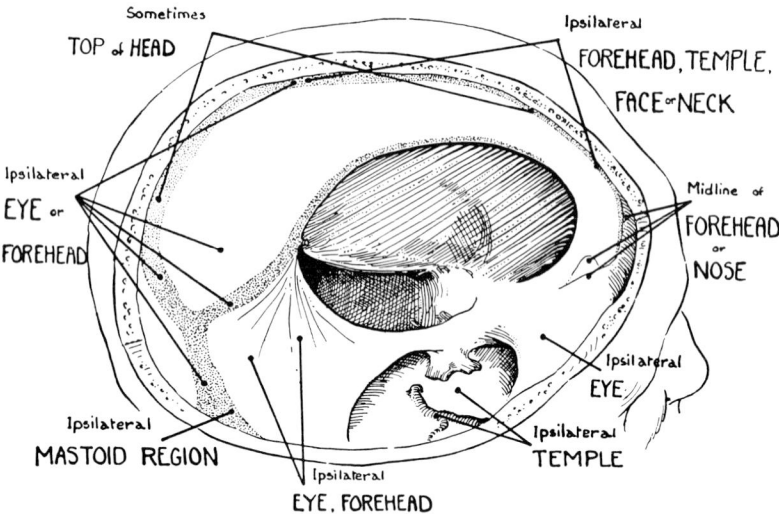

Sometimes
TOP of HEAD

Ipsilateral
FOREHEAD, TEMPLE,
FACE or NECK

Ipsilateral
EYE or
FOREHEAD

Midline of
FOREHEAD
or
NOSE

Ipsilateral
EYE

Ipsilateral
MASTOID REGION

Ipsilateral
TEMPLE

Ipsilateral
EYE, FOREHEAD

Fig. 19.2 This drawing indicates the areas of the cerebral dura mater which are usually found to be sensitive at operation, and the patient's localization of the pain produced. (From Penfield & McNaughton 1940.)

walls of the dural sinuses, and the attached cerebral veins. The pia-arachnoid and the cortical arteries in general were insensitive. However, traction or electrical stimuli applied to the larger arterial branches of the Circle of Willis, or the adjacent pia-arachnoid at the base of the brain sometimes caused pain.

Ray and Wolff reported similar findings from stimulation of intracranial structures above the tentorium. In the posterior fossa, they noted that the walls of the sigmoid sinus, the surrounding dura, the vertebral artery and some larger branches of the basilar artery were pain-sensitive. The pain evoked was usually localized behind the ear, in the occipital region, or down the neck on the same side.

When we compare the pattern of distribution of the dural nerves (as traced with osmic acid) with the pain-sensitive areas observed in the operating room, there is a surprising degree of correspondence (Fig. 19.3). The nerve supply to the middle meningeal artery apparently derived from all three divisions of the trigeminal nerve, is readily seen, as well as the periarterial sympathetic plexus, which enters with the artery through the foramen spinosum. We have not been able to trace the middle meningeal nerves back to their precise origin, but suspect that they may all come ultimately from the first trigeminal division.

The tentorial nerve of Arnold (1851), a recurrent branch of the first trigeminal division, is also shown, with its abundant distribution to

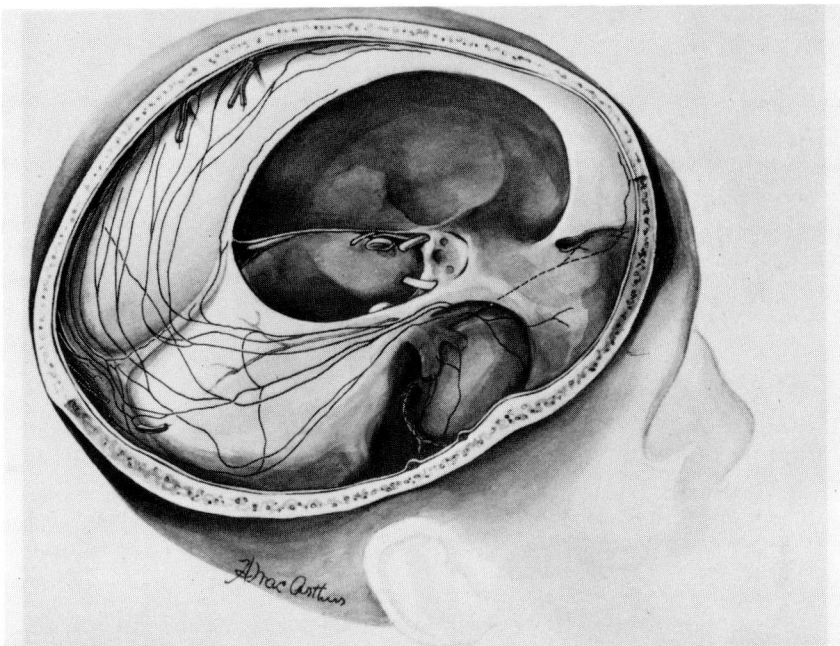

Fig. 19.3 Drawing of the interior of the skull, right side, showing the typical distribution of the dural nerves in the anterior and middle fossae. Note the branches of the trigeminal nerve to the middle meningeal artery, and the tentorial nerves from the first trigeminal division which are distributed to tentorium, falx, and dural sinuses.

tentorium, falx, the dural sinuses and their venous attachments. The recurrent course of the tentorial nerve is explained by the fact that the mesenchyme which will form the tentorium and posterior part of the falx migrates posteriorly during early embryonic development, with its trigeminal nerve supply. The consistent reference of pain from these structures to the forehead and eye is readily explained by its origin as a distinct branch of the first division.

To further demonstrate the tentorial nerve pathway in man, we will describe some observations made by one of us (W.F.) during craniotomy under local anaesthesia in patient T.L. The findings are summarized in Fig. 19.4.

In this patient, the sensitivity of points along the superior longitudinal sinus and on the falx in the parieto-occipital region was abolished by injection into the posterior part of the falx and the region of the torcular. After the injection, however, pressure or traction on the superior sagittal sinus produced pain referred to the forehead or the back of the head on the *opposite* side. In this instance, the most anterior of the sensitive points was

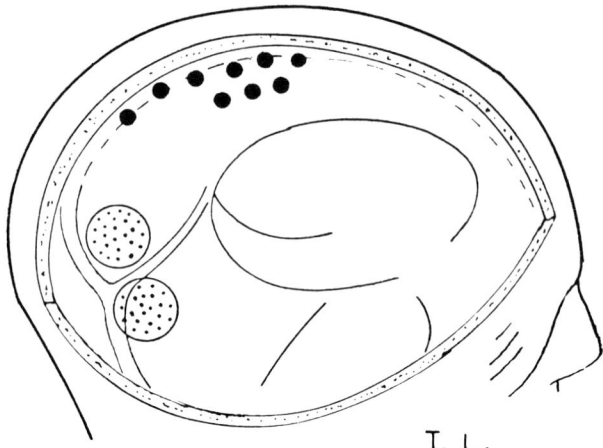

T. L.

Stimulation findings noted in case T.L.

Fig. 19.4 The stimulation findings noted in patient T.L. The black dots represent the sensitive points along the superior sagittal sinus. The larger stippled circles represent the approximate area of the falx and tentorium involved by the injection of Novocaine, which caused the superior sagittal sinus to become insensitive. (From Feindel *et al.* 1960.)

identified as being opposite the motor cortex. The persisting reference of pain to the opposite side of the head suggests that the Novocain in the tentorium was blocking most of the ipsilateral dural nerves, while the Novocain in the falx failed to block some of the sensory branches from the opposite tentorial nerve.

The dural nerves contain both myelinated and unmyelinated fibres. Dural nerve endings are difficult to demonstrate by silver stains. They include tree-like endings and a few encapsulated structures. Sensory endings have not been found in the walls of the dural sinuses. The pia-arachnoid does not appear to contain any sensory nerve fibres or endings.

Although the larger cranial arteries forming the Circle of Willis are sometimes found to be sensitive at operation, their intrinsic sensory nerve supply has not been firmly established by neuroanatomists, nor have many sensory-type endings been clearly demonstrated in the walls of either large or small arteries. There are vague reports in the older anatomical literature of trigeminal and other cranial nerve branches, which could be traced by dissection into the internal carotid plexus or to the Circle of Willis. We have not been able to demonstrate any nerves of this type, and the question of arterial sensory nerves clearly deserves further anatomical investigation.

The dural nerves within the posterior fossa (Fig. 19.5) as traced by osmic acid, appear to be mainly branches of the ninth, tenth and twelfth cranial

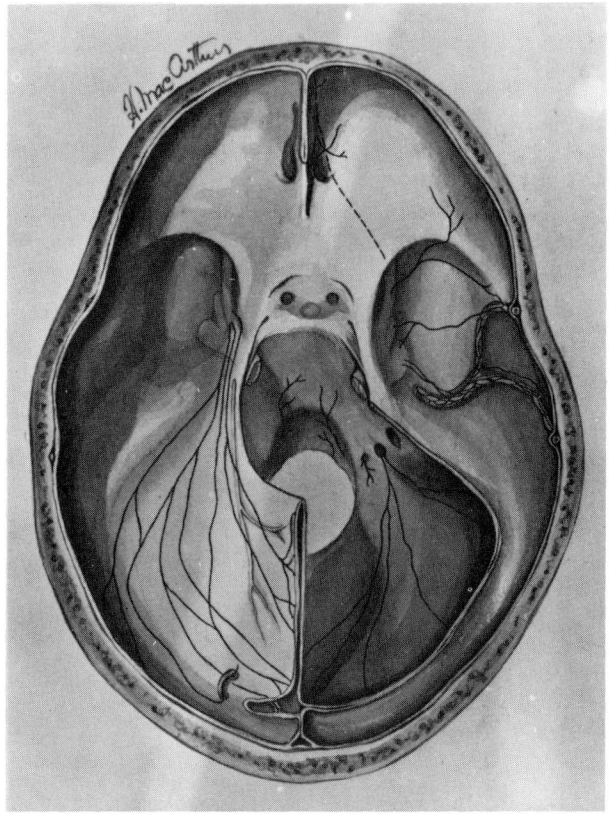

Fig. 19.5   Drawing of base of skull (as seen from above) to show the distribution of trigeminal sensory branches to middle meningeal artery (right side), tentorium (left side) and the dural nerves in the posterior fossa (right side). (From Feindel, *et al.* 1960.)

nerves, with a few small branches entering the dura of the posterior fossa through the foramen magnum. However, recent studies in the human embryo (Kimmell 1961) have shown that all nerves supplying the dura mater of the posterior cranial fossa have their origin in the first and second cervical nerves and the superior cervical sympathetic ganglia. Most nerve fibres are derived from a meningeal ramus of C2. They enter the posterior fossa as recurrent nerves through the foramen magnum, the jugular foramen and the hypoglossal canal.

In summary, we can state that the sensory nerve supply of the tentorium and supratentorial dura, the dural sinuses and their venous attachments, is derived from the trigeminal nerves. The sensory innervation of the arteries forming the Circle of Willis remains uncertain, but may ultimately prove to be trigeminal in origin. The dura and dural sinuses within the posterior fossa receive their sensory supply from the first and second cervical nerves, while the supply to vertebral and basilar arteries has not yet been clearly established.

The neural basis of headache

When we consider the abundant trigeminal nerve supply to supratentorial intracranial structures (dura, dural sinuses, arteries and veins) and also to pain sensitive extracranial structures (scalp, blood vessels and periosteum) it is not surprising that the trigeminal has been named 'the nerve of headache' by Vallery-Radot and Hamburger (1935)—('Le trijumeau est le nerf du mal de tête'). The sensory supply of posterior fossa structures appears to be of lesser importance as a pathway for headache.

Clinical experience in recent years has demonstrated that intractable unilateral headache due to migraine or other obscure intracranial causes can be relieved by trigeminal posterior root, or tract, section.

The experimental headache produced by intravenous histamine has been studied extensively as a model of vascular headache, with regard to the underlying pain mechanism and pain pathways (Schumacher, Ray & Wolff 1940). The pain appears to be produced by distention of the walls of the internal carotid arteries and their main branches, and not by distention of the middle meningeal arteries. The pain pathway is by way of the trigeminal nerve. As already reported, the main branches of the Circle of Willis are sometimes sensitive to direct mechanical stimulation, in patients undergoing craniotomy under local anaesthesia, though we have found difficulty in demonstrating a trigeminal sensory contribution to the internal carotid plexus, by anatomical methods. It is tempting to suggest that the pain produced by mechanical stimulation or distention of the larger cranial arteries is actually provoked by pressure or traction on adjacent pain-sensitive dural structures, such as the walls of the venous sinuses, and their venous attachments, which, as we know, receive an abundant trigeminal sensory supply.

In summarizing his extensive studies of intracranial pain, Wolff (1963) expressed the view that pain of intracranial origin is mediated by branches of the trigeminal and upper cervical nerves, and is produced by one or more of the following basic mechanisms.

(1) Traction upon pain-sensitive structures such as (a) veins entering the venous sinuses or (b) the sinus walls, (c) the middle meningeal arteries, or (d) the larger arteries at the base of the skull;
(2) distention and dilatation of intracranial arteries;
(3) inflammatory processes;

(4) direct pressure on sensory nerves of the cranium and upper cervical regions.

It will be of interest at this point in the discussion of headache mechanisms to refer to an early clinical paper by Gordon Holmes, entitled *Headaches of Organic Origin, and their Treatment*, which appeared in *The Practitioner* in the year 1913, when Holmes was an Assistant Physician at Queen Square (Holmes 1913). He was writing at a time when we lacked nearly all of the laboratory methods of investigation which are available today, and when Neurosurgery was in its infancy. Nevertheless, this paper makes excellent reading and displays Holmes' sound and practical approach to one of the most common and often most difficult diagnostic problems which the Clinical Neurologist still faces today, in spite of all our modern laboratory aids.

In discussing the headache caused by increased intracranial pressure, Holmes had this to say about headache mechanisms: 'The immediate cause of the pain in such cases has not definitely been settled, but there can be little doubt that it is due to the compression of the sensory fibres of the dura mater which come mainly from the trigeminal nerve. In meningitis, the mechanical factor is probably supplemented by involvement of the meningeal nerves.'

We can also go back again to Thomas Willis and compare his thoughts about headache mechanisms in the 17th century with current views. Undoubtedly, Willis would be gratified to find that modern studies have confirmed many of his own opinions.

Efferent nerves and the cerebral circulation

Having reviewed the afferent nerve supply of intracranial structures, let us consider briefly the *efferent* nerve supply (Fig. 19.6). As is well known, the entire arterial tree, both extra- and intracranial, is supplied with autonomic sympathetic nerves, whose cells of origin lie in the cervical sympathetic ganglia. Most of the intracranial nerves originate in the superior cervical ganglia or in scattered smaller ganglia within the internal carotid plexus and are distributed through a perivascular plexus which extends to pial and intracerebral arteries as small as 10 microns in diameter (Humphreys 1939).

There is also evidence for a parasympathetic vasodilator pathway to cerebral blood vessels by way of the facial nerve and its greater superficial petrosal branch to the internal carotid plexus. This was demonstrated anatomically (Chorobski & Penfield 1932) and physiologically (Cobb & Finesinger 1932). There has been abundant physiological confirmation of a vasodilator pathway since 1932, but to our knowledge, the exact anatomical pathway, as described by Chorobski and Penfield, has not been confirmed by other workers.

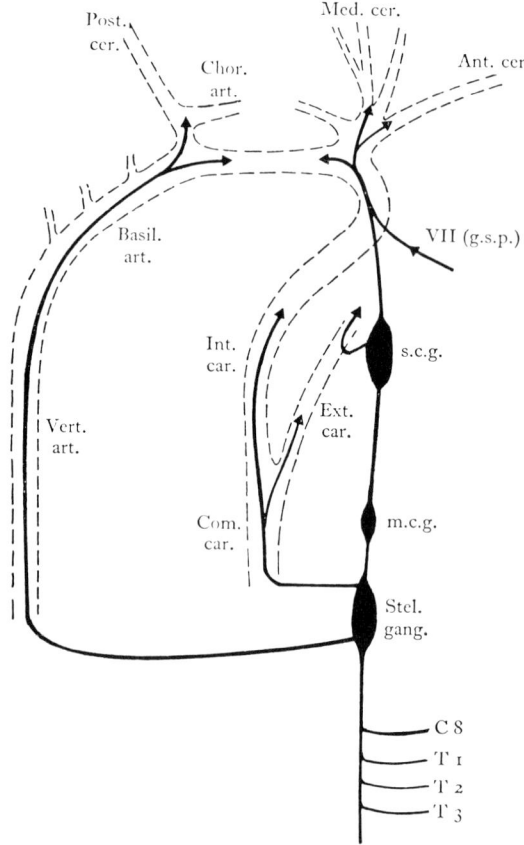

Fig. 19.6 A diagram summarizing the known efferent pathways to cerebral blood vessels. m.c.g. and s.c.g., middle and superior cervical ganglia. VII (g.s.p.) greater superficial petrosal nerve carrying vasodilator fibres from the intracranial portion of the facial nerve. (From Purves 1972.)

Recent interest in the secretory functions of the pineal body has led to renewed studies of its nerve supply by Kappers (1971) and others. The mammalian pineal body is innervated by the peripheral autonomic neuronal system. It receives noradrenergic postganglionic fibres from both superior cervical ganglia, which are distributed to the blood vessels and to the pineal cells. It also (in the macaque) receives preganglionic parasympathetic fibres (Kenny 1961) from the greater superficial petrosal nerve.

It should be mentioned here, also, that the chorioid plexuses are richly innervated, especially the venous vessels, and the fibres are well-demonstrated by the fluorescence technique for noradrenergic nerves. The function of these nerves in relation to the production of cerebrospinal fluid is still unknown.

When studying the distribution of the tentorial nerves, we noted that many of the finer branches could be traced to venous septa (The Cords of Willis) within the transverse sinuses and torcular, as well as along the veins entering the superior sagittal sinus (Fig. 19.7). It was not possible to say whether these were entirely afferent in function or whether they contained both afferent and efferent fibres. Le Gros Clark (1940) described a 'suprapineal arachnoid body' containing a sinusoidal plexus which appeared to be supplied by a nerve from the pineal body, and was located at the junction of the great vein of Galen and the straight sinus, where it might control the flow of venous blood entering the sinus. It is still not clear whether the branches from the tentorial nerves which we have traced along the walls of the straight sinus posteriorly are the same as those described by Clark, as being related to the pineal body. It seems possible that, apart from the pain

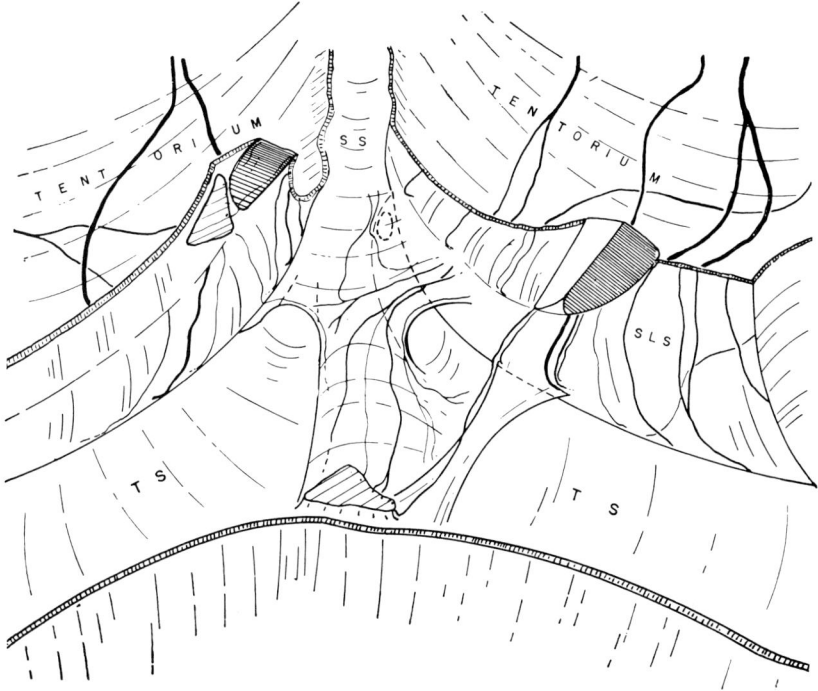

Fig. 19.7 Drawing of the torcular with the dura of the sinuses opened and viewed from behind. SS, straight sinus, SLS, superior sagittal sinus, TS, transverse sinus. Tentorial nerves run in the dural walls of the sinuses, and some arborize on the inner wall of the torcular. (From Feindel *et al* 1960.)

fibres, these rather abundant tentorial nerves may play some role in the control of intracranial circulation in man.

For many years following the demonstration of a vasomotor supply to cerebral blood vessels, there was a widely-held opinion that this was a vestigial vasomotor system of little or no physiological importance. However, the newer anatomical and physiological studies of recent years have shown beyond all doubt that this is part of an active and important vasomotor control system.

The motor endings in the muscular coat of the cerebral arteries have now been studied by electron microscopy and appear to be both noradrenergic and cholinergic in type (Nielsen *et al* 1971). With newer fluorescence techniques, it is now possible to demonstrate a dense terminal network of smooth and beaded fibres in the walls of cerebral arteries and veins (Peerless & Yasargil 1971) (Fig. 19.8). They are considered to be vasomotor in function. Further application of these fluorescence techniques (Fig. 19.9) has demonstrated widespread amine mechanisms of vascular control associated with post-ganglionic sympathetic nerve terminals, within the brain parenchyma, as well as adrenergic terminals from intracerebral sources such as the locus coeruleus (Owman *et al* 1974).

The increasing number of observations on intracerebral neuronal circuits specifically characterized by the presence of serotonin, dopamine, or

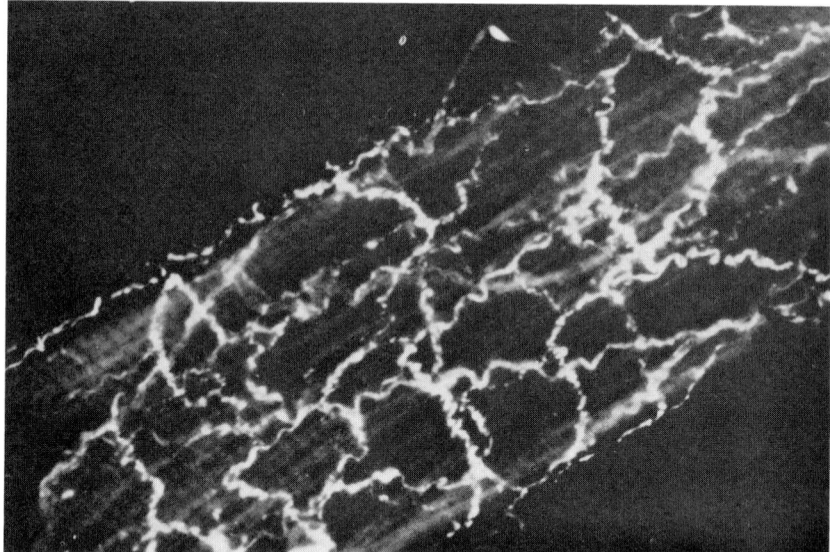

Fig. 19.8 Whole stretch preparation of a distal branch of the middle cerebral artery of a rabbit. The irregular, varicose white lines represent fluorescence from noradrenalin within nerve fibres and terminals. Fluorescence micrograph ×100. (From Peerless & Yasargil 1971.)

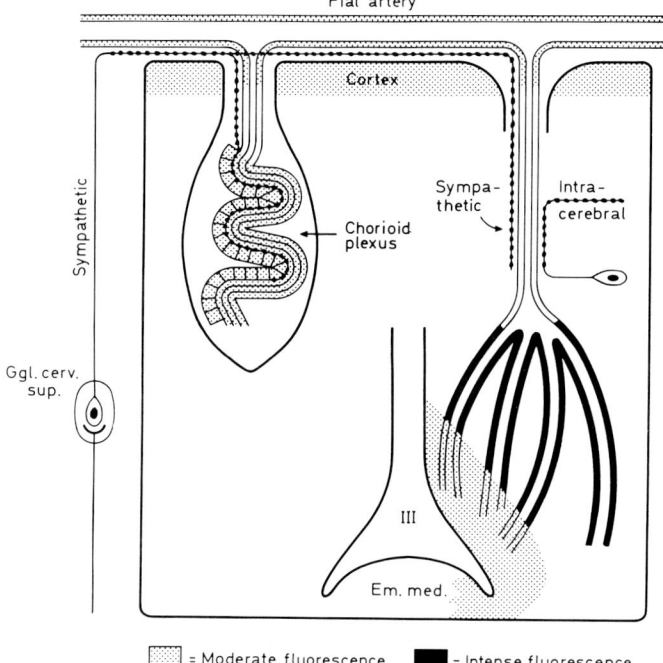

Pial artery

Cortex

Sympathetic

Sympa-
thetic

Intra-
cerebral

Chorioid
plexus

Ggl. cerv.
sup.

III

Em. med.

▨ = Moderate fluorescence   ■ = Intense fluorescence

Fig. 19.9 A schematic presentation of certain amine mechanisms in the brain. The pial arteries, small arteries and arterioles penetrating into the brain parenchyma as well as the arterioles supplying the chorioid plexus are innervated by post ganglionic sympathetic nerve terminals, having a characteristically beaded appearance. In addition, adrenergic terminals from intracerebral sources (e.g. locus coeruleus) run for a varying distance in close association with many of the cerebral arterioles.

When L-Dopa (or dopamine) is administered to experimental animals, formaldehyde-induced fluorescence becomes visible in the shaded areas, which include the pial arterial wall, the chorioid plexus, the brain capillary wall, and the brain parenchyma surrounding the median eminence (Em. med.). (From Owman, *et al* 1974.)

noradrenaline, suggests that the perivascular innervation of the cerebral vessels may well represent an integral part of a complex balance of neuronal systems that are activated or regulated by chemical transmitters.

A recent experimental study by Purves and Ponte (1975) also emphasizes the physiological importance of the innervation of intracranial vascular structures. They have shown that the well-established reflex, whereby a rise in systemic pressure is followed by vasoconstriction of cerebral arteries—is dependent upon the baroreceptors in the carotid sinus. Increasing evidence indicates that pathways from the receptors in the carotid sinus to the cerebral vessels provide a means for a coordinated response of the cardiovascular system, when the blood or oxygen supply to the brain is threatened.

The increasing importance of humoral factors in the control of cerebral circulation is also seen in the current approach to the vexing clinical problem of vasospasm of the cerebral arteries associated with subarachnoid haemorrhage. Much evidence involves chemical factors in fresh platelets such as serotonin and prostaglandins, in the onset and persistence of this excessive vasoconstriction. Prostaglandins are powerful constrictors of cerebral arteries, particularly those below 500 microns in diameter (Yamamoto *et al* 1972). An important gap in our view of vasospasm is that its identification until now has depended upon x-ray angiography, in which vessels of such small size cannot be seen. Thus, the correlation of the severity and duration of vasospasm as we recognize it on x-ray angiography with the clinical condition of the patient has often been quite unsatisfactory. The quantitative reduction of cerebral blood flow resulting from vasospasm in these small vessels should provide a better indication of the cerebral effects of vasospasm. The influence of noradrenergic perivascular nerves in vasospasm has been emphasized particularly by Peerless (Feindel 1971).

The role of humoral factors in controlling cerebral circulation should have a promising application in the study of migraine. For a long time, the phenomena of the migraine attack (particularly in its classical form) have been ascribed by clinicians to changes in intracranial circulation. The prodromal symptoms (visual disturbances, paraesthesias, etc.) have been explained on the basis of early vasoconstriction of cerebral arteries, and the headache on the basis of later vasodilatation, affecting both intra- and extracranial arteries. This is a plausible theory, but it has never been proven, and attempts to treat migraine by altering the vasomotor control of cerebral blood vessels have been a failure. As Lance (1973) states in a recent study of migraine, 'There is no convincing evidence that the neural control of blood vessels is impaired in migraine, that migraine is caused by an abnormal neural discharge, or that operation on nerve pathways will interrupt the course of the migraine attack'. The study of humoral agents in relation to migraine, particularly the biogenic amines, is already well under way, and may eventually provide the answer to a very old problem.

References

ARNOLD F. (1851) *Handbuch der Anatomie des Menschen*, Vol. 2. Freiburg.

CHOROBSKI J. & PENFIELD W. (1932) Cerebral vasodilator nerves and their pathway from the medulla oblongata. *Archs. Neurol. Psychiat.* (Chicago) **28**, 1257–89.

CLARK W.E. LE GROS (1940) A vascular mechanism related to the Great Vein of Galen. *Brit. med. J.* **I**, 476.

COBB S. & FINESINGER J.E. (1932) Cerebral circulation: XIX. The vagal pathway of the vasodilator fibres. *Archs. Neurol. Psychiat.* (Chicago) **28**, 1243–56.

FEINDEL W., PENFIELD W. & McNAUGHTON F. (1960) The tentorial nerves and localization of intracranial pain in man. *Neurology, Minneapolis* **10**, 555–63.

FEINDEL W. (1962) Thomas Willis (1621–

1675) the founder of neurology. *Canad. med. Ass. J.* **87**, 289–96.

FEINDEL W. (Ed.) (1965) *The Anatomy of the Brain and Nerves, by Thomas Willis, M.D.*, Vols. I & II. McGill University Press, Montreal.

FEINDEL W. (Ed.) (1971) Symposium on recent research in the cerebral microcirculation. *J. Neurosurg.* **35**, 123–80.

HOLMES G. (1913) Headaches of organic origin and their treatment. *Practitioner* **90**, 968–84.

HUMPHREYS S.P. (1939) Anatomic relations of cerebral vessels and perivascular nerves. *Archs. Neurol. Psychiat.* (Chicago) **41**, 1207–21.

KAPPERS J.A. (1971) The Pineal Gland, an introduction. In: Wolstenholme G.E.W. & Knight J. (Eds) *The Pineal Gland*, pp. 3–34. Churchill Livingstone, Edinburgh and London.

KENNY G.C.T. (1961) The 'nervus conarii' of the monkey. *J. Neuropath. & Exp. Neurol.* **20**, 563–70.

KIMMELL D.L. (1961) Innervation of spinal dura mater and dura mater of the posterior cranial fossa. *Neurology*, (Minneapolis) **11**, 800–9.

LANCE J. (1973) *Mechanism and Management of Headache*, 2nd edn. Butterworths, London.

MCNAUGHTON F. (1937) The innervation of the intracranial blood vessels and dural sinuses. *Res. Publs. Ass. Res. nerv. ment. Dis.* **18**, 178–200.

NIELSEN K.C., OWMAN C. & SPORRONG B. (1971) Ultrastructure of the autonomic innervation in the main pial arteries of rats and cats. *Brain Res.* **27**, 25–32.

OWMAN C., EDVINSSON L. FALCK B. & NIELSON K.C. (1974) Amine mechanisms in brain vessels, with particular reference to autonomic innervation and blood-brain barrier. In: Cervos-Navarro J. (Ed) *Pathology of Cerebral Circulation*, Ch. 2.

Walter de Gruyter, Berlin and New York.

PEERLESS S.J. & YASARGIL M.G. (1971) Adrenergic innervation of the cerebral blood vessels in the rabbit. *J. Neurosurg.* **35**, 148–54.

PENFIELD W. (1935) A contribution to the mechanisms of intracranial pain. *Res. Publs. Ass. Res. nerv. ment. Dis.* **15**, 399–416.

PENFIELD W. & MCNAUGHTON F. (1940) Dural headache and innervation of the dura mater. *Archs. Neurol. Psychiat.* (Chicago) **40**, 1–33.

PURVES M.J. (1972) *The Physiology of the Cerebral Circulation.* Cambridge University Press, London.

PURVES M.J. & PONTE J.C.M.R. (1975) The role of the carotid body receptors in the control of the cerebral blood vessels. In: Purves M.J. (Ed.) *The Peripheral Arterial Chemoreceptors*, pp. 409–26. Cambridge University Press, London.

RAY B.S. & WOLFF H.G. (1940) Experimental studies on headache. Pain sensitive structures of the head and their significance in headache. *Arch. Surg.* **41**, 813–56.

SCHUMACHER G.A., RAY B.S. & WOLF H. G. (1940) Experimental studies on headache. Further analysis of histamine headache and its pain pathways. *Archs. Neurol. Psychiat.* (Chicago) **44**, 701–17.

VALLERY-RADOT P. & HAMBURGER J. (1935) *Les Migraines.* Masson et Cie, Paris.

WILLIS T. (1683) *Two discourses concerning the Soul of Brutes.* Second Part, Chap. I, Of the Headache, p. 106. Dring, Harper & Leigh, London.

WOLFF H.G. (1963) *Headache and Other Head Pain*, 2nd edn, pp. 53–95. Oxford University Press, New York.

YAMAMOTO Y.L., FEINDEL W., WOLFE L.S., KATOH H. & HODGE C.P. (1972) Experimental vasoconstriction of cerebral arteries by prostaglandins. *J. Neurosurg.* **37**, 385–97.

STUDIES IN DICHOTIC LISTENING: CONTRIBUTIONS TO NEUROPHYSIOLOGY

ANTONIO DAMASIO AND HANNA DAMASIO

Introduction

Dichotic listening, i.e. auditory simultaneous stimulation or two-channel listening, designates the procedure whereby a subject is presented with a series of different but simultaneous auditory stimuli in both ears and is then asked to report what he heard. The technique dates back to the 1950s when Broadbent (1954, 1956) used it to investigate memory. The subject would listen to two different series of three digits fed simultaneously into the two ears and it was found that material heard in one was systematically reported first, followed by material from the opposite ear. Today, we confront the subject with a series of double stimulations and require him to report what he perceived after each presentation. The series may have variable length. The stimuli (words, digits, environmental sounds) are presented through high-fidelity earphones from a stereophonic tape, balanced for extraneous noise. The procedure takes place in a sound-proof room with minimal interference from other sensory modalities. The evaluation of performance, as followed in our own studies, is made by computing:

(1) the total number of correctly reported items,
(2) the amount of correct double reporting,
(3) the ratio between the correct right ear reporting and correct left ear reporting.

Interest in this neurobehavioural technique only developed in the 1960s, after Kimura (1961a, b) reported that, when different verbal stimuli are presented competitively in both ears, those coming from the side opposite the dominant hemisphere are more efficiently perceived and reported. These findings have been well replicated and the most widely accepted interpretation postulates that the crossed auditory pathway inhibits the ipsilateral one.

In subsequent studies, Kimura and co-workers (1962, 1964; Knox & Kimura 1970, King & Kimura 1972) demonstrated that when non-verbal stimuli were presented to both ears, again in competition, those that were fed in the ear opposite the non-dominant hemisphere would be more accurately perceived and reported. In other words, the reverse of the relationship described for verbal stimuli was observed. This means that, regardless of the fact that the auditory input system projects to both hemispheres via ipsilateral and contralateral pathways, it seems that the crossed component is functionally superior and probably inhibits the ipsilateral, with respect to the hemisphere that is presumably processing a given type of information. Since the left hemisphere is generally assumed to be the better processor of verbal information, it is natural to find that the right ear is the more efficient of the two, for it is the origin of the crossed channel that will more efficiently transport verbal stimuli to left hemisphere structures, while possibly inhibiting the pathway that originates in the left ear. Such ear preference is now described in the literature as 'right ear dominance for verbal material'. Conversely, since the right hemisphere is considered the major processor of non-verbal information, it is understandable that non-verbal stimuli coming from the left ear will be better perceived than those coming from the right, again as a result of functional prepotency of the crossed tract. 'Left-ear dominance for non-verbal material' designates this state of affairs.

Another concept that emerged from the early studies was that of the 'lesion effect'. This designated the extinction of stimuli presented in one of the ears, a finding which correlated with lesions of the auditory areas in the *contralateral* temporal lobe. For instance, extinction of the right-ear channel, i.e. extinction of material presented in the right ear, was associated with left temporal lesions, and lesions of the right temporal lobe became associated with extinction of the left channel. The preponderance by crossed prevailing over non-crossed pathways was also used to explain this finding.

The explanation was given added support by the work of Sparks and Geschwind (1968) and Milner and co-workers (1968) showing that patients with callosal section failed to report any verbal stimuli given in the left ear. Information that was being conveyed to the right hemisphere by the crossed pathway (since it was presented in the left ear) was being blocked in its further travel to the left hemisphere. The site of interruption was likely to be the transversal crossing of the callosum in the direction of the left auditory cortex. Interestingly, if the stimuli were given monaurally, with no competitition involved, the ipsilateral pathway from the left ear to the left auditory cortex would still be effective. These results substantially supported the suggestion that, under circumstances of competition, crossed pathways prevailed over ipsilateral.

In recent years there has been an effort to replicate and extend these findings. Dichotic listening has been widely used in the study of brain function, particularly in regard to the problems of cerebral dominance and handedness, and the techniques of diotic and monotic listening have been introduced to complement dichotic listening studies.

Since the callosal experiment is a central issue in the theory, we have tried to investigate the generality of these findings. In essence, we sought to determine whether the results applied to other types of disconnection between the two auditory cortices and were not limited to the surgical split of the callosum in patients with untractable epilepsy. For example, we found the same pattern of left-ear extinction in cases of lesions of the splenium of the corpus callosum, after infarction of the posterior cerebral artery, and in one case of deep left temporal glioma in which post-mortem examination clearly showed damage to the outflow from the callosum (Damasio *et al* 1976). The anatomical data in this study also supported the notion that the interauditory pathway crosses the callosum in the splenium, most probably in front of the intervisual connection and caudal to the intersomaesthetic. This is in keeping with experimental data in the rhesus monkey (Pandya *et al* 1971).

A considerable number of studies have added to knowledge of hearing behaviour. The experimental situations have been refined to include several types of stimuli—for instance, words of high and low ranks of frequency, meaningful and meaningless, artificially generated by computer; even musical elements have been studied (Borkowski *et al* 1965, Bartz *et al* 1967, Shankweiler & Studdert-Kennedy 1967, Spreen *et al* 1967, King & Kimura 1972). In regard to these, it has been suggested that the left ear is 'dominant' for musical stimuli (Spellacy 1970, King & Kimura 1972). This would be in keeping with the assumption that the right hemisphere is the more adequate mediator of non-verbal experience. Further experiments along this line have shown that 'musical dominance' varies with different aspects of musical language, namely melody and rhythm, and it has been suggested that the right ear may be dominant for rhythm whereas the left ear may be the best for the perception of chords and melody (Shankweiler 1966, Gordon 1970). This agrees well with the crude but useful concept that the left hemisphere may be a processor of time relationships and the right a processor of space relationships. But, to make things more complicated, it has also been recently suggested that these kinds of musical 'dominance' only apply to the 'musically naïve' and that the nervous system of 'musically sophisticated' subjects handles every aspect of music as it handles verbal language, that is, with the left hemisphere. We are referring to the experiments of Bever and Chiarello (1974) who reported marked ear differences between musicians and non-musicians using a monotic listening technique. The idea that dominance is a flexible aspect of brain function has also been given support by Shankweiler and Studdert-Kennedy (1975) in a study in which ear preference in a dichotic listening task was correlated with handedness measures.

Diotic listening studies derive from the problems posed by dichotic listening. Diotic listening is a much simpler procedure in which series of simultaneous and different stimuli are presented in the space that surrounds the subject and not directly to the ears. The two competing stimuli may be given in different hemispaces, or in the same, or one may be given in front of the subject in midline position and the other to the left or the right of the subject. Its purpose is to investigate whether or not the positioning of competing stimuli in the surrounding space, is a factor in the listening performance. From the results available (Morais & Bertelson 1973), it seems possible that right-ear dominance effect for verbal stimuli extends to the right hemispace of a normal subject. In other words, if verbal stimuli are competing within the 'right auditory field', they may have a better chance of being perceived correctly and recorded.

In spite of the considerable interest it has aroused and of the fascinating suggestions it has produced, several questions remain unanswered regarding the dichotic listening process. Its reliability as a neuropsychological test measure seems modest and certainly influenced by the degree of difficulty of the tasks. Age and level of education are also determinants of performance, as we have been able to demonstrate. Illiterates and elderly normal subjects perform at a lower level, reflected in the decrease of scores of both channels while the left/right ratios are maintained. These factors need to be taken into account when dichotic listening is being used as a clinical tool or for research purposes.

One other question that researchers have not addressed themselves to is the following: provided that temporal lobe and the auditory areas are vital for the listening process, what does the rest of the brain have to do with such performance? We will report here a study offering a preliminary answer to this problem.

Material and methods

Dichotic listening performances was studied in 200 non-selected brain-damaged patients who came consecutively for behavioural assessment to the Language Research Laboratory of the Centro de Estudos Egas Moniz, Hospital de Santa Maria, Lisbon. Two dichotic listening tasks were given to each patient. The first consisted of the reporting of 18 pairs of different Portuguese words of 2 and 3 syllables. In the second there were 19 pairs of different digits. The presentation of tasks conformed to the standard procedures of the Language Research Laboratory. Prior to the test period, the tasks were explained and trial runs were made. During the test period the patients had to report the stimuli received in both ears and were given unlimited time to do so, before the examiner proceeded to the next pair of items. The tapes used in the study were balanced for intensity and standardized on a control population consisting of several groups of normals with different age brackets and cultural levels. Prior to the experiments, hearing ability was tested with a Keeler type B pure tone audiometer and was symmetrical in both cases. Tapes were then played by means of K0–727B high fidelity earphones in a TEAC A-22 stereo cassette recorder.

Patients presenting with abnormal patterns were then selected according to the following criteria:

(a) reliable right handedness;
(b) absence of deficit or asymmetry in pure tone audiometry;
(c) presence of reliable focal pathology as evidenced by clinical data, neuropsychological assessment, electroencephalography, neuroradiology, neurosurgery and neuropathology when available.

Only 65 patients met these criteria. These were grouped according to locus of lesion. There were 21 with frontal lobe lesions, 12 with parietal lobe lesions, 9 with temporal lobe lesions, and 1 with a lesion of the corpus callosum. In 22 cases, the pathology involved contiguous regions, 11 cases being classified as fronto-parietal and 11 as parieto-temporal. Thirty-four patients had lesions of the left hemisphere and 30 had lesions of the right hemisphere.

Results

Five different patterns of abnormal dichotic listening performance were identified. Patterns 1 and 2 were designated as *total extinction of the right ear* or of the *left ear*, corresponding to a zero score on the respective channel. Patterns 3 and 4 were designated *partial extinction of right* or *left ear* and corresponded to a marked decrease in the score of the respective channel, below the level of controls matched for age and education. *Alternate extinction*, pattern 5, corresponded to a situation of no dichotic reporting, but where the extinguished channel was inconsistently the right or the left, within the same task, i.e. a patient would extinguish three consecutive stimuli coming from the left and then turn to extinguishing one or two stimuli coming from the right and then revert again to the left side extinction in an unpredictable sequence. To our knowledge this pattern has not been described previously in either normal or brain-damaged subjects.

The number of patients presenting with the above abnormal patterns was as follows:

(1) total extinction of the right ear: 5 patients;
(2) total extinction of the left ear: 11 patients;
(3) partial extinction of the right ear: 8 patients;
(4) partial extinction of the left ear: 23 patients;
(5) alternating extinction: 13 patients.

Table 20.1 Distribution of the different dichotic listening patterns according to locus of lesion

	Left hemisphere						Right hemisphere					
	Occipital	Temporal	Parieto-temporal	Parietal	Fronto-parietal	Frontal	Frontal	Fronto-parietal	Parietal	Parieto-temporal	Temporal	Occipital
Total extinction right ear		3	2									
Partial extinction right ear					1	7						
Alternate extinction		1			2	10						
Total extinction left ear*		1						5	5	3	1	
Partial extinction left ear		3	1	3			4	3	4	5		

* Including 1 patient with a lesion in the corpus callosum.

The relation between the several patterns and locus of lesion is shown in Table 20.1. As can be seen, total extinction of the right ear correlated with temporal and temporo-parietal lesion in 5 cases. On the other hand, total extinction of the left ear corresponded to lesions on the right hemisphere with a much wider distribution (frontal, parietal and temporal) in a total of 14 cases.

Partial extinction of the right ear mainly correlated with frontal lesions (in 7 cases) while partial extinction of the left ear appeared in relation to lesions on both hemispheres (temporal and parietal on the left hemisphere, in a total of 7 cases, frontal, parietal and parieto-temporal on the right hemisphere, in a total of 16 cases).

The pattern of alternate extinction only appeared in relation to the left hemisphere, particularly in 10 cases with frontal lesions (there were two other cases with fronto-parietal leasions and one with a temporal lesion).

Discussion

As expected there were no lesions of the occipital lobes in patients with abnormal dichotic listening patterns. However, lesions in the parietal lobes and particularly in the frontal lobes (without concomitant temporal lesions) did appear in relation to abnormal dichotic performance. Left frontal lobe lesions, in particular, correlated well with the disruption of the usual dichotic pattern and were associated with partial extinction of the right channel or with the curious pattern of alternate extinction. One may venture to say that lesions in the frontal lobe lower the ability to handle the task properly, although, unlike lesions in the temporal lobe, they do not make it systematically impossible to perform.

Another interesting suggestion from this data is that the placing of lesions of the left hemisphere associated with abnormal patterns is rather more precise than their counterparts on the right hemisphere. On the left side, lesions tend to cluster in the temporal and prefrontal regions. The lesions on the right hemispheres are distributed in a more scattered fashion. Also there is no alternate pattern of extinction in relation to right hemisphere pathology and the pattern of complete extinction of the left ear does not possess the same clear-cut association of the pattern of complete extinction of the right ear.

These results suggest that: (1) the hearing process, at least as tested in dichotic listening but probably in other tests as well, does depend on structures other than those where the auditory pathways terminate; (2) in regard to the handling of verbal stimuli, the left frontal lobe possibly plays a conducting role. In general, these preliminary findings support the notions of prevalence of crossed pathways for competition tasks, as well as that of the asymmetry of left and right hemisphere function in regard to verbal information.

Studies in dichotic listening have contributed to our idea of how the auditory pathways may function. By looking at their known anatomical substrate one would not expect them, necessarily, to operate in this fashion. Another contribution pertains to hemisphere function. Listening studies have, in general, supported the concept of dominance relating to verbal and nonverbal stimuli in association with opposite halves of the brain. But probably more important is the suggestion that specialized training, in regard to a given stimulus, may bring about a 'shift' of dominance and that dominance, though anchored in identifiable anatomical asymmetries of the hemisphere (Geschwind 1971, Geschwind & Levitsky 1968), is also dependent on learning and training and is therefore a dynamic rather than static condition. This is to be inferred, for instance, from the different performance of musicians as compared to the musically uneducated, as reported by Bever and Chairello (1974).

This is also reflected in one of our studies (Damasio *et al*, 1977) in which we played the usual different verbal stimuli but selected words of similar phonetic structure thereby complicating the task of pattern discrimination. A strong trend toward reversal of the dominance pattern in the direction of left-ear superiority was observed. In addition, this reversal was more or less marked according to the educational level of the subjects: highly educated subjects showing the trend less strongly than illiterate subjects.

These results imply that the brain is capable of handling different types of information with different approaches and that this is possibly related to specific training regarding (1) a particular stimulus, and (2) level of education in general. This is not to refute the idea of left and right hemisphere specialization but rather to say that: (a) the nervous system processes information in a flexible manner so that operations that theoretically might be directed by one hemisphere may actually be controlled by the other, and (b) one can postulate a gradient between two extreme forms of operation of the opposite hemispheres, so that certain stimuli, in certain circumstances, will be processed with a mixed strategy that does not conform exactly to what is presumed to be the 'typical' right or left hemisphere functioning.

Acknowledgements

The author thanks Drs. A.C. Caldas, J. Ferro, J. Grosso and N. Antunes for their cooperation in the gathering of data.

References

BARTZ W.H., SATZ P., FENNELL E. & LALLY J.R. (1967) Meaningfulness and laterality in dichotic listening. *Journal of Experimental Psychology* **73**, 204–10.

BEVER T.G. & CHIARELLO R.J. (1974) Cerebral dominance in musicians and non-musicians. *Science* **185**, 537–9.

BORKOWSKI J.G., SPREEN O. & STUTZ J.Z. (1965) Ear preference and abstractness in dichotic listening. *Psychonomic Sciences* **3**, 547–8.

BROADBENT D.E. (1954) The role of auditory localization in attention and memory span. *Journal of Experimental Psychology* **47**, 191–6.

BROADBENT D.E. (1956) Successive responses to simultaneous stimuli. *Quarterly Journal of Experimental Psychology* **8**, 145–52.

DAMASIO H., DAMASIO A.R. & CASTRO-CALDAS A. (1977) *Reversal of Ear Dominance Pattern for Phonetically Similar Words* (in preparation).

DAMASIO H., DAMASIO A.R., CASTRO-CALDAS A. (1977) *Reversal of Ear Dominance Pattern for Phonetically* spheric disconnection. *Neuropsychologia* **14**, 247–250.

GESCHWIND N. (1971) Some differences between human and other primate brains. In: Jarrard L.E. (Ed.) *Cognitive Process of Non-Human Primates*. Academic Press, New York.

GESCHWIND N. & LEVITSKY W. (1968) Human brain: Left–right asymmetries in temporal speech region. *Science* **161**, 186–7.

GORDON H.W. (1970) Hemispheric asymmetries in the perception of musical chords. *Cortex* **6**, 387–98.

KIMURA D. (1961a) Some effects of temporal lobe damage on auditory perception. *Canadian Journal of Psychology* **15**, 156–65.

KIMURA D. (1961b) Cerebral dominance and the perception of verbal stimuli. *Canadian Journal of Psychology* **15**, 166–71.

KIMURA D. (1964) Left-right differences in the perception of melodies. *Quarterly Journal of Experimental Psychology* **16**, 355–8.

KIMURA D. (1967) Functional aysmmetry of the brain in dichotic listening. *Cortex* **3**, 163–78.

KING F.L. & KIMURA D. (1972) Left-ear superiority in dichotic perception of vocal non-verbal sounds. *Canadian Journal of Psychology* **26**, 111–16.

KNOX C. & KIMURA D. (1970) Cerebral processing of non-verbal sounds in boys and girls. *Neuropsychologia* **8**, 227–37.

MILNER B., TAYLOR L. & SPERRY R.W. (1968) Lateralized suppression of dichotically presented digits after commissural section in man. *Science* **161**, 184–6.

MORAIS J. & BERTELSON P. (1973) Laterality effects in dichotic listening. *Perception* **2**, 107–11.

PANDYA D.N., KAROL E.A. & HEILBROMM D. (1971) The topographical distribution of interhemispheric projections in the corpus callosum of the rhesus monkey. *Brain Research* **32**, 31–4.

SHANKWEILER D.P. (1966) Effects of temporal lobe damage on the perception of dichotically presented melodies. *Journal of Comparative Physiology and Psychology* **62**, 115–19.

SHANKWEILER D. & STUDDERT-KENNEDY M. (1967) An analysis of perceptual confusion in identification of dichotically presented CVC syllables. *Journal of the Acoustic Society of America* **41**, 1581.

SHANKWEILER D. & STUDDERT-KENNEDY M. (1975) A continuum of lateralisation for speech perception. *Brain and Language* **2**, 212–15.

SPARKS R. & GESCHWIND N. (1968) Dichotic listening in man after section of neocortical commissures. *Cortex* **4**, 3–16.

SPELLACY F. (1970) Lateral preferences in the identification of patterned stimuli. *Journal of the Acoustic Society of America* **47**, 574–8.

SPREEN O., BORKOWSKI J.G. & BENTON A.L. (1967) Auditory word recognition as a function of meaningfulness, abstractness and phonetic structure. *Journal of Verbal Learning and Verbal Behaviour* **6**, 101–4.

SOME OBSERVATIONS OF CLINICAL INTEREST ON
THE PATHOPHYSIOLOGY OF EPILEPSY

ROBERT B. AIRD

In his Saville Oration, published in the *Lancet* in 1927, Gordon Holmes emphasized one of the basic properties of cortical grey matter that underlies its convulsive activity, namely '. . . the occurrence of any physiological event in it (grey matter) facilitates the recurrence of that event'. Goddard and his co-workers have only recently capitalized on this point in their studies of the 'kindling' phenomenon (Goddard *et al* 1969). One can but wonder how fresh and spritely the following comments will seem to others fifty years hence.

It would be impossible to cover the pathophysiology of epilepsy in a short chapter. Much of this subject remains obscure, but the following observations, based upon an analysis of present knowledge of epilepsy, should prove of interest to clinicians.

In a study made on the propagation of discharge from gross, cerebral foci as determined by special electroencephalographic (EEG) techniques in human subjects (Aird & Garoutte 1960), limited conclusions were made but, in retrospect, one or two additional points that we failed to recognize are worth discussing.

From a review of 1300 EEG records, 151 were obtained with definite foci which showed exacerbations characterized by the spread of abnormal activity that developed either spontaneously or as the result of activating procedures. The selection of records was based upon EEG criteria and at the time we had no knowledge of the clinical data; the original pool of EEG records was obtained on patients selected from the files of the University of California Hospital in order to assure the availability of complete and adequate clinical and laboratory studies for the entire group. Only after we fully agreed upon the findings in these 151 records did we correlate the EEG data with the clinical findings.

By using a system of EEG recording which permitted a direct comparison of many homologous tracings that were obtained simultaneously and side-by-side, we were able to study the development and propagation of discharge from human, cerebral foci in the following ways: (1) local cortical spread, presumably involving short internuncial cortical neurons; (2) spread to the contralateral homologous region (mirror focus) via transcallosal or other interhemispheric pathways; and (3) diffuse spread in the form of bilaterally synchronous and equal slow wave activity, which neurophysiological studies suggest is mediated by corticofugal pathways to the mesencephalon where, by involvement of the reticular formation, the spread is projected to both hemispheres. Although this study had obvious limitations in that it could not follow many of the subcortical details of propagation as revealed by animal research, it did, nevertheless, demonstrate the following points:

(1) When EEG and clinical findings were correlated, it became apparent that differentiation could not be made between epileptic and nonepileptic patients on the basis of the EEG findings. It was clear that the routes of discharge shown by this study were essentially identical in both groups. The evidence suggested that focal discharge spreads by whatever routes are available to it and that the distinction between epileptic and nonepileptic must depend upon other neurophysiological factors (presumably subcortical) than those demonstrated by this approach.

(2) Since gross generalized EEG changes developed in many of these patients, whether epileptic or not and when the patients were conscious and relatively alert, it was obvious that the inhibitory mechanisms were still operating effectively to protect them. Two conclusions might be deduced from this. Firstly, one must differentiate between gross generalized EEG activity and clinical epilepsy. This was a point that was strongly emphasized by Holmes in his last paper on epilepsy written just 30 years ago (Holmes 1946). Secondly, and more importantly, the inhibitory processes referred to constitute a primary protective mechanism for the maintenance of normal CNS function and it is on this basis that differences between the epileptic and nonepileptic presumably occur. Neurophysiological studies have shown that generalized tonic-clonic seizures develop only when subcortical, extrapyramidal centres are substantially involved in the epileptic discharge (Wilder & Schmidt 1965). This, of course, could not be discerned in our human EEG studies.

(3) Definite activation of the contralateral homologous region, i.e. the development of a 'mirror focus', was found in nearly one-half of the group selected and suggestively occurred in another 29%. Since such mirror foci appeared predominantly in the nonepileptic group and in nonepileptic patients whose primary focus was marked and chronic, we have always doubted the great significance attached by many authorities over the past fifteen years to such mirror foci. This does not mean to say that mirror foci and other secondary foci may not be important in the propagation of epileptic discharge in some patients. This probably is true when such secondary foci involve pathological changes as are so common with the diffuse and often bilateral pathology usually associated with epilepsy.

Another possibility concerns the 'kindling' phenomenon already mentioned. Even here, however, considerable variations in the physiological evidence have been found and underlying differences in genetic factors and the associated epileptic susceptibility probably must be taken into account.

In accordance with our EEG studies on humans, more recent neurophysiological evidence suggests that mirror foci indeed are not as important in epilepsy as was formerly considered to be the case. Morrell (1969) has now shown that input into such foci from a second source is necessary before they can assume the proportions of an independent focus and that the callosal pathway alone is not enough. As discussed elsewhere (Aird & Woodbury 1974), I suspect that there is still more to it than this.

A corollary of this point is that the corpus callosum is not a major route for the propagation of epileptic discharge (Jasper 1969). This, also, was suggested by the relatively poor results obtained by Van Wagonen long ago (Van Wagonen & Herran 1940) as a result of sectioning the corpus callosum in patients with intractable epilepsy. In spite of this, there is still an occasional resurgence of interest among neurosurgeons in this approach.

In our EEG studies of focal discharge, there were many instances of temporal lobe epilepsy. This is a condition of special interest in that it usually shows a temporal focus by EEG (Gibbs *et al* 1948) and frequently is initiated by temporal aurae (Penfield & Jasper 1954). On this basis the International Classification of the Epilepsies has equated temporal lobe seizures to 'partial seizures of complex symptomatology'. However, the fully developed temporal lobe attack, which is characterized by loss of contact, automatic activity and amnesia, does not have focal characteristics and in its more brief forms is frequently confused with *absence*. This raises an issue of major clinical importance: what is the significance of focal activity in different forms of epilepsy? The predominant thought has been to emphasize the importance of focal findings, whether clinical, EEG, isotopic or roentgenographic. Since spreading epileptic discharge has been said to be the beginning of the attack and in fact part of the seizure itself, such focal activity has been ascribed a major role in epilepsy. Our clinical studies, correspondingly, have been aimed at finding such focal characteristics and this has been greatly emphasized because of the importance of such findings for purposes of neurosurgical intervention. However, the results of countless studies of this type over the years now make it abundantly apparent that foci are to be found almost as commonly in association with seizures which are generalized from the start as with the more obvious focal forms of epilepsy. This has led many authorities to believe that there is a focal ictus in all forms of epilepsy. The more recent findings of Bancaud, Talairach and their co-workers using a stereo EEG technique, have especially emphasized the frequency of deep foci, unsuspected by routine EEG, or by clinical and other forms of study (Bancaud *et al* 1967). Such foci have been found in patients with *absence*, for example, in such varied sites as prefrontal, orbital and medial frontal cortex, cingulate cortex and the parasagittal and temporal regions (Penfield & Jasper 1946, Tükel & Jasper 1952, Ralston 1961, Walker & Morello 1967, Waltregny *et al* 1969). This represents a very considerable extension of our old thinking in regard to the *absence variant* form of epilepsy associated with deep pathology. Essentially the same picture has emerged with generalized tonic-clonic seizures that clinically appear to be generalized from the start. In many seizures generalized from the start such foci have been shown to be neurophysiologically significant and it is now generally conceded that a clear distinction cannot be made between this type of seizure and the more obvious focal forms of epilepsy (Bancaud 1969, 1971). The same point has been made from an EEG standpoint, e.g. that it frequently is not possible to distinguish between what have been designated as 'primary' and 'secondary' bilaterally synchronous, spike and wave patterns (Steward & Dreifuss 1967).

The evidence quoted is not as confusing as it might at first appear. While focal findings obviously are still of great importance, it is now clear that, except in limited focal forms of epilepsy, such foci do not determine the clinical character of the seizure that they trigger. Sustained clinical forms of seizure clearly depend upon the circuits of the CNS that each involve. Focal seizures as a rule are easily determined on the basis of clinical, EEG and other laboratory studies. Generalized tonic-clonic seizures also are obvious, regardless of the foci that may serve to trip them off. In this case we have a fully generalized seizure that involves the entire CNS and the peripheral neuromuscular elements as well. *Absence* attacks, on the other hand, involve little or no motor activity, nor again the psychomotor, psychosensory, or automatic activity of temporal lobe epilepsy. Without going into all of the interesting background of neurophysiological studies that have been made on *absence* (Hunter & Jasper 1949, Williams 1953, Guerrero-Figueroa *et al* 1963, Marcus *et al* 1968, Gloor 1968), it is now clear that in *absence* we are dealing with a limited seizure pattern that involves primarily the corticoreticular system from the rostral portion of the reticular formation and thalamic nuclei to the cortex, bilaterally. The principal clinical manifestation of *absence* is loss of consciousness, a symptom that can be produced by the pathophysiological involvement of the upper brain stem and diencephalic portion of the reticular formation. There is evidence to suggest that the slow wave component of the spike and wave discharge, typical of *absence*, represents an inhibitory influence as opposed to the excitatory effect of the spike component. In any case, from a clinical standpoint it is obvious that in *absence* we are dealing with a highly inhibited form of epilepsy. The attacks are brief, not fully generalized as mentioned before, and can be interrupted by strong sensory stimulation. Thus, in *absence* we have a seizure type that involves bilateral, but nevertheless limited, regional portions of the nervous system. Regardless of how it may be initiated, it is the bilateral, corticoreticular circuits of *absence* that determines its clinical manifestations. In spite of its classification as a generalized seizure, *absence* is only generalized in the sense of involving bilateral corticoreticular circuits. It is not fully generalized in the sense of generalized clonic-tonic seizures with their involvement of the deeper structures of the brain and entire central nervous system.

It is of interest to examine temporal lobe epilepsy in this same light. As already indicated, our concepts of temporal lobe epilepsy as a focal form of seizure have been developed as a result of EEG evidence, chiefly obtained during interictal periods, and the association of temporal aurae that often initiate these episodes. For the reasons already enumerated the question remains—are these evidences of the focal initiation of attacks to be accepted as proof that the subsequent temporal lobe seizure is also focal in character? The following points have raised doubt on this score:

(1) The clinical manifestations, e.g. automatic activity associated with amnesia and sometimes behavioural and autonomic aberrations, are not focal in the usual sense of unilateral or localized seizures.

(2) At the start of many temporal lobe spells, the EEG is 'suppressed' in the temporal areas (Feindel *et al* 1952). Temporal spiking disappears and is replaced by either low voltage, fast activity or a relatively flat tracing. This is followed by a gradual build-up of higher voltage, slow wave activity that appears bilaterally. These findings strongly suggest that bilateral subcortical activity is involved in temporal lobe seizures and may be associated with a relative normalization of the cortical activity.

(3) EEG foci in temporal lobe epilepsy may be limited to one anterior temporal region, may appear simultaneously in both temporal areas, or even alternate from one side to the other (Gibbs *et al* 1948, Jasper *et al* 1951, MacLean & Arellano 1950). Stoll *et al* (1951) obtained considerable neurophysiological evidence which strongly suggested that the unilateral or bilateral spiking, and again the rhythmic discharges, in the EEG from the temporal poles represent 'a secondary conducted disturbance and need not necessarily indicate a primary cortical lesion'.

(4) In the electrocorticograms of temporal lobe patients developing automatisms, Jasper reported the invariable spread of the epileptic discharge to both temporal lobes and a significant spread to temporoparietal cortex and often frontal cortex as well (Jasper 1964). These changes occurred without convulsive movements and might have been explained as an 'EEG activation' or diffuse spread phenomenon in the sense previously described, except for the fact that these patients were confused or out of contact.

(5) The neurophysiological evidence, however, is far more convincing than

the EEG evidence. The Montreal school (Feindel & Penfield 1954, Feindel & Gloor 1954, Jasper 1964) has shown that epileptic activation of the amygdala or hippocampus alone does not produce an automatism. It was only when the discharge spread to the diencephalon, upper midbrain and to the opposite amygdalohippocampal complex that such attacks developed. This involvement of bilateral and widespread subcortical structures has been explained by the direct and synaptic connections of the amygdala and hippocampi (Green & Shimamoto 1953, Feindel & Gloor 1954, Feindel & Penfield 1954, Gloor 1955, Nauta 1961, Jasper 1964). Discharge from the amygdalohippocampal complex to the thalamus and fornix system with its diffuse connections to extrapyramidal and other subcortical and brain stem structures no doubt also explains the development of generalized tonic-clonic seizures in some patients. These and other studies (Ajmone-Marsan & Stoll 1951) have also shown how discharge from foci in the tip of the temporal horn, orbital surface of the frontal lobe, cingulate gyri, uncus and temporoinsular cortex quickly spreads to activate the amygdalohippocampal complex.

The evidence thus supports the thesis that the automatisms of temporal lobe epilepsy depend upon the involvement of subcortical and bilateral structures. The circuits involved, although relatively diffuse and bilateral, as was the case in *absence*, are actually regional in character and by no means involve the whole CNS as in generalized tonic-clonic seizures. The regional involvement in temporal lobe epilepsy concerns the amygdalohippocampal complexes and their physiologically related, subcortical structures in the mesial diencephalon and upper brain stem. It is the involvement of these so-called 'limbic system' structures that explain the behavioural, automatic, autonomic and amnesiac characteristics of temporal lobe epilepsy.

The question may logically be raised in patients experiencing temporal aurae as to whether such episodes should be termed temporal lobe epilepsy in contradistinction to the automatisms previously discussed. The answer would be yes, if we also are prepared to designate different forms of epilepsy to the aurae that precede generalized tonic-clonic seizures and other forms of epilepsy. Some of these might qualify under the guise of focal epilepsy going on to 'grand mal'. However, this still leaves a problem with respect to the frequent occurrence of minor lapses in temporal lobe epilepsy. For years I have included questions with regard to such episodes in my history-taking of patients suspected of epilepsy. These include questions of slight lapses unnoted by family or friends, unless they are directly engaged in conversation. The patient is aware of such episodes since he may miss the thread of a conversation or lecture. Again, if reading or studying, he may have to reread a passage several times before grasping its significance. It usually is possible to distinguish these episodes from 'day dreaming' and *absence*. As a rule they are associated with other evidences of temporal lobe epilepsy. Such episodes form a gradual spectrum ranging from aurae alone, through short periods of confusion, to minor lapses and on to obvious automatisms. Since all of these may occur at different times in the same patient, it becomes an unrewarding exercise of differentiation to assign the designation of temporal lobe epilepsy to the symptoms recognized by the patient and automatisms to the more definite lapses. Also, because the treatment is the same for all, it is more practical to designate the entire complex as temporal lobe epilepsy. The only difference between temporal lobe epilepsy and other forms of epilepsy in this respect concerns the great number, type and variety of focal symptoms, which are indicative of focal temporal discharge and which feed into the bilateral, regional circuits that are involved in fullblown temporal lobe attacks.

To summarize the points I have made: when viewed from the standpoint of the predominant and essential cerebral circuits that are involved in epilepsy, it becomes apparent that there are three basic types of seizures. First, there are the focal or partial seizures. Although our studies show that these often involve contralateral homologous regions ('mirror foci') and some generalized effects as judged by EEG evidence, from both clinical and neurophysiological standpoints their predominant involvement remains localized or at least unilateral and are not generalized. Secondly, there are what may be termed 'bilateral regional' seizures, involving primarily the limbic system in the case of temporal lobe epilepsy and the corticorreticular system in the case of *absence*. Epileptogenic foci may be important in both, but it is the bilateral and regional circuits that determine the clinical character of these seizure types. While both involve bilateral cerebral structures, the involvement is limited and regional in comparison with truly generalized seizures of the tonic-clonic type, which constitutes the third category. When viewed in this way, the regional and bilateral structures that are involved in *absence* should not be considered generalized and in the case of temporal lobe epilepsy should not be considered focal, as defined in the first category mentioned.

In conclusion, I would urge that as clinicians we take stock of our past preoccupation with the focal aspects of epileptic phenomena. As important as they are, we should develop a new perspective with respect to the now well-documented neurophysiological basis for the circuitry patterns underlying the different clinical forms of seizures. Only in this way can we fully understand them, and in this I would include such aspects as their genetic differences and differences in response to therapy. However, these latter are involved subjects which cannot be discussed within the limits of this presentation. I would like to conclude with a statement that Sir Gordon Holmes in his last paper on epilepsy in 1946 quoted from Oliver Wendell Holmes: 'If I wished to show a student the difficulties of getting at the truth from clinical experience, I would give him the history of epilepsy to read'.

References

AIRD R.B. & GAROUTTE B. (1960) Propagation of epileptic discharge as revealed by activated EEG. *Epilepsia* **1**, 337–50.

AIRD R.B. & WOODBURY D.M. (1974) *The Management of Epilepsy*, pp. 22–4. Charles C. Thomas, Publishers, Springfield, Illinois.

AJMONE-MARSAN C. & STOLL J. JR. (1951) Subcortical connections of the temporal pole in relation to temporal lobe seizures. *Arch. Neurol. Psychiat.* (Chicago) **66**, 669–86.

BANCAUD J., BONIS A., COVELLO L. & CROIZE B. (1967) The EEG in complicated and symptomatic migraine. *Electroenceph. Clin. Neurophysiol.* **23**, 502.

BANCAUD J. (1969) Physiopathogenesis of generalized epilepsies of organic nature (Stereo-encephalographic study). In: Gastaut H., Jasper H., Bancaud J. & Waltreguy A. (Eds) *Physiopathogenesis of the Epilepsies*, Chap. 14. Charles C. Thomas, Publishers, Springfield, Illinois.

BANCAUD J. (1971) The role of the cerebral cortex in 'generalized' epilepsy of organic origin. Contribution of stereo-electro-encephalographic studies to the 'centrencephalic' concept. *Presse Méd.* **79**, 669–73.

FEINDEL W. & GLOOR P. (1954) Comparison of electrographic effects of stimulation of the amygdala and brain stem reticular formation in cats. *Electroenceph. Clin. Neurophysiol.* **6**, 389–402.

FEINDEL W. & PENFIELD W. (1954) Localization of discharge in temporal lobe automatism. *Arch. Neurol. Psychiat.* **72**, 605–30.

FEINDEL W., PENFIELD W. & JASPER H. (1952) Localization of epileptic discharge in temporal lobe automatisms. *Trans. Am. Neurol. Assoc.* **77**, 14–17.

GIBBS E.L., GIBBS F.A. & FUSTER B. (1948) Psychomotor epilepsy. *Arch. Neurol. Psychiat.* **60**, 331–9.

GLOOR P. (1955) Electrophysiological studies on the connections of the amygdaloid nucleus in the cat (I & II). *Electroencephal. Clin. Neurophysiol.* **7**, 223–64.

GLOOR P. (1968) Generalized cortico-reticular epilepsies. Some considerations on the pathophysiology of generalized bilaterally synchronous spike and wave discharge. *Epilepsia* **9**, 249–63.

GODDARD G.V., McINTYRE D.C. & LEECH C.K. (1969) A permanent change in brain function resulting from daily electrical stimulation. *Exper. Neurol.* **25**, 295–330.

GREEN J.D. & SHIMAMOTO T. (1953) Hippocampal seizures and their propagation. *Arch. Neurol. Psychiat.* **70**, 687–702.

GUERRERO-FIGUEROA R., BARROS A., DE BALBIAN VERSTER F. & HEATH R.G. (1963) Experimental 'petit mal' in kittens. *Arch. Neurol.* **9**, 297–306.

HOLMES G. (1927) Local epilepsy (Saville Oration). *Lancet* **i**, 957–62.

HOLMES G. (1946) Evolution of clinical medicine as illustrated by the history of epilepsy. *Brit. Med. J.* **2**, 1–4.

HUNTER J. & JASPER H.H. (1949) Effects of thalamic stimulation in unanesthetized animals: The arrest reaction in petit mal-like seizures, activation patterns and generalized convulsions. *Electroencephal. Clin. Neurophysiol.* **1**, 305–24.

JASPER H.H. (1964) Some physiological mechanisms involved in epileptic automatism. *Epilepsia* **5**, 1–20.

JASPER H. (1969) Mechanisms of propagation: Extracellular studies. In: Jasper H., Ward A.A. & Pope A. (Eds) *Basic Mechanisms of the Epilepsies*, Chap. 16. Little, Brown & Co., Boston.

JASPER H.H., PERTUISET B. & FLANIGIN H. (1951) EEG and cortical electrograms in relation to surgical therapy of patients with temporal lobe seizures. *Arch. Neurol. Psychiat.* **65**, 270–90.

MacLEAN P.D. & ARELLANO Z.A.P. (1950) Basal lead studies in epileptic automatisms. *Electroenceph. Clin. Neurophysiol.* **2**, 1–16.

MARCUS E.M., WATSON C.W. & SIMON S.A. (1968) An experimental model of some varieties of petit mal epilepsy. Electrical-behavioral correlations of acute bilateral epileptogenic foci in cerebral cortex. *Epilepsia* **9**, 233–48.

MORRELL F. (1969) Cellular pathophysiology of focal epilepsy. *Epilepsia* **10**, 495–505.

NAUTA W.J.H. (1961) Fibre degeneration following lesions of the amygdaloid complex in the monkey. *J. Anat.* **95**, 515–31.

PENFIELD W. & JASPER H. (1946) Highest level seizures. *Res. Publ. Assoc. Res. Nerv. Ment. Dis.* **26**, 252–71.

PENFIELD W. & JASPER H. (1954) *Epilepsy and the Functional Anatomy of the Human Brain*. Little, Brown & Co., Boston.

RALSTON B.L. (1961) Cingulate epilepsy and secondary bilateral synchrony. *Electroenceph. Clin. Neurophysiol.* **13**, 591–8.

STEWART L.F. & DREIFUSS F.E. (1967) Centrencephalic seizure discharges in patients with focal hemispheral lesions. *Electroenceph. Clin. Neurophysiol.* **23**, 292–3.

STOLL J., AJMONE-MARSAN C. & JASPER H.H. (1951) Electrophysiological studies of sub-cortical connections of anterior temporal region in cat. *J. Neurophysiol.* **14**, 305–16.

TÜKEL K. & JASPER H. (1952) The electro-encephalogram in parasagittal lesions. *Electroenceph. Clin. Neurophysiol.* **4**, 481–94.

VAN WAGONEN W.P. & HERREN R.Y. (1940) Surgical division of commissural pathways in corpus callosum; relation to spread of epileptic attack. *Arch. Neurol. Psychiat.* (Chicago) **44**, 740–59.

WALKER A.E. & MORELLO G. (1967) Experimental petit mal. *Trans. Amer. Neurol. Assoc.* **92**, 57–61.

WALTREGUY A., REGIS H., DRAVET C. & GASTAUT H. (1969) The contribution of intracarotid sodium amytal tests in physio-pathogenic study of petit mal variant. (Lennox Syndrome). In: Gastaut H., Jasper H., Bancaud J. & Waltreguy A. (Eds) *Physiopathogenesis of the Epilepsies*, Chap. 24. Charles C. Thomas Spring-field, Illinois.

WILDER B.J. & SCHMIDT R.P. (1965) Propagation of epileptic discharge from chronic neocortical foci in monkey. *Epilepsia* **6**, 297–309.

WILLIAMS D. (1953) A study of thalamic and cortical rhythm in petit mal. *Brain* **76**, 50–69.

AXOPLASMIC TRANSPORT AND ITS PATHOLOGICAL
IMPLICATIONS

J. C. SLOPER

To Emeritus Professor W. Bargmann on his 70th birthday

It is now widely accepted, not only that nervous impulses are transmitted along axons, but also that axons and, indeed, dendrites too, transport materials along their length (see reviews by Sloper 1966, Dahlström 1971). At least in the case of the axon, this transport is bidirectional. Thus organelles such as vesicles have been visualized moving in both directions; and there is evidence that inclusions such as viruses can move centripetally, as can injected materials such as horse-radish peroxidase (which can be visualized in electronmicrographs). The main site of metabolic synthesis, however, is the neuronal cell-body. Substances such as dopamine and vasopressin are synthesized here, loculated into vesicles, and transported down the axon. There is suggestive evidence that other substances are similarly handled, although it is possible that some are transported in extravesicular form. Among the former are potential or actual neurotransmitters, their precursors, and related enzymes; that is, substances including acetylcholine, choline acetyltransferase, GABA and 5HT. Protein and glycoprotein are also transported down the axon, thus subserving the maintenance of the axolemma and of organelles such as microtubules, neurofilaments, mitochondria and 'synaptic' vesicles. The carriage of 'trophic factors', for example concerned with the maintenance of skeletal muscle, has also been postulated. This emphasis on the perikaryon as the main site of metabolite synthesis is not to deny that some protein synthesis is conducted in the axon—for mitochondria can fulfil this role. Again, as Vogt (1953) suggested years ago, considerable modification of metabolites may occur, for example in the nerve ending, where metabolites are known too to be taken up from the circulation. Curiously enough, however, no attention has been paid to the flow or transport of water.

The rates of transport of substances in axons vary between less than 10 mm per day to several 100 mm per day. When it is realized that axons may be over 1000 mm in length and in general less than 10 μm in width, it will be appreciated that the axonal transport of metabolites and organelles is almost certainly susceptible to profound disorders, disorders which, by analogy with the cardiovascular system, are likely to play a considerable role in nervous diseases, not least those associated with senility. Our duty is to unravel these disorders of transport or flow. Just as current cardiovascular pathologists have devoted the last hundred years to clarifying the implications of Harvey's discovery of the circulation of the blood, so we must now analyse the implications of Weiss' work on the *cellulifugal* flow of axoplasm and Bargmann's discovery of the *transport* of metabolites along the axon.

Historical aspects

The concept of axoplasmic transport or flow is complementary to that of the carriage of nervous impulses but requires one to look on the nervous system as much as a soup-kitchen as a telephone exchange. Although Scott (1906) speculated on the possibility of axoplasmic flow or transport of metabolites, we largely owe the discovery of axoplasmic transport to Bargmann, an anatomist, and his collaborators (Bargmann 1954) (Fig. 22.1).

This is not to decry the brilliant earlier work of Weiss and J. Z. Young. It was the latter (1942) who inferred that the flow of axoplasm played a part in the growing-out of the injured axonal stump; it was Weiss (1944), (Weiss & Hiscoe 1948) who established that the growth of such axons 'furnished a steady supply-stream to replenish peripheral macro-molecular systems, including proteins, lost by metabolic degradation' (Weiss 1959). As recently as 1972 he emphasized that this slow axonal flow was 'cellulifugal *of* the axon, not *in* the axon'.

These observations are to be contrasted with those made by Bargmann and his school in Kiel between 1949 and 1953, years in which it was established that neurohormones were transported along axons of the tractus hypophyseus to be released from their nerve terminals in the posterior pituitary. The concept of axoplasmic *transport* we thus owe primarily to Bargmann, that of axoplasmic flow to Weiss and J. Z. Young. It should be added that the properties of the secretory neurons of Bargmann and Scharrer were rather neglected in the 1950s by those concerned with nerves which were not, at that time, regarded as 'secretory'. It must now be accepted, however, from the work of many, including in particular Cross and his co-workers (see Cross *et al* 1975) that these secretory neurons can transmit nervous impulses. Bargmann's discoveries are thus of general significance in the central and peripheral nervous system. This attribution of priority in the field of axoplasmic transport to Bargmann should not belittle the major contributions made by other workers in the field, in particular by Ernst and Bertha Scharrer, Speidel, Collin, Hanström, Popjak and Stutinsky (see Sloper

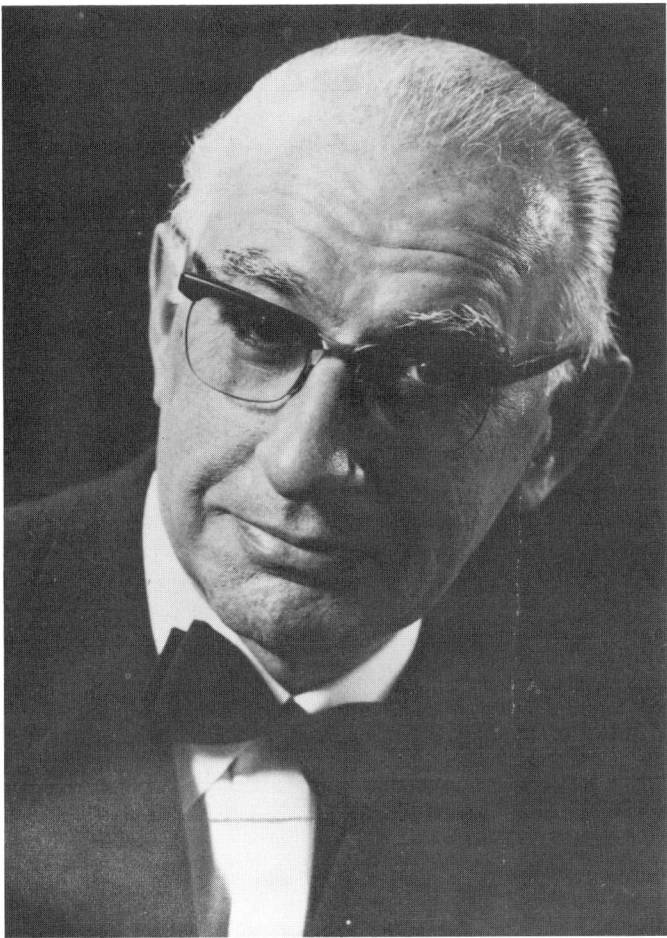

Fig. 22.1 Professor Emeritus W. Bargmann.

1958a). The beautiful comparative anatomical observations of Ernst Scharrer undoubtedly paved the way to the general acceptance of the findings of Bargmann and his school.

It was Bargmann's 70th birthday on 17 January 1976. Nearly thirty years ago Fraülein Jakob (his chief technician) stained a section of a Teleost hypothalamo–neurohypophysial system by a technique used by Gomori for the beta cells in the pancreatic islets. The minute that Bargmann saw this preparation he realized that he had demonstrated neuro-secretory material (NSM) along the entire hypothalamo–neurohypophysial tract (HNS). Waving his rather noisome cigar—laboratory tradition has it—he leapt from his seat crying, 'Donnerwetter!'. Within four years he and his colleagues, and in particular Hild, Ortmann, Schiebler and Zetler, a pharmacologist, had shown,

(1) that they could selectively stain the HNS in a wide variety of vertebrates;
(2) that where in the system there was stainable NSM, there one could also find high neurohormonal activity (oxytocic or vasopressor activity);
(3) that interruption of the tractus hypophyseus led alike to the aggregation of neurohormonal activity and of NSM on the cell-body side of the cut end;
(4) that an appropriate stress (dehydration or saline administration in the case of vasopressor activity) led alike to the depletion of NSM and of vasopressor activity from the HNS.

Without, initially, the use of electronmicroscopy, Bargmann was unable to decide where in the axon these substances were conveyed. It was left to Palay (1955) to show that they were probably carried in vesicles some 100 nm in diameter, work soon confirmed by Bargmann; and to Heller and Lederis (1961) to establish that ultracentrifugate fractions made from the posterior lobe of the pituitary characterized by high vasopressor and oxytocic activities, were also characterized electronmicroscopically by such vesicles. Bargmann in fact originally thought that his NSM was a glycoprotein bearer substance. It was for me to show, in 1954, that it was more probably a polypeptide exceptionally rich in cystine and probably devoid of lipid, and therefore akin to the neurohormones themselves.

This work has been corroborated since by the use of similar histochemical techniques for the demonstration of oxytocin and vasopressin *in vitro* (Rodeck 1959a, b, Gutierrez & Sloper 1969). Moreover Uttenthal and co-workers succeeded in 1967 in preparing antibodies against neurophysin and were able to show that these antibodies were labelled with fluorescent markers which could demonstrate material in the same distribution as our cystine-rich NSM. The neurophysins, which are also exceptionally rich in cystine, are either precursors or carriers of the octapeptide neurohormones.

The next step was the calculation of the rate of transport of these substances down the tractus hypophyseus by the injection of S^{35} DL-labelled cysteine into the *subarachnoid* space (Sloper 1958a, b). It was shown in autoradiographs that isotope accumulated within minutes in the cell-bodies of SON and PVN, but not until some hours later in the infundibular process of the posterior pituitary, where the nerves of the tractus hypophyseus end; this delayed arrival of isotope in the posterior pituitary was confirmed by the estimation of radioactivity in tissue samples. The two techniques are complementary. Sample measurement has the disadvantage that preparations of posterior pituitary necessarily include large amounts of tissue such as the glandular pars intermedia.

This technical shortcoming of sample measurement was stressed too by Weiss (1959) when he assessed what he regarded as the first really conclusive evidence of axonal transport. Earlier work had involved isotopic measurements of samples of peripheral nerves from animals injected with radioisotope either intraperitoneally (Samuels *et al* 1951) or into the spinal cord (Ochs & Burger 1958), and this Weiss regarded as suggestive but inconclusive. He held as conclusive, however, his own observations (Weiss 1959) made with Waelsch and Lajtha on autoradiographs on the lateral line nerve of axolotls; these involved the intraperitoneal injection of C^{14}-labelled aminoacids. These workers on peripheral nerves possibly disregarded our earlier work on the HNS on the grounds that secretory nerves were not true nerves, a view that must now be dismissed in the light of the demonstration, e.g. recently by Cross *et al* (1975), that such nerves undoubtedly conduct nervous impulses. It follows that, by Weiss' criteria, we must regard our early estimations of rates of transport in the tractus hypophyseus as not only the first to be made in the field of neurosecretion but also as the first 'conclusive' evidence of transport in not only the central but also the nervous system as a whole. The term 'conclusive' should still, however, be used with some reservation: for all radioisotopic work to date on axoplasmic transport has been based on the premise that the labelled material found in axons following the injection of labelled aminoacids largely reflects the presence of polypeptides synthesized in the neuronal cell-body; i.e. that there is not free diffusion of these labelled aminoacids across the axolemma to organelles such as mitochondria which have some capacity for protein synthesis.

At all events, by the Second International Symposium on Neurosecretion in 1957 (Sloper 1958a) I provided evidence, which at that time seemed improbable, that cystine-rich polypeptides traversed the tractus hypophyseus in a matter of hours. It was clear, too, that I had devised a means of biosynthesizing labelled vasopressin; this Sachs (1960) later achieved. A critical step was the *subarachnoid* (or intraventricular) injection of radioisotope, a step missed by several later workers in their initial studies. Detailed calculations suggesting rates of transport of labelled neurophysins (precursor or carrier polypeptides), vasopressin and oxytocin, of about 100 mm a day, have since been made by Pickering and co-workers (Jones & Pickering 1969, and see Cross *et al* 1975) and by Norström and Sjöstrand (1971), in Bristol and Gothenburg respectively.

Physiopathology of axonal transport

In these early years it became apparent to those few people working in the field of neurosecretion that all nerves might be regarded as secretory, but some more so than others. At this time, too, Vogt (1953) established the presence of high concentrations of dopamine, adrenaline and noradrenaline in the hypothalamus, work since extended brilliantly to 5-hydroxytryptamine, GABA and other potential neurotransmitters. Dopamine is a particularly suitable model, in view of its physiological role in striatal activity.

Just as most of these potential transmitter substances appear to be carried along axons, so too is it probable that the hypothalamic 'release hormones' (e.g. CRH, TRH) are secreted in the same way. It should be emphasized, however, that evidence sufficient to satisfy all the Kiel criteria has rarely been proffered.

A period spent in 1955 in Aarhus with Einarson, a pioneer in the study of neuronal nucleic acid metabolism, convinced me of the importance of looking on the neuron as a rather complex epithelial cell and of studying it pathologically from this viewpoint. We already knew from work on motor-nerves how injured axons could bud-off axons and thus form new endings on skeletal muscle. The envelopment of islands of pars tuberalis by axons in the residual pituitary stalk of hypophysectomized humans strongly suggested that a similar process might occur in the central nervous system, thus explaining the curious reformation of a neurohormone storage region in the residual neurohypophysis in the median eminence of long-hypophysectomized humans (Sloper & Adams 1956, Sloper & King 1963). Currently, neuropathologists are engaged in the ultrastructural analysis of such problems: in this field there are many little-understood pitfalls, largely reflecting the fact that tissue samples are so tiny (see Sloper 1972, p. 138).

An equally interesting pathological problem was to decide whether the 'loss' of Nissl substances (and NSM) from apparently enlarged cell-bodies in the SON of dehydrated rats or rats given hypertonic saline, stresses which lead to the secretion of antidiuretic hormone, was a pathological change. This was a theory in line with the classical neuropathological concept of tigrolysis. At this time, too, many felt that neurons in the SON devoid of stainable NSM were 'inactive' or degenerating. Both tenets were wrong. For, by using ^{35}S-methionine (a good marker of protein synthesis) and ^{35}S-cysteine, I was able to show that neurohormone transport probably increased in animals given hypertonic saline, which depletes the posterior pituitary alike of vasopressor activity and stainable neurosecretory material. It became clear that the neuronal, nuclear and nucleolar *enlargement* seen in the SON of suitably stressed animals and the depletion of their nerve terminals of hormone NSM and neurosecretory vesicles, material normally stored there, could be interpreted as a *work*-hypertrophy, a view totally at variance with the concepts of 'degeneration' mooted at that time.

More recently we have shown that in rats given hypertonic saline there is a statistically significant increase in the least diameter of axons in the tractus hypophyseus (Grainger & Sloper 1974), the first evidence of a 'work-hypertrophy' of axons yet provided. This same work allowed us to deduce the presence of up to some 80,000 axons in the pituitary stalk of the rat. Since their *mean* diameter was 330 nm (that is, below optical resolution −500 nm) it will be appreciated that estimations of this kind have had to await the electronmicroscope. One can in fact approach such problems by counts of perikarya, but this takes no account of the division of axons.

In the light of these findings, it is rather useful to visualize the secretory system in the HNS in terms of small water-tanks leading by pipes to taps feeding baths (the nerve terminals). In these, neurohormone is stored, and released through small plug-holes. Nerve terminals in the infundibular process of the stressed animal I liken to baths with the plugs out and the taps running fast. This concept has been useful, not least in the interpretation of a curious form of diabetes insipidus recently discovered by Valtin (see below) where the neurons of the HNS can form oxytocin but not vasopressin; these neurons seem in fact to be undergoing a 'frustration' hypertrophy. The crucial point is that a system can be highly active, despite the depletion of its stores of, e.g. neurohormone, and current workers concerned with dopamine-levels in the striatal system might find this analogy helpful.

I have emphasized the plasticity of secretory neurons because this concept is foreign to classical neuropathology. I should, however, also emphasize that the perikarya we have studied certainly seem unable to divide after birth: indeed in our studies with ^{3}H-thymidine we have found that cell-division in the perikarya of the SON must stop by the 13th day of the 20-day period of gestation in the fetal mouse. Yet our observations on the injured pituitary-stalk in man indicate a capacity for axonal regrowth, thus confirming the work of Stutinsky and others in animals. Neuroglial cells related to secretory neurons also show significant changes. Thus as early as 1951 Ortmann observed in osmotically stressed animals the increased mitotic activity of the interstitial glial cells of the posterior pituitary. The function of these cells is unknown. It seems likely, indeed, that glial-cell multiplication may be a common concomitant of a work-hypertrophy of secretory neurons, and thus may perhaps—with measurements of, say, nuclear diameter in the perikaryon—provide useful parameters for the study of secretory activity elsewhere in the brain.

In these early years (see Sloper 1966) we studied the effects of various forms of injury on the HNS. Curiously enough, high doses of irradiation caused no measurable disturbance in transport. The effects of compression on flow or transport had long been studied, in particular by Weiss (see Weiss & Pillai 1965), and *in vivo* first by Thomsen (1954). It was, in fact, the observation of an accumulation of NSM in the tractus hypophyseus of hypophysectomized humans, who died 32 hours after hypophysectomy (Sloper & Adams 1956) which first drew my attention to the probable rapidity of axoplasmic transport.

More recent pharmacological studies involving the administration of toxic substances such as acrylamine, triorthocresyl phosphate (TOCP) and diisopropyl phosphorofluoridate (DIFP), which can cause peripheral neuropathies, have since been made by others and particularly by Bradley and Austin (see Bradley & Williams 1973, Austin *et al* 1975). In TOCP-treated cats, slower rates of axonal transport seemed particularly affected. Similarly, in murine and avian inherited neuromuscular diseases (suspected of being motor neurone disease or forms of muscular dystrophy respectively), Bradley and Jaros (1973) and again Austin and others (1975) have shown disturbances in certain aspects of axonal transport. This work is still in the pioneer stage, but should clarify the pathogenesis of a wide variety of neuropathies.

My own interest has more recently centred on a remarkable disease of the CNS which I believe may well have human counterparts. This is a form of congenital diabetes insipidus (Valtin 1967) inherited as a recessive gene in rats. No vasopressin is formed, although oxytocin (a very similar octapeptide) and its neurophysin are secreted. The only morphological abnormality yet found in the SON and PVN is the presence of enlarged neuronal cell-bodies, which closely resemble those seen in stressed or dehydrated animals, a point confirmed by autoradiographic studies (Valtin *et al* 1965). Similarly, as in dehydrated animals, the infundibular process is enlarged and depleted of NSM (oxytocin has some slight antidiuretic activity): nerve endings are enlarged and contain scanty neurosecretory vesicles. What is secreted besides oxytocin is still unknown; but to me the simplest hypothesis is that neurones in the SON and PVN are exhibiting a form of frustration hypertrophy, perhaps due to excessive osmotic stimulation, due to their failure to form vasopressin.

In adult animals the microtubular content ($23 \cdot 27 \pm 1 \cdot 76$) of axons in the tractus hypophyseus in these animals is grossly enlarged (Sloper & Grainger 1974) but in newborn animals, born from parents homozygous for diabetes insipidus, the count is normal, increasing significantly by the fourth day after birth (Grainger & Sloper 1976). If it can be accepted that polypeptide transport is increased above normal (see Jones & Pickering 1969, Pickering & Jones 1971, Cross *et al* 1975) then it does seem likely that microtubules play a significant role in transport. This is the more probable since in normal rats given hypertonic saline (which increases the secretion of vasopressin) there is a significant ($12 \cdot 48 \pm 1 \cdot 26$) but lesser increase in microtubular number. Microtubule counts could indeed be a method of studying activity (and disease states) in other systems, for example the striatal system in animals with experimental striatal disease. Our own studies are the first to be made in physiologically stressed or diseased subjects.

The mechanisms of transport

It is possible that there are many and different transport mechanisms. Thus the rates of transport are diverse as are the varieties of organelles and substances transported. Again, axons differ markedly in size and length and structure. Some are myelinated, some unmyelinated: some have neurofilaments, some have not. This diversity suggests, in its turn, variations in the susceptibility of axons to toxic and other disease processes. What we must do is determine the nature of, and morphological basis for, the underlying transport mechanisms.

Just as the concept of axoplasmic flow stemmed from the study of axonal regeneration, so Weiss' early deductions centred around the belief that flow was derived from the forces resultant on the synthesis of substances in the perikaryon. In the early years the possibility was also considered that pulsation of the axolemma contributed to transport. For my part, mindful of Dorothy Russell's belief in the pulsation of oligodendroglia, I wondered if pituicytes by pulsating could similarly contribute to transport in the unmyelinated nerves of the hypophysis. No positive evidence has been found in favour of these views, although cell-body synthesis of axoplasma could well be responsible for the centrifugal flow of newly formed axoplasm in regeneration. Conversely, in a brilliant series of experiments centring on transport in peripheral nerves, Ochs (see e.g. 1971) has established the importance of transport mechanisms *within* the axon. His major feat was to establish (using tritiated aminoacids) that transport could occur independently of any propulsive force exerted from the soma (perikaryon); that the mechanism of transport appeared to be present all along the length of the axon; and that fast transport was rapidly blocked by oxidative blocking agents. Ochs is now firmly convinced of the significance of oxidative phosphorylation in the transport process.

The morphological basis of transport is still obscure, but centres on the submicroscopic constituents of the axon (see Fig. 22.2). These include neurofilaments (some 9 nm in diameter), microtubules (19–24 nm in diameter), vesicles and saccules derived from the endoplasmic reticulum (30–60 nm in diameter), whisps of material commonly seen in relation to microtubules, mitochondria, and vesicular structures of varying size, many with electron-dense content. Those between some 60 and 200 nm in diameter include at the lower range so-called synaptic vesicles in which substances such as acetylcholine are segregated. Catecholamines tend to be in slightly larger vesicles, vasopressin and oxytocin with their neurophysins in vesicles 100–200 nm in diameter. Microtubules are derived from dimers which group themselves to form a close-packed helical structure, the wall of the microtubule.

A unitary theory of structure must explain how water, macromolecular

MICROGRAPHS   AT   35,000   MAGNIFICATION

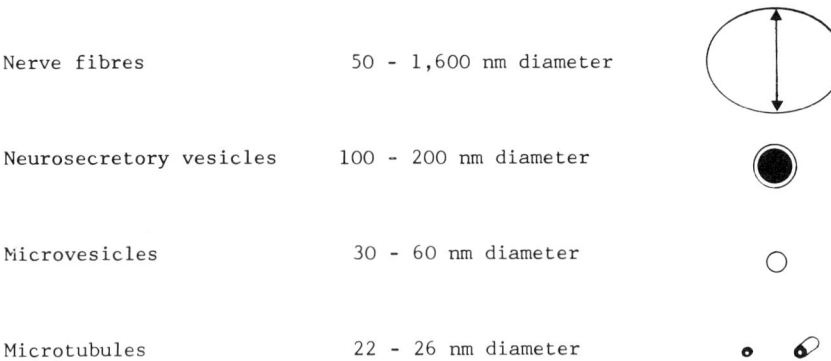

Nerve fibres   50 - 1,600 nm diameter

Neurosecretory vesicles   100 - 200 nm diameter

Microvesicles   30 - 60 nm diameter

Microtubules   22 - 26 nm diameter

Fig. 22.2   Diagrammatic representation of profiles of some constituents of axons.

substances, and vesicles and mitochondria, can be conveyed in both directions along structures varying between 50 and 10,000 or more nm in diameter, and along distances up to a million nm long. The problem is the more complex, in that transport mechanisms could well be different in myelinated and unmyelinated, and therefore presumably more distensible, axons. Equally, we know singularly little about the viscosity of the axoplasm, which could well be an extremely important factor, especially in the very fine axons (50 nm upwards in diameter) which we have studied recently in the tractus hypophyseus. I should add that information on axonal diameter and number in specific tracts is almost entirely lacking, and yet this should be the first required information in most neuropathological problems. In the tractus hypophyseus of the rat, our recent counts have indicated up to some 80,000 axons in the lower part of the pituitary stalk. In normal animals the mean least diameter of axons is $331 \pm 15 \cdot 6$ nm, the range from 50 to 2100 and more nm. These unmyelinated fibres seem to *lack* neurofilaments. Mean microtubular count per fibre is $8 \cdot 74 \pm 1 \cdot 22$. We did not count the profiles of endoplasmic reticulum. The only relevant data are those derived by Friede and Samorajski (1970) on the pooled findings from measurements on 80 peripheral axons from three rats, one an adult. This emphasis on measurement is not pedantry. The heterogeneity of the average fibre tract is astounding, but not really appreciated until one begins to make counts at a magnification of 36,000. Moreover, in systems now under close examination, such as the striatal system so brilliantly analysed by Hassler (see Kataoka *et al* 1974), Hornekiewicz (1972, 1973), and by Kanazawa (Kanazawa & Toyokura 1974), experimentation is going to be difficult without quantitative analyses comparable with those we have provided for the tractus hypophyseus, and are now preparing on motor nerves to the peroneal muscles of the rabbit.

Pharmacological experiments on the mechanisms of transport stem from the observations of Wiśniewski & Terry (1967) and Wiśniewski *et al* (1968) which indicated that colchicine disrupted microtubules in which the nerves had also inhibited the transport of labelled metabolites. However, as Wisniewski would be the first to stress, colchicine and other similar substances which can interfere with microtubules or microfilaments are known to have many other effects. It follows that microtubular disruption could be coincidental rather than causative. Further evidence for this is the fact that aminoacid transport in the tractus hypophyseus can be blocked by very high doses of colchicine without any apparent change in microtubular content (Norström *et al* 1971, Flament-Durand & Dustin 1972). It should be emphasized that the doses of colchicine used were all but lethal in these particular experiments. Such experiments do not, therefore, exclude the contribution of microtubules to transport; this is likely, for, as previously mentioned, we have seen in the tractus hypophyseus of rats statistically significant increases of microtubular number in two situations where there is evidence of increased axonal transport of polypeptide; that is, in rats given hypertonic saline and in rats suffering from congenital diabetes insipidus, a condition characterized, as noted earlier, probably by frustration hypertrophy of the secretory neuron. Ochs and others (Ochs 1971, 1974) postulated that the transport mechanism which he had shown to be ATP-dependent, might involve microtubules and/or neurofilaments and be capable of carrying polypeptides, and presumably vesicles. A rough analogy has been drawn to the relative movement along each other of myosin and actin filaments in skeletal muscle. Such a model is plausible enough; but in a system such as the tractus hypophyseus (which lacks neurofilaments) one must suppose that the whispy structures which one sees occasionally in relation to microtubules, correspond in some way with the neurofilaments which are so conspicuous in (say) peripheral nerves. Whatever the case, the size of the neurosecretory vesicles in the tractus hypophyseus is such (100 nm) that I feel tempted to suppose that peptides are transported, in part at least, outside these vesicles. The closely packed microtubules we see in the axons of stressed animals tie in with this theory, as does the observation, perhaps artefactual, that much hormone, especially in stressed animals, is not apparently associated with vesicles (Barer *et al* 1963), but is extravesicular.

Another way of explaining vesicle and solute transport is in terms of a new hypothesis advanced by Gross (1975), who works primarily on a piscine olfactory nerve, which contains numerous very fine unmyelinated axons. His belief is that an energy source along the microtubule diminishes locally the viscosity of the axoplasm, thus potentiating transport of materials along a viscosity gradient. What we clearly require is a means of measuring the axoplasmic viscosity in these fine axons.

Another and equally interesting hypothesis is that of Droz and his colleagues (Droz *et al*, 1973, 1975, Droz & Koenig 1971). They made a fundamental advance by studying transport (in the nerves of the avian ciliary ganglion) by autoradiography in *electronmicrographs*. Compression experiments suggest that fast-transported labelled proteins and glyco-proteins were *within* the saccules of the endoplasmic reticulum. Undoubtedly we must now think of compartmentalization in transport, thus perhaps explaining bidirectional transport. Perhaps a major side of fluid flow is not only within the endoplasmic reticulum but also within microtubules. Whatever the case, only when we are clearer as to the mechanisms of transport will we be properly equipped to analyse the role of disturbances in transport in neurological disease.

References

Austin L., Komiya Y. & Tang B.Y. (1975) Axoplasmic flow of protein and phospholipids in dystrophic mice. In: Bradley W.G., Gardner-Medwin D. & Walton J.N. (Eds) *Recent Advances in Myology. Proceedings of the Third International Congress on Muscle Diseases*, pp. 224–8. Excerpta Medica, Amsterdam.

Barer R., Heller H. & Lederis K. (1963) The isolation, identification and properties of the hormonal granules of the neurohypophysis. *Proc. Roy. Soc.* **B.158,** 388–416.

Bargmann W. (1954) *Das Zwischenhirn-Hypophysensystem.* Springer, Berlin.

Bradley W.G. & Jaros E. (1973) Axoplasmic flow in axonal neuropathies. II. Axoplasmic flow in mice with motor neuron disease and muscular dystrophy. *Brain* **96,** 247–58.

Bradley W.H. & Williams M.H. (1973) Axoplasmic flow in axonal neuropathies. 1. Axoplasmic flow in cats with toxic neuropathies. *Brain* **96,** 233–46.

Cross B.A., Dyball R.E.J., Dyer R.G., Jones C.W., Lincoln D.W., Morris J.F. & Pickering B.T. (1975) Endocrine neurons. In: Pincus G. (Ed.) *Recent Progress in Hormone Research* Vol. 31, pp. 243–94. Academic Press, New York and London.

Dahlström A. (1971) Axoplasmic transport (with particular reference to adrenergic neurons). *Phil. Trans. Roy. Soc. Lond.* **B.261,** No. 839, 325–8.

Droz B., Bennett G., Giamberardino L.Di, Koenig H.L. & Rambourg A. (1975) Contribution of electron microscopy to the study of the axonal flow. In: *VIIth International Congress of Neuropathology*, p. 73. Excerpta Medica, Amsterdam.

Droz B. & Koenig H.L. (1971) Dynamic condition of protein in axons and axon terminals. *Acta neuropath. (Berl.)* Suppl. V, 109–18.

Droz B., Koenig H.L. & Giamberardino L. Di (1973) Axonal migration of protein and glycoprotein to nerve endings. I. Radioautographic analysis of the renewal of protein in nerve endings of chicken ciliary ganglion after injection of (^{3}H) lysine. *Brain Res.* **60,** 93–127.

Flament-Durand J. & Dustin P. (1972) Studies on the transport of secretory granules in the magnocellular hypothalamic neurons. I. Action of colchicine on axonal flow and neurotubules in the paraventricular nuclei. *Z. Zellforsch.* **130,** 440–54.

Friede R.L. & Samorajski T. (1970) Axon caliber related to neurofilaments and microtubules in sciatic nerve fibers of rats and mice. *Anat. Rec.* **167**, 379–87.

GRAINGER FELICITY & SLOPER J.C. (1974) Correlation between microtubular number and transport activity of hypothalamo-neurohypophyseal secretory neurons. *Cell Tiss. Res.* **153**, 101–13.

GRAINGER FELICITY & SLOPER J.C. (1976) Microtubular number in the tractus hypophyseus of newborn rats and newborn rats with congenital diabetes insipidus. *Cell Tiss. Res.* **69**, 405–14.

GROSS G.W. (1975) The microstream concept of axoplasmic and dendritic transport. In: Kreutzberg G.W. (Ed.) *Advances in Neurology* Vol. 12, pp. 283–96. Raven Press, New York.

GUTIERREZ M. & SLOPER J.C. (1969) Reaction *in vitro* of synthetic oxytocin and lysine-vasopressin with the pseudoisocyaninchloride technique used for the demonstration of neurohypophysial secretory material. *Histochemie* **17**, 73–7.

HELLER H. & LEDERIS K. (1961) Density gradient centrifugation of hormone-containing subcellular granules from rabbit neurohypophyses. *J. Physiol. (Lond.)* **158**, 27–9p.

HORNYKIEWICZ O. (1972) Dopamine and its physiological significance in brain function. In: Bourne G.H. (Ed.) *Structure and Function of Nervous Tissue* Vol. VI, pp. 367–410. Academic Press, New York.

HORNYKIEWCIZ O. (1973) Dopamine in the basal ganglia. Its role and therapeutic implications (including the clinical use of L-DOPA). *Br. med. Bull.* **29/2**, 172–8.

JONES C.M. & PICKERING B.T. (1969) Comparison of the effects of water deprivation and sodium chloride inhibition on the hormone content of the neurohypophysis of the rat. *J. Physiol.* **203**, 449–58.

KANAZAWA I. & TOYOKURA Y. (1974) Quantitative histochemistry of GABA in the human substantia nigra and globus pallidus. *Confinia Neurologica (Basel)* **36**, 273–81.

KATAOKA K., BAK J.J., HASSLER R., KIM J.S. & WAGNER A. (1974) L-glutamate decarboxylase and choline acetyltransferase activity in the substantia nigra and the striatum after surgical interruption of the strio-nigral fibers of the baboon. *Exp. Brain Res.* **71**, 77–92.

NORSTRÖM A., HANSSON H.-A. & SJÖSTRAND J. (1971) Effects of colchicine on axonal transport and ultrastructure of the hypothalamo-neurohypophyseal system of the rat. *Z. Zellforsch.* **113**, 271–93.

NORSTRÖM A. & SJÖSTRAND J. (1971) Axonal transport of proteins in the hypothalamo-neurohypophysial system of the rat. *J. Neurochem.* **18**, 29–39.

OCHS S. (1971) The dependence of fast transport in mammalian nerve fibers on metabolism. *Acta neuropath. (Berl.)* **Suppl. V**, 86–96.

OCHS S. (1974) Systems of material transport in nerve fibers (axoplasmic transport) related to nerve function and trophic control. *Ann. N.Y. Acad. Sci.* **228**, 202–23.

OCHS S. & BURGER E. (1958) Movement of substance proximo-distally in nerve axons as studied with spinal cord injections of radioactive phosphorus. *Amer. J. Physiol.* **194**, 499–506.

ORTMANN R. (1951) Über experimentelle Veränderungen der Morphologie des Hypophysen-Zwischenhirnsystems und die Beziehung der sog. 'Gomorisubstanz' zum Adiuretin. *Z. Zellforsch.* **36**, 92–140.

PALAY S.L. (1957) The fine structure of the neurohypophysis. In: Waelsch H. (Ed.) *Ultrastructure and Cellular Chemistry of Neural Tissue*, pp. 31–49; *Progress in Neurobiology* vol. 2 Korey S.R. & Nurnberger J.I. (Eds) Hoeber, New York.

PICKERING B.T. & JONES C.W. (1971) The biosynthesis and intraneuronal transport of neurohypophysial hormones: preliminary studies in the rat. *Mem. Soc. Endocr.* **19**, 337–51.

RODECK H. (1959) Zusammenhange zwischen Neurosekret und den sogenannten Hypophysenhinterlappenhormonen. III. Untersuchungen zur färberischen Darstellung von synthetischem Oxytocin; IV. Untersuchungen an schwefelhaltigen Aminosären. *Z. ges. exp. Med.* **132**, 122–35; 225–35.

SACHS H. (1960) Vasopressin biosynthesis. I. *In vivo* studies. *J. Neurochem.* **5,** 297–303.

SAMUELS A.J., BOYARSKY L.L., GERARD R.W., LISBET B. & BRUST M. (1951) Distribution, exchange and migration of phosphate compounds in the nervous system. *Am. J. Physiol.* **164,** 1–15.

SCOTT F.H. (1906) On the relation of nerve cells to fatigue of their nerve fibres. *J. Physiol.* **34,** 145–62.

SLOPER J.C. (1954) Histochemical observations on the neurohypophysis in dog and cat with reference to the relationship between neurosecretory material and posterior lobe hormone. *J. Anat. (Lond.)* **88,** 576.

SLOPER J.C. (1958a) The application of newer histochemical and isotope techniques for the localisation of protein-bound cystine or cysteine to the study of hypothalamic neurosecretion in normal and pathological conditions. In: Bargmann W., Hanström B. & Scharrer E. (Eds) *Zweites Internationales Symposium über Neurosekretion*, pp. 20–5. Springer, Berlin.

SLOPER J.C. (1958b) Hypothalamo-neurohypophysial neurosecretion. *Int. Rev. Cytol.* **7,** 337–89.

SLOPER J.C. (1966) The experimental and cytopathological investigation of neurosecretion in the hypothalamus and pituitary. In: Harris G.W. & Donovan B.T. (Eds) *The Pituitary Gland* Vol. 3, pp. 131–239. Butterworth, London.

SLOPER J.C. (1972) The validity of current concepts of hypothalamo-neuro-hypophyseal neuroscretion. In: Kappers J. Ariëns & Schade J.P. (Eds) *Progress in Brain Research* Vol. 38, pp. 124–43. Elsevier Scientific Publishing Co., Amsterdam.

SLOPER J.C. & ADAMS C.W.M. (1956) The hypothalamic elaboration of posterior pituitary principle in man. Evidence derived from hypophysectomy. *J. Path. Bact.* **72,** 587–602.

SLOPER J.C. & KING BARBARA C. (1963) Activity and degeneration in secretory neurones of the hypothalamus and posterior pituitary of the rat. *J. Path. Bact.* **86,** 179–97.

THOMSEN ELLEN (1954) Studies on the transport of neurosecretory material in *Calliphora erythocephalia* by means of ligaturing experiments. *J. exper. Biol.* **31,** 322–30.

UTTENTHAL L.O., LIVETT B.G. & HOPE D.B. (1971) Release of neurophysin together with vasopressin by a Ca^{2+} dependent mechanism. *Phil. Trans.* **B.261,** 379–80.

VALTIN H. (1967) Hereditary hypothalamic diabetes insipidus in rats (Brattleboro strain). *Amer. J. Med.* **42,** 814–27.

VALTIN H., SOKOL H.W., SAWYER W.H. & HARRINGTON A.R. (1965) Possible synthesis of a 'defective polypeptide' in a strain of rats with hereditary hypothalamic diabetes insipidus. *Excerpta Medica Internat. Congr. Ser.* **No. 83,** Vol. 2, 1267.

VOGT M. (1953) Vasopressor, antidiuretic and oxytocic activities of extracts of the dog's hypothalamus. *Brit. J. Pharmacol.* **8,** 193–6.

WEISS P. (1959) Evidence by isotope tracers of perpetual replacement of mature nerve fibers from their cell bodies. *Science* **129,** 1290.

WEISS P.A. (1972) Neuronal dynamics and axonal flow: axonal peristalsis (time-lapse phase-contrast cinematography). *Proc. Nat. Acad. Sci. USA* **69/5,** 1309–12.

WEISS P. & PILLAI A. (1965) Convection and fate of mitochondria in nerve fibres: axonal flow as vehicle. *Proc. Natn. Acad. Sci. (Wash.)* **54,** 48–56.

WIŚNIEWSKI H., SHELANSKI M.L. & TERRY R.D. (1968) Effects of mitotic spindle inhibitors on neurotubules and neurofilaments in anterior horn cells. *J. Cell Biol.* **38,** 224–9.

WIŚNIEWSKI H. & TERRY R.D. (1967) Experimental colchicine encephalopathy. I. Induction of neurofibrillary degeneration. *Lab. Invest.* **17,** 577–87.

YOUNG J.Z. (1942) Functional repair of nervous tissue. *Physiol. Rev.* **22,** 318–74.

INDEX